WITH ADDITIONAL CHAPTERS BY

ALAN JENNINGS
M.B., B.S., F.A.N.Z.C.P., D.P.M.
Late Director for the Mentally Handicapped,
Health Commission of N.S.W.

AND

SUSAN WILLIAMS
B.Soc.Wk.,
Deputy Social Worker in Charge,
Royal Prince Alfred Hospital, N.S.W.

FOREWORD BY
W. H. TRETHOWAN
Professor of Psychiatry, University of Birmingham

ILLUSTRATED BY
BERNARD HESLING

Psychiatric Nursing

BY

DAVID MADDISON
M.B., B.S., F.R.A.C.P., F.A.N.Z.C.P., D.P.M.
Dean of the Faculty of Medicine and Professor of
Psychiatry, University of Newcastle, N.S.W.
Late Director of Nursing Training,
New South Wales Division of Psychiatric Services

PATRICIA DAY
R.M.N., R.G.N.
Late Chief Instructor, Nursing Training School,
Gladesville Hospital, N.S.W.

BRUCE LEABEATER
B.A.
Principal Clinical Psychologist
Broughton Hall Psychiatric Clinic

FOURTH EDITION

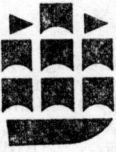

CHURCHILL LIVINGSTONE
EDINBURGH LONDON AND NEW YORK
1975

CHURCHILL LIVINGSTONE

Medical Division of Longman Group Limited

Distributed in the United States of America by
Longman Inc., 72 Fifth Avenue, New York,
N.Y. 10011 and by associated companies,
branches and representatives throughout
the world.

© Longman Group Limited 1975

All rights reserved. No part of this publication
may be reproduced, stored in a retrieval system,
or transmitted in any form or by any means,
electronic, mechanical, photocopying, recording
or otherwise, without the prior permission of the
publishers (Churchill Livingstone, 23 Ravelston
Terrace, Edinburgh).

First edition - - 1963
Second edition - 1965
Reprinted - - - 1967
Third edition - - 1970
Reprinted - - - 1971
Reprinted - - - 1973
Fourth edition - 1975

ISBN 0 443 01311 X

Library of Congress Cataloging in Publication Data

Maddison, David.
    Psychiatric nursing.

    Bibliography: p.
    Includes index.
    1. Psychiatric nursing. I. Day, Patricia, joint author. II. Leabeater, Bruce, joint author. III. Title. [DNLM: 1. Mental disorders. 2. Psychiatric nursing. WY160 M179p]
RC440.M213   1975   610.73'68   75-9908

Printed in Great Britain

When we step into the family, by the act of being born, we do step into a world which has its own strange laws, into a world which could do without us, into a world which we have not made.

From *Heretics*, by G. K. CHESTERTON.

FOREWORD

WHEN the senior author of this book returned to Sydney in 1957 from a visit to overseas psychiatric centres one of the first tasks he was asked to undertake was to organise the training of psychiatric nurses. In addition to his University appointment, therefore, he became the first Director of Nursing Training in the New South Wales Division of Mental Hygiene, as it was then called. Under his auspices a new training school for psychiatric nurses was founded at Gladesville Hospital. This was one of several matters needing attention as part and parcel of the much overdue development of the State's psychiatric services. Years of unenlightened administration, lack of finance, chronic shortage of staff of all kinds and grades, had led to the treatment of the mentally ill in New South Wales falling woefully behind a standard appropriate to the mid-twentieth century; this, in an otherwise progressive and health conscious community. Morale in the mental hospitals was low; the conditions under which the majority of psychiatric patients were treated savoured far too much of custodial care. Indeed, these were not so much hospitals as anachronistic institutions, ruled by lock and key and pervaded by an air of therapeutic hopelessness and inertia.

However, here as elsewhere, a psychiatric revolution was on its way. The training of medical officers was proceeding with enthusiasm; psychologists and social workers were being recruited; far-reaching administrative changes were foreseen and finally effected and the out-dated Lunacy Act was undergoing a thorough and much needed revision.

What of the psychiatric nurse? From all these new and exciting developments, a reassessment of her status could not be excluded. While she had always been looked upon as a member of the team, little more than lip service had been paid to this concept of her role. Both at home and abroad it began to be realised that her proper function did not begin and end merely with her supervision, in a general kind of way, of the daily lives of the patients in her charge. No longer could she be thought of as no more than the handmaiden of the medical officer, responsible only for putting his prescriptions into effect.

FOREWORD

The evolution of the mental hospital, from its antiquated prison-like function into a therapeutic community free from the trappings of seclusion and restraint, has necessarily made ever increasing demands on the nurse's skill and, with their fulfilment, has added to her professional stature. It has, indeed, become quite apparent that the success of this evolutionary process depends as much, if not more, on the nurse as on any other member of the psychiatric team.

The orientation of the Gladesville school was dynamic from the start but, like other innovators, its director and his two principal allies soon discovered that when teachers set out to teach an old subject in a new way, a serious handicap to progress may be the lack of an up-to-date text. From this dilemma they chose the most arduous but only satisfactory means of escape: hence this book.

While today's output of literature on psychiatry and related subjects is more than embarrassingly large, the appearance of a modern text-book on psychiatric nursing can still be considered a major event; the more so, in this instance, because the principles which the authors have so clearly established are by no means only relevant to their place of origin but can be seen to have a world-wide application.

W. H. TRETHOWAN.

1963

PREFACE TO THE FOURTH EDITION

SINCE this text first appeared there have been some outstanding developments in psychiatry and psychiatric nursing, so that major changes were required in the third edition and, to a lesser extent, in this present edition. A much greater emphasis is now laid on the practice of psychiatry in the community, with particular stress on the roles and responsibilities of the nurse. The chapter on psychiatric social work has been completely re-written for this present edition, once more emphasising the substantial diffusion of psychiatric practice from institutional to community settings.

The chapter on physical treatment has been radically revised, with decreasing emphasis on less frequently used therapies such as cerebral surgery, continuous narcosis and insulin treatment. Numerous minor revisions have been undertaken in order to introduce concepts or syndromes which are more important now than they were a decade or so ago, but these additions have been made without any significant change in the overall length of the text.

It is a special pleasure to draw attention to changes in the tense employed in various sections of the book, particularly those dealing with inpatient treatment; in other words, it is now possible to point to certain undesirable practices in psychiatric hospitals as being things of the past, rather than emphasise the need to alter them, as seemed necessary in 1963.

We are deeply indebted to several senior colleagues who read various sections of the book at our request and advised us on their modification. Dr. Ross Holland, whose post as Senior Specialist Anaesthetist in the New South Wales Department of Public Health has given him unrivalled experience in the technical aspects of electrotherapy, provided much detailed material which has been incorporated into the revised section on this topic, and also prepared the relevant illustration. Dr. David Bell made a major contribution to the re-writing of the section

PREFACE

on epilepsy. In bringing the reading list up to date we have received substantial help from Professor I. Pilowsky, Dr. B. J. Hughson and Miss P. Alexander. Dr. Beverley Raphael, Mrs. Susan James and Mr. John Birch gave a great deal of their spare time to the tasks of proof-reading and an extensive revision of the index.

D. C. M.
P. D.
B. L.

1975.

CONTENTS

Chapter		Page
1	THE HISTORICAL BACKGROUND OF PRESENT DAY PSYCHIATRY	1
2	THE ROLE OF THE NURSE IN THE PSYCHIATRIC HOSPITAL	16
3	THE DEVELOPMENT OF HUMAN BEHAVIOUR	33
4	ADULT LIFE, MIDDLE AND OLD AGE	65
5	THE DYNAMICS OF HUMAN BEHAVIOUR	77
6	PSYCHIATRIC SYMPTOMS AND SIGNS	104
7	FACTORS IN THE DEVELOPMENT OF PSYCHIATRIC ILLNESS	133
8	CLASSIFICATION OF PSYCHIATRIC ILLNESS	153
9	NEUROTIC REACTIONS	166
10	NEUROTIC REACTIONS (contd.)	196
11	FUNCTIONAL PSYCHOTIC REACTIONS	219
12	ORGANIC REACTIONS	253
13	CHILD PSYCHIATRY	283
14	MENTAL RETARDATION	299
15	PSYCHOSOMATIC REACTIONS	313
16	PSYCHIATRIC TREATMENT: PSYCHOLOGICAL METHODS	327
17	PSYCHIATRIC TREATMENT: PHYSICAL METHODS	352
18	REACTIONS TO ILLNESS AND HOSPITALISATION	378
19	THE PSYCHIATRIC HOSPITAL AS A THERAPEUTIC COMMUNITY	397
20	METHODS OF OBSERVING AND RECORDING BEHAVIOUR	413
21	RELATIONSHIP OF THE NURSE TO THE PATIENT'S RELATIVES	428
22	NURSING CARE IN SPECIAL SITUATIONS	438
23	OCCUPATIONAL, RECREATIONAL AND SOCIAL THERAPIES	457
24	CONVALESCENCE AND REHABILITATION	471
25	THE NURSE IN THE COMMUNITY	481
26	PSYCHIATRIC SOCIAL WORK	494
27	CLINICAL PSYCHOLOGY	505
	RECOMMENDED READING	512
	INDEX	517

1
THE HISTORICAL BACKGROUND OF PRESENT DAY PSYCHIATRY

TODAY psychiatry is a respectable branch of medicine, a recognised part of medical knowledge which is steadily gaining in status and prestige. With its growth, psychiatric nursing has become a major branch of the nursing profession and the psychiatric nurse all over the world is recognised as an especially important person in the care and treatment of the mentally ill. A great deal of thought and attention is now given to the selection of men and women suitable for a psychiatric nursing career and the nurse's training has the standard and scientific background which fit her to talk on equal terms to her colleagues, the general and the obstetric nurses. All this is really very new—much newer than the nurse might suppose, as the following pages will show.

MENTAL ILLNESS AND MAGIC

For very many centuries, both before and after the birth of Christ, the little thought that was given to mental disturbance was entirely in terms of magic, spirits and demons. Happenings which we now recognise as due to activity of the brain were regarded as "supernatural", that is, not capable of being explained by any of the laws of nature. "Bad" or "sick" behaviour was seen as the result of the possession of the individual by evil spirits and many and varied were the steps taken to try to drive these spirits from the body of the afflicted person. Primitive medicine men, often themselves mentally abnormal, carried out fantastic rites in an attempt to cure both mental and physical diseases. In other civilisations holes were bored into the skull to encourage the evil demon to emerge. Conversely, it was sometimes believed that the mentally ill were in some way sacred and that harm would befall anyone who attempted to interfere with them.

There is no doubt that forms of mental illness did exist even in these early times. From early Egyptian writings (around 1500 B.C.) one can recognise descriptions of alcoholic states, severe bouts of depression, some neurotic illnesses and the mental changes of old age. But even during the highly developed Greek civilisation such an intelligent and knowledgeable writer as **Homer** believed that emotional disturbances were produced by the rages of the Gods.

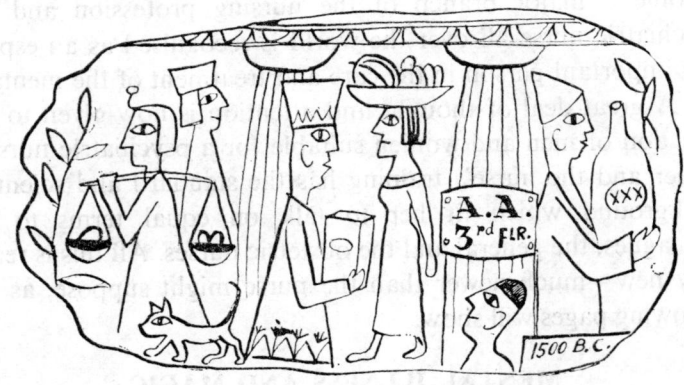

FIG. 1
Alcoholism was a problem in ancient Egypt.

The earliest known person to take what we would now call a scientific view of human nature and mental illness was the Greek physician **Hippocrates** (about 460-377 B.C.). At a time when his colleagues were still clinging to the old supernatural beliefs he insisted that human health and sickness must be looked at in terms of the usual laws of nature. He pointed out that the brain was responsible for thoughts and feelings, not the heart or diaphragm as had previously been suggested. Through careful observation of sick people he came to certain conclusions about physical and mental illnesses which are as true today as when he made them—for example, he recognised some connection between attacks of depression and of extreme cheerfulness, an original observation about the form of mental disorder now described as manic-depressive psychosis (p. 242). His writings contain descriptions of insanity occurring after child-birth and of mental confusion developing during severe infections and after brain haemorrhage. He saw that some people were more likely than others to develop mental illness and suggested that hereditary influences might be at work in some cases. Many of his theories, as might be expected, were quite wrong—he thought, for instance, that the type of neurotic behaviour we now call hysteria was due to the " wandering " of the uterus throughout the body. (It was on account of this theory that the term " hysteria " came into being, derived, like the word " hysterectomy ", from the Greek word for the uterus.) But in view of the emphasis today on the importance of sexual conflicts in the causation of mental disorder he was perhaps not as wrong as he might have been in prescribing marriage and pregnancy as a cure for hysterical girls, a remedy which is too simple but which is based on a fragment of truth. Despite his several errors Hippocrates introduced into medicine a fundamental principle which has never altered and which remains the basis of all proper medical and nursing care—the principle that diagnosis, understanding and treatment must always be based primarily on the observation of one's patient.

The basically scientific ideas of Hippocrates found little support in his own time and even less in the succeeding centuries. Various forms of treatment were employed for abnormal mental states but these were based on notions which we would now consider absurd. For example, many Greek physicians used a plant known as Hellebore, employing the black variety if the patient were hearing " voices " of a gloomy nature, the white variety if the " voices " were cheerful! With the coming of the so-called **Dark Ages** (from 200 A.D. onwards), any progress that might have sprung from Greek and Roman civilisations was completely lost. For many centuries any type of scientific investigation was frowned on by the Christian Church, whose ministers returned to the insistence that what we now regard as mental illness could only be evidence of possession by the Devil. Even in physical illnesses treatment was largely confined to various types of faith-healing and even this could only be practised by Churchmen or, at certain periods, by Kings. If one believed sufficiently in the power of the faith-healer to bring about cure, then cure occurred; lack of improvement obviously indicated that the patient's faith was insufficiently strong! Ideas of this type, totally without logical foundation, persist for example in the practices and beliefs of present day Christian Scientists.

WITCHCRAFT

A specially ugly chapter in the history of psychiatry is concerned with witches and witchcraft. The execution of alleged witches was practised throughout the Dark Ages, but reached its peak at an even later period during the fifteenth and sixteenth centuries, at a time when men generally were developing rather more progressive ideas about science and medicine. A book on witch-hunting, describing in detail the peculiar and unpleasant habits of witches, was written in 1486 and shows clearly how many of these unfortunate persecuted women were in fact mentally ill. Anyone showing the slightest sign of mental deviation ran the risk of being branded as a witch or a magician. Otherwise eminent men of the time recommended that people afflicted in this way should be at once burned to prevent their creating further havoc as agents of the Devil, witches being infallibly recognisable by such miscellaneous signs as a hooked nose and a preference for sexual intercourse on Thursdays, Fridays and Saturdays! The witchcraft theory became a justification for all sorts of mischief—" married men are bewitched " (so it was said) " to use other men's wives and to refuse their own ". Nonsensical though these ideas appear to us today, under the influence of mass popular opinion at the time many thousands of women " confessed " to a state of devil-possession and were tortured and executed as a result, all in the name of God and using the alleged authority of the Bible. One German executioner is said to have personally burned alive 700 old women for this reason. Even such an enlightened monarch as Queen Elizabeth I made witchcraft a crime punishable by death and men were employed during her reign to track down witches, receiving a fee for each one detected. Such was the fate of a large number of mentally ill people during a substantial period of our history.

Though such practices no longer occur in any civilised community, two aspects of the witchcraft era are important for us today. Public opinion about mental illness has certainly changed radically during this present century—and particularly during the last 25 years—but one need not look far to find, even in our own community, relics of the same sort of attitude towards psychiatric patients, even though it be expressed in a totally different way. Some otherwise highly intelligent and well-educated people are clearly still reluctant to look at mental illness in any scientific rational manner, feeling more comfortable if they see psychiatric patients as members of a race apart, " afflicted " by some mysterious malady; such people are still thinking of mental illness in terms very similar to those which their ancestors used 500 years ago. The second point is another aspect of the first—primitive theories about the origin of mental illness still persist amongst uncivilised native peoples, many of whom still accept entirely " supernatural ", magical explanations of the cause of both physical and mental diseases. These have not in fact completely died out, however, even in our own culture, especially among the least educated section of our society. The nurse will find not a few of her patients or their relatives who insist on seeing mental illness as a punishment by God for wrong-doing, rather than looking for natural understandable causes. A certain section of the population still believes that masturbation causes blindness or insanity, or that an individual's mental condition is influenced by the phases of the moon (the term " lunacy ", still not completely abandoned, is derived from this old-fashioned belief). We are not perhaps, as a society, quite as scientific in our thinking about mental illness as we would like to believe; the persistence of superstitions and prejudice about psychiatry is still a substantial obstacle to the work of the psychiatric nurse and the adequate rehabilitation of her patients.

THE DEVELOPMENT OF THE PSYCHIATRIC HOSPITAL

Hospitals for the mentally ill are known to have existed in Egypt and the Middle East during the period of time (roughly from 700 to 1200 A.D.) when Arabian cities were virtually the only centres in the world practising any scientific type of medicine. When in the fifteenth century the focus of the medical world shifted to Spain, new mental institutions were built there. Only in 1547 was the first mental hospital provided in London, the hospital of **St. Mary of Bethlehem**. But for several centuries thereafter the treatment of the patients confined therein was primitive and brutal, no real distinction being made between the requirements of the mentally sick and those of the criminal. " Treatment " consisted almost entirely of punishment and was in the hands of warders, not doctors or nurses. There were no beds, no toilets, and no adequate food. Recommendations were made that the patient should be closely guarded in " a chamber where there is little light " and that he should be kept in permanent fear of his " keeper ". It was said that " maniacs often recover much sooner if they are treated with torture and torments in a hovel instead of with medicaments ". The underpaid " keeper " added to his income by collecting small sums from fashionable Londoners who came at week-ends to stare at this apparently fascinating spectacle, as people gaze on animals in a zoo. (The public exhibition of the mentally ill was still a feature of life in Vienna as recently as 1853.) Small wonder that the name " Bethlehem " was quickly shortened to " Bedlam ", a word which has survived in our language to describe situations of chaos and uproar.

Little change took place in this unsavoury picture until the end of the eighteenth century (only a little over 150 years ago).

BACKGROUND OF PRESENT DAY PSYCHIATRY

In 1791 a Frenchman, **Philippe Pinel,** became chief of a mental hospital near Paris; immediately following the French Revolution, the atmosphere of the time was favourable to a new recognition of the rights and dignity of man, and Pinel at once set about a series of reforms which changed the whole spirit of care for the mentally ill. He ordered that patients should no longer be chained to posts, punishment was completely forbidden and isolation of patients in single rooms was restricted to a brief period and then only when ordered by the doctor. Study of the patient's personality was declared to be essential for his understanding. Patients for the first time were housed in various wards depending on their degree of mental disturbance, with separate accommodation for those who in addition were physically sick. Above all, Pinel insisted on the necessity for kindness in the management of the mentally ill and saw the personalities of the doctors and nurses as the single most important factor in bringing about a cure. In implementing these changes he received invaluable help from the man whom we would now call his Superintendent of Nursing (or Chief Male Nurse), Jean-Baptiste Pussin, who had preceded Pinel to the hospital, and who together with his wife played a vital part in the prevention of cruelty to patients and the institution of humane methods of care.

Pinel's example was quickly followed in other parts of the world. **William Tuke** in 1796 founded the York Retreat in England which set out to use the methods of Pinel under the term " moral treatment ". Encouragement and kindness were to form the basis of hospital care, coupled with routine work and the abolition of fear. The traditional medical treatments for mental disorder, for example, bleeding, purgatives and so on, were regarded, quite correctly, as useless. (Even Benjamin Rush, an otherwise progressive American doctor with a special interest in psychiatry, had in 1783 recommended beatings, frequent blood-lettings and planned insults as useful methods of " treatment ".)

So the mental hospital began to develop up to the point at

PSYCHIATRIC NURSING

which we know it today. Later in this book (Chapter 19) the nurse will find that it is still believed, as Pinel believed, that the atmosphere of the psychiatric hospital is a most important, perhaps *the* single most important, factor in the patient's progress. She will unfortunately, even today, find occasional people who believe that punishment is a good method of controlling the psychiatric patient and who have failed to realise the everlasting importance of Pinel's reforms. But she will find a much larger number of persons concerned with examining the hospital staff and its spirit in order to develop to the full its potential value to her patients.

A word should be said about the direction in which the psychiatric hospital is now moving in its development. Many nurses may have grown up with the belief that admission to a mental hospital is the only possible step, indeed the only desirable step, for any patient with a significant degree of mental illness. On the contrary, there is now an increasing realisation that admission to a mental hospital is a highly significant and possibly harmful procedure which must only be arranged when all other avenues of help have been exhausted or are obviously unsuitable. The hospital is now tending to become the vital centre point of the psychiatric service for the community in a given area, but providing in addition some or all of the following facilities to the surrounding neighbourhood:

(1) An **outpatient service** for early diagnosis and treatment.

(2) A **day hospital,** where patients attend during the day for treatment, sometimes for four or five days each week, but return to their homes at nights and week-ends.

(3) Supervised **after-care** of the patient discharged from hospital, both through the outpatient department and through associated **hostels** and **rehabilitation centres.**

(4) A **domiciliary service,** giving consultation and treatment in the home where such a course is warranted, and providing a further agency for after-care when the patient is unable or unwilling to use the services at the hospital (p. 485).

BACKGROUND OF PRESENT DAY PSYCHIATRY

(5) **A consultative service,** designed to be utilised by those various agencies in the community whose day-to-day work is intimately concerned with psychiatric illness and with the mental health of the population generally—schools and baby health centres are only two of the many examples of such agencies (p. 487).

In addition, patients with psychiatric illness are being treated in increasing numbers in **general hospitals,** usually in special psychiatric units but in some instances in general medical beds. This is an important development, not only because of the implications for patient care and for the more comprehensive education of doctors and nurses, but because it provides skilled psychiatric help for many physically ill people (as described in Chapter 15) who would not be likely to use the facilities of the psychiatric hospital itself.

The nurse will find herself, during her training and subsequently, involved in all these activities to a greater or lesser extent; the scope and breadth of psychiatric nursing have greatly increased in recent years, and the keen nurse of today will be involved in several types of rewarding experience in patient care. Moreover the senior nurse is likely to become attached to hospital services which provide domiciliary, consultative and preventive programmes. Much more attention is given to these developments, and the nurse's role in them, in Chapter 25.

SCIENTIFIC DEVELOPMENTS OF THE LAST CENTURY

By 1860 the methods of caring for the mentally ill were in general rather more humane and civilised. **John Conolly,** another pioneering British medical superintendent, had by 1839 completely forbidden the use of restraint in his hospital and achieved in this way a surprisingly high recovery rate among his patients. Nevertheless there was still an almost complete lack of understanding of the nature and causes of mental disease. In this Victorian age psychiatric illness was still regarded by the general public, and by many physicians, as " sinful " and a scientific approach to problems of abnormal thinking and behaviour developed only very gradually over the next 100 years.

Charcot, a French doctor, may be regarded as the first physician to extend the concept of mental illness beyond the obvious forms of frank " madness ". He recognised the importance and frequency of neurotic illness and, from 1878 onwards, gave special attention to the condition known as hysteria (described in this book as " conversion reaction ", p. 184) and demonstrated how it could be modified by hypnosis, a form of treatment until then regarded as suitable for use only by quacks and frauds, although it had been known in ancient times.

Kraepelin. This famous German professor gave us the first clear descriptions of the various forms of psychiatric illness. His text-book, first appearing in 1883, grouped together various mental symptoms as characteristic of the reaction now known as schizophrenic (p. 219), others as manic depressive (p. 242), others again as typical of organic brain damage (p. 253). He emphasised that understanding of the patient could only be achieved by a study of his whole life history. His theories concerning the causes of mental illness paid little attention to psychological and emotional disturbance and are therefore out of line with a great deal of modern thought. But he was certainly the first person to introduce any order and system into our study of psychiatry.

Freud. With the first publications on psychiatric topics by Sigmund Freud, who lived from 1856 to 1939, a completely new light was thrown on the nature of mental processes. The appearance in 1900 of his first major work, " The Interpretation of Dreams ", led to the development of a radically different approach to the study of human behaviour, a technique of investigation and treatment known as **psychoanalysis**. Many aspects of Freud's theories will be referred to during the course of this book, but there can be listed here three major contributions which he made to our understanding of mental illness:

(1) his insistence that all mental processes, like physical ones,

BACKGROUND OF PRESENT DAY PSYCHIATRY

had causes and could be understood if enough were known about the life and development of the individual;
(2) his discovery that a large part of human mental activity took place outside of the individual's own awareness— his description, that is to say, of unconscious mental processes (p. 78);
(3) his emphasis on the very great importance of the early years of life for the development of personality and for the later occurrence of mental illness.

All these ideas were revolutionary and even now are not fully accepted, either by the general public or by the medical and nursing professions. They have provided however the first system of ideas from which an understanding of psychiatric illness can be developed and have given very numerous leads towards the treatment of psychiatric patients, including nursing care.

Freud's later followers have branched out in several different directions and founded numerous " schools ", each adding something to the basic theory of psychoanalysis or laying stress on a different aspect of it. The particular contributions of **Sullivan** and **Laing** are considered in Chapter 7.

THE DEVELOPMENT OF PHYSICAL TREATMENTS

Freud's work, though it led to a much richer understanding of the nature of mental illness, did not bring about any significant alteration in the condition of the vast number of people sufficiently disturbed to require treatment in a mental hospital. **Bromides** were introduced to medicine in 1857 and **barbiturates** in 1903; both groups of drugs were valuable in the control of disturbed behaviour but had no direct effect on the course of mental illness. Treatment of brain disease due to syphilis by physical means (artificial fever and drugs) was introduced between 1890 and 1920 and was further improved by the use of penicillin in 1941.

The substantial improvement in the discharge rates of patients from mental hospitals did not however begin until the introduction of the various forms of treatment known loosely as " shock treatment ". In the late 1920's states of unconsciousness deliberately brought about by large doses of **insulin** were first used in psychiatric hospitals. Later it was found that artificially produced fits greatly hastened the recovery of some psychiatric patients; these were first brought about by drugs (1933) but later by the use of electrical currents passed through the brain (1938). **Electro-convulsive therapy,** as it came to be called, was without doubt a very great advance and is still a valuable tool in the psychiatric hospital today; early claims, however, that it would lead to an almost complete emptying of mental hospitals proved quite unjustified.

Roughly similar statements can be made about the new **tranquillising drugs.** The first of these, " Largactil " (chlorpromazine), has been very widely used since 1954, and has been followed by a whole host of rather similar drugs, all sharing the common property of quietening disturbed behaviour and lessening tension whilst avoiding the sedative effects of drugs such as barbiturates. Naturally these have provided a further major step forward in treatment, both in acute and chronic forms of mental illness; they have helped to shorten the course of acute psychiatric illness and to bring many of the more disturbed chronic patients under control and into better contact with their surroundings. Even more recently a large number of drugs have been produced which are sometimes of substantial help in the treatment of patients with severe forms of depressive illness.

But these drugs have not reduced the need for skilled psychiatric nursing, nor have they made less real the importance of the relationships between nurses and their patients which will be constantly referred to throughout this book. On the contrary, the wise use of drugs gives many patients the chance of better contact with the nurse, of a kind which might not otherwise have been achieved in the time available. The easy availability of these, and of the other forms of physical treatment previously described, does not permit the nurse to see herself merely as a technical assistant to the psychiatrist. Nor should she ever look on them unwittingly as yet another form of " restraint "—for to replace the old-fashioned mechanical restraint by chemical restraint, while less brutal, is to go back in effect to the time before the reforms of Pinel and Conolly.

THE PROFESSION OF PSYCHIATRIC NURSING

It has already been indicated that the care of the mentally ill was kept, over many centuries, in the hands of completely untrained persons, gaolers rather than nurses, lacking any kind of scientific knowledge and usually, as far as we are aware, unsympathetic and often deliberately cruel to their unfortunate charges. Their only technique for the handling of disturbed behaviour was either direct punishment or the use of various restraining devices ranging from chains to strait-jackets. No doubt the brutalising conditions in which patients were housed aggravated any violent tendencies, and these would have been even further provoked by the inhuman methods of control. We surely need not envy those whose task it was to work in such an atmosphere.

Various nursing groups had accompanied the Crusaders in the eleventh, twelfth and thirteenth centuries. From that time on nurses of a sort began to appear in hospitals, but were completely lacking in any form of training. In Roman Catholic hospitals, both for the physically and mentally ill, the nuns provided relatively good food and rest and attempted to create an atmosphere of spiritual calm for their patients—but again of course without any knowledge of the particular nursing skills now so familiar to us. However the name of one nun, Sister Nicole, of the Order of the Daughters of Charity at the Petites-Maisons in Paris, may be mentioned in view of what we know of her enlightened care of insane patients, as early as 1655. By accepting aggressive behaviour without resentment she contributed to what would now be called a permissive environment, something that must have been extremely rare in those times. During the same period the Brothers of the Order of St. John of God began to provide services for the mentally ill at Charenton, also in France, and this hospital still exists, as do many similar hospitals founded by the Order all over the world.

Elsewhere nurses were of low status, often women of poor reputation and drunken habits. As recently as 1857 the *London Times* described nurses in London hospitals in the following terms: " Lectured by committees, preached at by Chaplains . . . scolded by matrons, sworn at by surgeons . . . grumbled at and abused by patients, insulted if old and ill-favoured, talked flippantly to if middle-aged and good-humoured, tempted and seduced if young and well-looking..."[1] It scarcely sounds an attractive life (though perhaps not *totally* unrecognisable even to the nurse of today).

It was during the nineteenth century that there first took hold the view that nurses should be selected and trained for their responsible duties. The idea was first developed in Germany, discharged female prisoners receiving the initial courses of instruction but soon being followed by more conventional young ladies, of whom **Florence Nightingale** was one of the first (1836). Under her influence the first British training school for general nurses was established at St. Thomas's Hospital in 1860. But a system of education for mental nurses had been set up even prior to this; in 1854 the Crichton Royal Hospital in Scotland began " a full, if popular discussion of insanity in the different forms, intelligible by the shrewd and sensible if somewhat illiterate class of persons employed as attendants and nurses ".[2] In Britain at any rate an examination and a certificate for psychiatric nurses were established (1891) long before similar requirements were demanded from their colleagues in general hospitals.

The development of mental nursing in Australia during the nineteenth century followed roughly similar lines, and is

---

[1] Haggard, H. W. (1929). *Devils, Drugs and Doctors.* New York: Blue Ribbon Books.
[2] Easterbrook, C. E. (1940). *The Chronicle of Crichton Royal.* Dumfries; quoted by Hunter, R. A. (1956), *Lancet* **1,** 98.

BACKGROUND OF PSYCHIATRIC NURSING

particularly associated with the name of Thomas Digby, an Englishman who came to Australia in 1836 to become Superintendent of the first mainland asylum, at Tarban Creek, New South Wales (now Gladesville Hospital). Assisted by his wife as Matron, Digby (a former attendant) devoted his time and energy to establishing the best possible conditions for his patients, instituting regulations for the behaviour of the "keepers" which attempted to ensure that treatment would be along humane lines.

Since that time the status of the psychiatric nurse has risen, then fallen, and in the period since World War II has again risen, quite dramatically so in recent years. Hunter, in the article cited above, has suggested that the decline in status of the psychiatric nurse began in the 1930's and was directly related to the increasing use of the various forms of physical treatment; the importance of the nurse-patient relationship was lost sight of and the frequently powerful effects of electrotherapy and drugs led the psychiatrist to the temporary belief that he and he alone was of significance in the restoration of mental balance. Now, however, this unfortunate trend has been completely reversed; more and more the invaluable role of the well-trained psychiatric nurse has been acknowledged. New emphasis has been laid on old truths—that, for instance, however well staffed the psychiatric hospital may be in other ways, the patient spends by far the greatest part of his time in contact with nurses, whose attitudes and behaviour will have a crucial effect on him. Conolly's words of 1856 are recognised as still true today: "The physician . . . well knows that the attendants are his most essential instruments. . . . They may often be considered, indeed, his best medicines." The nurse has moved back to where she belongs, as a vital, indeed indispensable, member of the hospital team; her education and training are given at least as much thought and attention as the education and training of the general nurse. Her place in the team, and the essential principles underlying her task, are taken up in the next chapter.

2

THE ROLE OF THE NURSE IN THE PSYCHIATRIC HOSPITAL

THERE are more patients requiring psychiatric treatment today than ever before, even though more is understood about mental illnesses and despite the fact that more research is being carried out. It is an exciting and interesting time for the nurse engaged in this branch of nursing, as there is at present an upsurge of hopefulness about the future of psychiatric patients.

In all branches of medicine the overwhelming value of skilled nursing is increasingly realised and nowhere is this more true than in the practice of psychiatry. In the psychiatric hospital the number of nurses, compared with the number of the other members of the team, is proportionately so large that they must inevitably have an extremely great influence on the patient's behaviour and well-being. Moreover, the nature of the nurse's contact with the patient ensures that her relationship with him will be an intimate and close one. Throughout this book emphasis will be placed on the importance and the complexity of the relationships which nurses develop with their patients; it will be seen how this relationship must be different in every instance, for no two patients are ever the same and therefore no situation is ever experienced in quite the same way. Also, no two nurses are ever the same; even the one nurse's personality will change and mature during the process of training and she will grow in understanding as a result of experience, so that she relates to patients in a quite different way at the end of her training from the way in which she related at the beginning.

The psychiatric nurse will also find that many of the principles and practices which she learns during her hospital training are capable of a wider application in home and community settings. Today's emphasis is, wherever possible, on prevention rather than cure, so that the nurse's role includes learning the components of mental health, guarding her own and her family's adjustment and making positive efforts to promote in the families and friends of patients ideas about mental health and mental illness which can favourably influence the community's attitudes.

THE PRINCIPLES OF PSYCHIATRIC NURSING

The Importance of the Patient's Total Personality. First and foremost the psychiatric nurse must realise that every individual patient is a complicated person, with multiple needs derived from a variety of sources. There are no easy answers available for the student of human behaviour, whether this behaviour be healthy or sick; most of society's glib statements about the causes of psychiatric illness she will find to be incorrect. The patient's personality has numerous aspects and numerous factors which go to make it up—he has a physical life, a mental life, a social and community life, economic and spiritual needs. His environment and life experiences, as well as his hereditary endowment, all in some measure will have contributed to and influenced his illness.

The Significance of Personal Relationships. Psychiatric nursing care is based fundamentally on an understanding of **interpersonal relationships,** that is, the patterns of feeling which develop *between* people. As part of her training the nurse learns to promote these relationships in ways which will be helpful. The patient, with his unique and many-sided individuality, has to be observed and known in as close and as intimate a contact as is felt to be in his best interests. Obviously the nurse must be seen by him as helpful and not intimidating, so that her approach to him in many instances needs to be careful and slow, though his capacity for closeness may change substantially as he improves.

The nurse herself also has a unique and individual personality which she requires to understand. Unless and until she sees for herself why she behaves in certain ways and how her own mental life operates she cannot use herself as an instrument of treatment as effectively as she might. Her own personality and the use which she makes of it are the most important pieces of equipment for the nursing care which she will provide; the most powerful drugs and the highest degree of technical skill lose their full efficacy if the nurse is not also using herself intelligently. In bathing or dressing patients, in offering them tablets or administering intramuscular injections, her approach to them and her feeling about them will vitally affect their responses.

At the same time, the nurse is not the only one who can help the patient and in some instances may not be the best one to do so; she may therefore be called upon to promote his relationship with some other person who can help him more. Every patient requires a variety of contacts and will almost certainly need different types of relationship at different stages of his treatment. Though the nurse may wish to continue a relationship which offers him maximum support and which gives her personal satisfaction she will find that at some point she must guide him towards independence.

Recognition of the Patient's Needs. Nursing care in psychiatry in the final analysis consists of recognising and responding to the patient's needs. It may be extremely difficult to discover what his inner needs really are, yet the quality of the nurse's care depends upon uncovering them and then proceeding to find ways in which to deal with them. Some of the needs which he expresses may of course not be rational and it may therefore not be in his best interests to satisfy them—for example, he may want her to agree that the voices he hears are real and have a magical power over him.

Less than in other branches of medicine, a precise diagnosis (which may be made with difficulty even by the psychiatrist) is a poor guide for effective action. Much more importantly,

THE ROLE OF THE NURSE

whatever his diagnosis, the nurse is required to learn what are the patient's assets and liabilities, what are his basic problems and what it is that he lacks which successful nursing care might restore. It is much less important for her to know that Tom Smith has been diagnosed as suffering from a " schizophrenic reaction " than for her to see that he is not eating because he believes that his food is being poisoned and that therefore it is her task to find some way to encourage him to eat it. Later, if all goes well, she is able to relinquish the patient's dependence on her and allow him to see for himself what he must do to answer his own needs.

The Importance of Unconscious Motivation. Freud's idea of unconscious mental life has already been briefly referred to in Chapter 1 (p. 11) and is taken up more fully in Chapter 5 (p. 78). Here it need only be said that all of the patient's behaviour does have meaning in terms of his wishes, guilts and fears, but that some of these aspects of his life are hidden even from his own awareness. In some instances his unconscious needs may be fairly obvious to the nurse though not to the patient himself and it may at times be hard for her to accept that what is so clear to her is hidden from him. In other cases the depth and complexity of his unconscious problems may be such that they are not really clear even after many hours of treatment with a psychiatrist. In general terms, however, the nurse will be successful in her role in proportion to the extent to which she can understand motives which are outside the patient's awareness. It is not suggested for one moment that she should tell the patient what she feels his needs are or what his behaviour means; this course of action in all probability will cause him to retreat still further from any uncovering of his inner self. If the patient's behaviour does require interpreting to him, then the psychiatrist is usually the only person who is qualified to do so and who knows when the patient is ready to accept and benefit from such an interpretation.

The Attitudes of a Psychiatric Nurse. Certain attitudes are necessary for any nurse who aims to make a success of her dealings with psychiatric patients.

ACCEPTANCE. The patient must be accepted as he is, as a sick person, regardless of colour, creed or behaviour. Whether he is likeable, tantalising or socially objectionable should ideally make no difference to her attitude; in fact the more perverse his behaviour the greater his need for acceptance, for the less likely is it to be accepted by others. She accepts, while not necessarily agreeing with, his cultural and religious beliefs; she does not moralise nor measure him by a rigid set of standards; on the contrary, she acknowledges that he has grown to be the sort of person that he is as a result of his experiences. At the same time the nurse must learn also to accept her colleagues and, finally, to accept herself.

UNDERSTANDING. She requires to develop the capacity to understand people and their needs, however these needs may be expressed. This constant requirement poses a tremendous challenge; it is so much easier for her to criticise and to theorise than to understand.

RELIABILITY. She must be truthful and honest, acknowledging if necessary her lack of ability or her mistakes, prepared to learn the answers and not cover up her ignorance. She must be sure of her facts, not relying on hospital gossip, but having the courage of her convictions when sure that they are soundly based. She must be consistent, holding a reasonable control over her emotions so that she can be someone on whom the patient can rely, even at times when she has worries in her own private life.

RESPONSIBILITY. She will learn to accept responsibility at first in minor and perhaps menial tasks, gradually increasing her participation until she is equipped to handle more serious burdens. Yet she must never be too proud to seek help when this seems necessary.

HUMILITY. Psychiatry is a powerful discipline to teach a person his own limitations. The nurse will need to acknowledge that something new can be learnt from any other person, however mentally ill. In her hands more than in others rests the vital task of maintaining human dignity, which can only be based on the realisation that mentally ill patients, whatever form their illness takes, are human beings, like herself in many ways, though with less fortunate life experiences behind them.

INTELLIGENCE. The good nurse uses her intellectual capacity to the full, not only maintaining the required standard of education but aiming to increase it. While retaining a healthy respect for rules and regulations, she will aim to understand them so that she may use them constructively. The more she is eager and willing to learn, the more she will see problems in their correct perspective and will be able more efficiently to employ her time and talents.

PROFESSIONALISM. Psychiatric nursing is a professional role and carries with it professional responsibilities. Good manners and good appearance are important, for the nurse's own physical and mental health will make her someone of particular value to the uncertain and insecure patient. She listens willingly to his point of view and is tactful and sincere. She maintains a high degree of respect for the patient's confidences and his often quite sensational life history.

PSYCHIATRIC AND GENERAL NURSING COMPARED

Both psychiatric and general nursing are parts of the all-embracing nursing discipline; in fact an increasing number of countries in recent years have decided that general nursing training must include some experience with psychiatric patients. In such programmes the general nurse is taught a good deal about emotional and intellectual development and is given some understanding of human motivation, so that she may better understand the non-rational behaviour which may be shown by her physically ill patients when under stress. There are many factors which are common to both branches of the profession—for example, each type of nurse requires an adequate basic grounding in the structure and function of the body and in the nursing of bodily diseases. Though efficiency of a purely technical kind is of more vital importance to the general nurse, nevertheless it is still essential for it to be of a high standard in the psychiatric hospital, for here also the nurse cannot afford to make technical mistakes nor to be careless in physical treatments.

But in many respects the differences between the two segments of the profession are greater than the similarities. The psychiatric nurse is required in her training to know a great deal more about personality development and to understand the significance of the relationships between people and of the many influences, personal and social, which can affect these. The trained general nurse or trainee nurse working in a psychiatric ward for the first time is usually surprised to find the majority of the patients up and about, entering into obviously important but clearly very complicated relationships with the staff and with other patients in the wards. It is often hard to grasp the fact that some of these patients, looking so fit by general hospital standards, have an illness which is shown entirely in their mood and behaviour and attitudes, whereas in the general hospital wards psychological peculiarities are usually regarded as incidental, rather than basic, to the major illness. Moreover some psychiatric patients do not appreciate the need to be in hospital, do not wish to accept the fact and are therefore unable to make efforts to help themselves—a far cry from the typical general ward patient who realises that he is sick, who is prepared to stay in bed out of harm's way and who usually is fully co-operative and anxious to give what help he can.

When treatment is considered different goals, different methods and different limitations are inherent in the programme for the psychiatric patient. It is stressed later in this book (p. 154) how much the illness of the psychiatric patient grows out of his personality and reflects the whole of his life history, so that his management requires always to be individualised; because two cases of appendicitis are nursed in much the same

THE ROLE OF THE NURSE

way, the nurse with experience in a general hospital may assume that two cases of schizophrenia can also be nursed in the same way, which will be a fundamental and serious error. Many general medical and surgical illnesses can be dealt with by treatment directed specifically towards a single cause, and within reasonable limits it is likely that the results of this treatment can be predicted with a fair degree of confidence. Moreover, treatment in the general hospital can often be quite effective without any real communication of a personal kind between nurse and patient. The personality of the general nurse is important insofar as it may make the patient's stay in hospital pleasant or otherwise, and it is certainly true that in chronic, disabling or life-threatening illnesses, where the period in hospital is prolonged, she can play an invaluable supportive role. But when the illness is an acute one the nurse's technical skills are the prime consideration, and the relationship between nurse and patient is of relatively minor importance.

The causes of a psychiatric disturbance, however, are invariably multiple, complex, and in some instances very difficult to discover at all. It is also relatively difficult to make accurate predictions about the outcome of treatment or its duration. In a psychiatric ward a successful result may come about very slowly, in almost imperceptible stages, so that a great deal of patience and perseverance are commonly required; moreover, for a variety of reasons which will be considered later, goals have to be set at a realistic level within the limits of the patient's capacities. Successful treatment will probably involve certain modifications in his personality; he is likely, for instance, to change some of the ways in which he expresses his feelings and needs. Above all treatment in psychiatry involves the personalities, not only of the patients, but of all the members of the treatment team, including the nurse; the feelings the patients have towards the nurses, and the response these feelings may provoke, may be all-important. Even more than in general nursing, moreover, the team approach is essential, for without this the helpful influence of one person may be completely undone by the contradictory approach of another team member. Each discipline has much to learn from the other and in special areas the patient's maximum well-being requires a combination of the skills of both. Very obviously, there are many areas in which the psychiatric nurse follows the lead of the general nurse—in operating theatre technique, in the care of medical and surgical illness and so on. But the psychiatric nurse has also a great deal to offer her general colleagues in those situations where illness disturbs the patient's personal relationships, where it is necessary to keep sickness in its right perspective in a person's life, or in any instance where personality problems are either part of the reason for the illness or are affecting its outcome. With an increasing realisation that psychiatry has a great deal to offer to general medicine, there is a parallel recognition of the increasingly valuable contributions of the psychiatric nurse.

THE OTHER MEMBERS OF THE HOSPITAL TEAM

The treatment team in a psychiatric hospital is now regarded as extending more widely than the traditional five professionals —the **psychiatrist,** the **psychologist,** the **psychiatric social worker,** the **occupational therapist** and the **nurse.** Recreational therapists are assuming more comprehensive roles, while still working closely with the occupational therapists, and nurses themselves are among those who are receiving special training in these skills. Hospital chaplains and some visiting clergy are becoming more involved in certain aspects of patient care, often taking an active part in ward groups, conducting discussions for trainee nurses and extending their activities to include plans for patients in the community. Industrial officers in hospital sheltered workshops (p. 464) also have an important role, particularly through their close and prolonged contact with long-term patients. In addition, many hospitals are establishing orientation and training programmes for voluntary workers. All these professional and lay people are therefore working closely together, towards the same ends, sometimes finding that their functions are combined and overlapping, yet with each having a special significance, which is nevertheless insufficient in isolation.

The nurse will lessen the burden on the patient and will render his treatment more efficient if she has a full knowledge of the other team members' functions and makes full use of their abilities and if she has satisfactory relationships with them as individuals. A group of North American research workers has shown, for example, that personal tensions between staff members working on a ward can lead to an increase in the amount of disturbed behaviour shown by the patients. All team members, like pieces of a jig-saw puzzle, only make a consistent impression when built into a harmonious whole. The good team, " Focussed on a common problem, operates like an orchestra where each instrument does not compete but contributes to the performance of the whole composition " (Frank).[1]

The Psychiatrist. The psychiatrist is a medical graduate, who has additionally undergone a lengthy period of post-graduate training in the special field of psychiatry. He is the only member of the team who has a substantial education in the biological sciences, and is therefore the only member empowered to prescribe drugs or other physical treatments. On the other hand, his medical training has often provided him with very little background in psychological and social aspects of health and disease. Because of his medical background he is traditionally (though not always) the leader of the team; he is the person who is likely to carry the greatest responsibility when things go wrong, and it is therefore usual for him to take the final decisions concerning diagnosis and treatment. It is increasingly recognised, however, that he takes such decisions only after full consultation with other members of the team, and in some instances his leadership function has been entirely delegated to other staff members. The psychiatric nurse will do well to recognise, without being over-awed by, the broad perspective which

[1] Frank, L. K. (1957). *J. Soc. Issues*, Suppl. Series 10.

the psychiatrist is likely to have because of his very lengthy and many-sided training programme, and she will be able to learn a great deal from him in formal lectures, informal discussions and case conferences, at which he will communicate his aims for particular patients and for the team in general. On the other hand, she must adapt his ideas to her own situation, and must recognise that her own unique opportunity for contact with the patient will frequently provide her with information which she should bring forward in order that his recommendations should be based on understanding which is as complete as possible. He will certainly come to acknowledge her as a competent professional once she has given satisfactory evidence of her professionalism, and he will then learn to rely on her technical and interpersonal skills within the ward; he will certainly hope to be able to trust her judgement and respect her ability to make her own contributions towards patient management. The more successful the relationship, the less will the psychiatrist require to supervise her in her day-to-day activities, and the nurse will find that he will increasingly entrust her with vitally significant aspects of patient and ward management.

The Clinical Psychologist. From the psychologist, who also has a special and more elaborate training than she has in the understanding of human development and behaviour, the nurse can also learn a great deal. She should take every opportunity to derive new information from his lectures and discussions and from the observation of the relationships which he develops with patients. In Chapter 27 the aims and methods of clinical psychology are considered in some detail, but the psychologist also is incapable of functioning alone and will be greatly aided in his task if the nurse is able to reassure the patient, build up the latter's confidence and allay whatever doubts and fears he may have about mental testing or other procedures in which he is participating with the psychologist. The nurse may be called upon to arrange times and places for interviews and to see that interruptions do not occur; also if she is wise and able to do so she will prepare the patient for the event, though not discussing the details of the tests which the psychologist may be administering nor their purpose. As with the psychiatrist, she aims to use intelligent observation to pass on relevant information about the patient and to report to the psychologist any after-effects of the patient's contact with him. She will later find that the information derived from the psychologist's procedures, when it is shared with her, will help her towards a much greater understanding of the patient's intellectual potential and personal conflicts.

The Psychiatric Social Worker. The special skills and orientation of the psychiatric social worker are described in Chapter 26. All members of the team need to be aware of her special role so that they can provide the encouragement which may be necessary to guide a patient in her direction. A word of reassurance on a quiet evening, pointing out that the social worker needs to get to know him, his financial and employment situation, in order that the hospital may more effectively assist him back to health, is often enough to remove doubts in the patient's mind. A difficult situation at home (for example, concern about her children when a young mother is admitted to hospital), fear of losing accommodation, financial worries, anxiety about contacting an employer—problems of this kind are often first raised with a nurse, who should be able to bring them to the notice of the social worker so that the patient's level of anxiety may be lowered by knowing that appropriate action is being taken on his behalf. From the social worker the nurse in return will gain a more complete picture of her patient, as she comes to understand the complexities of his family life, his social and community relationships. As psychiatric nurses, however, become increasingly involved in social and community aspects of psychiatry, there may arise a substantial (and sometimes confusing) overlap between the roles of the social worker and the nurse, an overlap which may need frank discussion.

Occupational and Recreational Therapists. The contact between the nurses and the members of the occupational and recreational therapy teams tends to be closer than with any of the others; there is a greater opportunity for them to be in a close working relationship and a greater similarity in their aims and techniques. It is important for the nurse to find out what the occupational therapist can and cannot be expected to do and to see that every opportunity exists for sharing significant knowledge, either about technical skills or about the patients themselves. Frequently patients leave the ward for occupation and recreation and this can easily lead to a feeling of division and competition between these two important partners; much of this will be avoided if the nurse and the occupational therapist come to know each other in a personal way. She should work hard to avoid any possible rivalry which could lead either the occupational therapist or the nurse to regard herself as the person most likely to help the patient. Part of the nurse's task will be to gain some knowledge of arts, crafts and games which can be used in the wards, for in the large hospitals it is usually only a limited number of patients who can be accommodated in the occupational departments and, as will be seen in Chapter 23, the nurse should be able to take over, particularly with the most disturbed patients, some of the occupational therapist's functions. Similar remarks apply to the necessity for personal contact and sharing of information with those people in the hospital who provide recreational and social therapy.

In actual fact the hospital team is even larger than has been indicated in this section. The nurse could not function without the men who stoke the boilers, who run the switch-board and who deliver the mail and it should not be forgotten that every single staff member can be regarded as a contributor to the therapeutic atmosphere. Patients may be considerably helped by members of the hospital lay staff with whom they work—for example, the librarian, gardener, laundress or storeman. Wherever it is indicated the nurse may need to explain to such a person, in a limited fashion suitable for non-professionals, something of the patient's problems and may need to put him in the picture about the aims of treatment in the particular case.

THE OBJECTIVES OF HOSPITAL CARE

The psychiatric hospital exists primarily in order to restore to the sick person his maximum mental and physical health and to send him out of hospital equipped as far as possible with understanding of himself and his illness and with a greater maturity of personality than when he entered. In Chapter 19 it is discussed in detail how easy it is for the hospital to lose sight of this **therapeutic role** and to slip quietly into patterns of **custodial care,** that is to say, the provision of an environment, however kindly, which aims merely to protect the patient from himself and to protect the community from him, rather than to use all the available resources to treat him. Ideally the patient should leave the psychiatric hospital better able to realise his potentialities in work and in play, more capable of gaining satisfaction from normal life and more able to withstand the strains and stresses of his existence.

Though it has already been indicated in the previous chapter that modern methods of psychiatric treatment seek wherever possible to avoid hospitalisation and to arrange care at an outpatient level or in a day hospital, nevertheless many situations do arise which involve the patient's leaving the community and entering the special hospital environment.

Symptomatic Treatment. There is in many instances an urgent need to relieve the symptoms and signs of the patient's illness and to minimise his distress by using any of the available treatments appropriate in the particular case—psychological and physical treatments, nursing care, occupational, recreational and social therapies. Whatever other factors enter into the picture the relief of the patient's personal discomfort must always be the dominant consideration in the nurse's mind.

Special Tests and Investigations. Some patients are admitted to hospital for special investigations of a complicated kind or to enable the medical staff to confirm a doubtful diagnosis. In this latter instance the observations and findings of the nurse will be of particular importance.

Establishment of Drug Therapy. The early stages of treatment with special drugs, such as tranquillisers or antidepressants, are often best carried out while the patient is under observation in hospital and in some instances this is absolutely essential. It may be desirable to have some epileptic patients in hospital to stabilise them on a regime of drugs.

Establishment of Psychotherapy. Some patients who are assessed as being suitable for management by psychological means, individually or in groups, may yet be required initially to enter hospital for a period in order to assist them to cope with the difficult early problems which frequently crop up in these treatments. Other patients, who are receiving psychotherapy at an outpatient level, may occasionally require admission to hospital, even if only for very brief periods, at a time when extremely anxiety-provoking conflicts are being brought to the surface and causing them considerable distress.

Relief of Environmental Stresses. Many patients require admission to hospital because it is felt that it will not be possible for them to begin to improve while they remain in an environment which is clearly stressful for them and which is in part causing or maintaining their illness. Particularly in the case of child patients, but with adults as well, it may be more practicable to modify the pathological environment while the sick person is temporarily removed from it.

Provision of Relief for Relatives. The care of mentally ill patients in the family setting, whilst often very rewarding and ultimately in the patient's best interests, can prove very trying to the relatives to whom this care is entrusted. In particular the management of mentally retarded individuals and the care of senile patients may be virtually continuous and extremely exhausting both mentally and physically. In some instances day hospital care is required rather than full psychiatric hospital admission; alternatively, admission may be arranged for brief periods to permit the patient's family a temporary respite from their burden.

Treatment of Intercurrent Disease. Psychiatric patients may require admission to hospital for the treatment of co-existing physical illnesses such as diabetes and tuberculosis.

Protection of the Patient and the Community. Some mentally ill persons require hospitalisation for their own protection, either because of the direct suicidal threat which they present or because their mental illness is such that they do not take adequate care of themselves; they may be drinking to excess, neglecting proper diet, spending money recklessly, or wandering around in a vagrant manner. Other patients may require to be hospitalised for the protection of the community, though this number is far smaller than the average person believes. Nevertheless there is a small minority of people with psychiatric illnesses who constitute a danger to other persons in their environment, either through violence or abnormal sexual behaviour, and who require treatment in hospital before they can be regarded as fit to live in the general community again.

Permanent Care and Protection. Some patients with psychiatric illnesses require care in hospital on a permanent basis, or at least for a very prolonged period. It is probably true that the number of such patients is a great deal smaller than has been previously thought; the poor quality of many hospital environments in past years has itself created many of these chronic problems (p. 399). The decision that a patient falls into this category should never be one which is reached lightly and should only be arrived at when a full study of the patient's assets and liabilities shows that it is highly unlikely or impossible that he will ever be able to live outside the hospital environment. Many of these patients have some variety of brain damage, either arising in very early life or brought about by some disease process in the middle or later years. Some patients with so-called functional psychotic reactions, especially schizophrenic reactions (see Chapter 11), also come into this category. For these people the hospital serves a special function which is considered in detail in Chapter 22 (p. 439).

It is repeated that, when care in hospital is regarded as unavoidable or as preferable under the circumstances, the central objective remains—namely, that the whole treatment resources of the hospital staff, using the special skills of each member of the therapeutic team, shall be brought to bear on his problems in an effort to achieve his discharge from hospital as soon as it appears that he can manage adequately in the community, either entirely on his own resources or using in addition the continued help which the hospital should be able to give.

3

THE DEVELOPMENT OF HUMAN BEHAVIOUR

IN our daily lives we all meet people who show themselves to be confident or insecure, relaxed or tense, meek or aggressive, happy or sad; as a result of our observations, we say that these people have "different personalities". There is Joan, aged 21, who faints at the sight of blood; Tom, a 17-year-old boy who stutters at work—but only when talking to his boss; there is

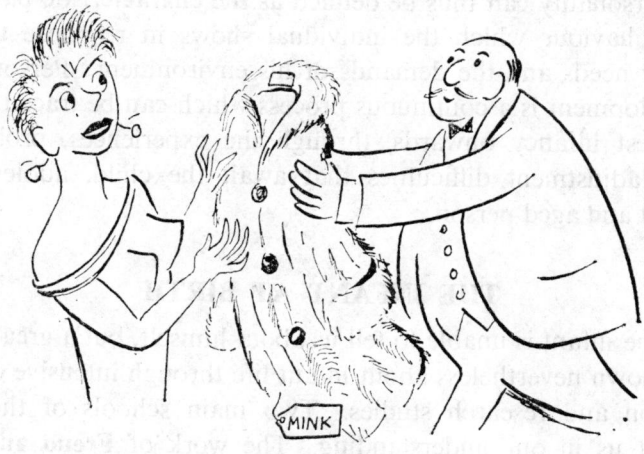

FIG. 2
Afraid of all furry things.

baby Jane aged 16 months, who screams at the touch of any furry object whether this be the family cat, a toy bear or the household rug. The conventional reaction is—" isn't it odd that they behave that way?" If we have additional information this sense of oddness disappears—we find that Joan faints because the experiences of her life have caused her to associate bleeding with extreme fear, that Tom has always stuttered in the presence of males in authority, that baby Jane was scratched by a cat in her fourteenth month but now links the fur, not the cat's claws, with the pain she experienced and has therefore become afraid of all furry things (Fig. 2).

Each of these examples demonstrates two basic features of personality. Firstly, personality patterns are influenced by each individual's past experiences; secondly, behaviour is not made up of accidental and meaningless occurrences but is determined by the personality structure of the individual. It is not that Joan, Tom and baby Jane are " just looking for attention " or " just being hard to get on with " when they act this way; their past experiences have determined that these particular reactions will occur in circumstances which they see as threatening.

Personality can thus be defined as the characteristic patterns of behaviour which the individual shows in response to his inner needs and the demands of his environment. Personality development is a continuous process which can be traced from earliest infancy onwards, through the experiences, problems and adjustment difficulties that await the child, adolescent, adult and aged person.

THE INFANT AT BIRTH

The infant is unable to tell us about himself, but a great deal is known nevertheless about infant life through intensive observation and research studies. Two main schools of thought assist us in our understanding. The work of **Freud** and the later psychoanalysts has given us a great knowledge of the emotional life of the infant and its influence on personality development, whereas the research of **Piaget** and his followers has given us a basis for understanding the development of thinking and the ways in which the baby comes to learn about himself and his surroundings.

The infant arrives in this world in a totally dependent and helpless state; his body, brain and nervous system are not yet fully developed or co-ordinated. This immature nervous system does not allow him to have a complete picture of himself and

THE DEVELOPMENT OF HUMAN BEHAVIOUR

his surroundings. The adult, through past experience, has come to recognise that he is someone separate and distinct from the other people and objects in his environment and can recognise that his internal thoughts and feelings are his and his alone and are not part of the external world. The baby begins life without this capacity—he does not know what is himself and what is not himself. In the very early months, when experiencing a pain, he is unable to distinguish whether the pain comes from inside himself or not.

At birth the infant is a bundle of undeveloped capacities which have been determined by his hereditary background. If all goes well these capacities steadily mature and he comes to sit up, walk, talk and make contact with people. This development will be influenced by his experiences; just as acquired physical disease may prevent proper motor co-ordination or speech, unhealthy emotional influences can delay or prevent his acquiring the feeling of security necessary for personality growth and social adjustment.

The development of his emotions or feelings also arises out of his experiences. He is born with a set of biological needs, for example, water, food, oxygen, warmth and survival. There is increasing evidence that he is also born with a primary need for attachment to his mother, quite apart from the gratifications (shortly to be described) which good mothering brings him. When these needs are requiring satisfaction there is set up a physiological reaction of unpleasant sensations and he is quickly driven to seek relief from these feelings. His emotional life is dominated by these powerful drives which require immediate gratification; this insistence on seeking his own pleasure through the removal of unpleasant tensions, regardless of other people's wishes, Freud has called the **pleasure principle** (p. 82). For example, he grows hungry because there is a need in his tissues for nourishment which is experienced by him as an unpleasant sensation. As a result he cries, he is fed, the need is satisfied, the unpleasant sensations are replaced by pleasant ones, following which he shows his contentment. We see that his first emotions arise out of primary needs; he will become anxious and angry when they are not met, happy and friendly when they are. The continuous repetition of this pattern allows him to learn that the unpleasant feelings will be removed and, since this removal is brought about by mother, she develops increasing meaning and importance for him. Therefore the atmosphere of the mother-child relationship contributes extensively to the shaping of the emotional development of the individual.

MOTHERING, SUCKLING AND WEANING

Through all of the infant's experiences with his mother, through each feeding situation, in " mothering " periods and in later weaning and toilet-training, she is the person who provides his first sustained social contact with another human being. (She need not in fact be his real or natural mother, as the role can be adequately filled by the right sort of person acting as a mother-substitute from an early age—for example, when a very young baby is adopted.) By the second month her presence, touch or voice from a distance will bring signs of recognition and contentment in him. He starts to build up a picture of what she is like and will later tend to transfer this same picture on to other people as they are introduced into his world. If experience has allowed him to feel satisfied by his mother and secure with her then his approach to other people will tend to be one of confidence; if the reverse of this has occurred he is likely to approach new people and new experiences with hesitancy and insecurity. The " good mother ", who accepts and is satisfied with her baby, is readily able to give him her love in her emotional and physical contacts with him.

Initially the feeding and suckling situation satisfies the needs for nourishment and provides the stimulation necessary to promote the development of the infant's primitive nervous system But the good mother does more than satisfy the needs of his tissues; she satisfies his dependence, she soothes him with her gentle voice and rhythmical movements, she comforts him with the warmth and softness of her body, she replaces the unpleasant hunger pains with feelings of " goodness ". She is gradually recognised by him as the person who gives " good feelings " and takes away " bad feelings ". He begins to trust mother who, through this trust, becomes the object of loving feelings. The capacity to love thus develops out of the satisfactions of this early relationship; it is certain that the infant who has met unsatisfactory mothering experiences will become the child and adult who, partly or wholly, finds it difficult to have or to express loving feelings towards another person.

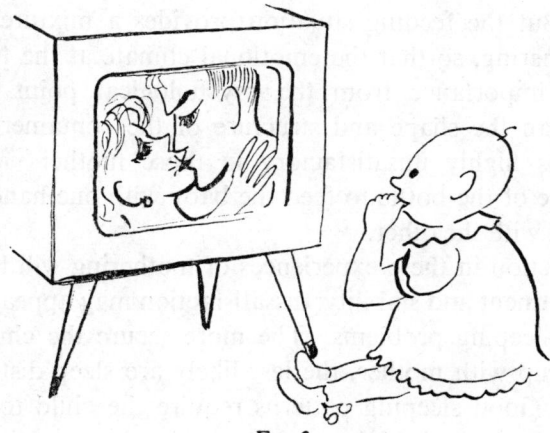

Fig. 3
The oral phase of personality development.

Because the infant's first feelings of goodness and comfort are obtained through feeding and suckling, food becomes linked with love and both become associated with lip and mouth sensations. In other words, the infant's mouth provides him with his first " taste " of the world and its people. Because of the great importance of the mouth, this period is referred to as the **oral phase** of personality development. This importance is clearly shown by the habit of thumb-sucking, carried on by all children to some extent; if food were all that were required, he would quickly remove his thumb when he found that it produced no milk—obviously he enjoys the sensations produced by sucking for their own sake. In later life traces of oral behaviour persist in quite normal people—in smoking, in the use of the mouth in love-making, in the common experience that anxiety and depression can sometimes be relieved by a good meal. One of the factors in the causation of drug dependence (see Chapter 10) is the relief of tension obtained by putting substances into the mouth.

A word should be said about the controversy over the relative merits of breast and bottle feeding. It is undeniable that natural breast-feeding can provide the mother with bodily and mental satisfactions which are reflected in contented handling of the infant. But the feeding situation provides a mixture of food and mothering, so that the emotional climate at the time is of primary importance from the psychological point of view, rather than the shape and structure of the container. Bottle-feeding is highly unsatisfactory in those mothers who take advantage of the bottle to feed the baby with one hand and do the beans with the other.

Satisfaction in these experiences of mothering will be shown in contentment and stability; dissatisfaction may appear in feeding and sleeping problems. The more secure the child in his relationship with mother, the less likely are sleep disturbances to arise. Good sleeping patterns require the child to develop the capacity to be left alone; if uncertain about mother, going to sleep may be felt by him as a rejection and her continued presence is required to reassure him. Unless the child has a physical illness, the amount of waking at night is greatest in those children who have had the least " mothering " during the day. Disturbed patterns of eating may also indicate emotional stress; the refusal of food often appears related to the feeling that the world and its people are bad and hurtful and consequently that food given to him from the world is also bad and hurtful. Many of the mentally ill adults who refuse to eat, stating that the food is poisoned, behave in the same way and for a similar reason.

But even when the relationship is proceeding smoothly and

there is contentment on both sides, sooner or later there come along the disruptive events of **teething** and **weaning**. Teething brings sore gums and the occurrence of angry biting feelings; through this biting the baby tries to discharge his feelings about the pain. He may become insecure and tense as the pleasure principle is frustrated; the mother's ability to take away his pain is no longer complete—moreover, due to the inadequate recognition of what is himself and what is not, the pain may be seen as coming from mother rather than as something arising inside himself. Weaning may occur about this time; the disappearance of the breast or bottle is a major loss for him—up to this point one or the other had been an essential part of his very existence and its removal threatens the stability of his little world. Since he sees this loss, and the consequent frustration of his oral needs, as the result of his own angry biting impulses, he is frightened by his own feelings of anger and aggression; at the same time he is further angered by the mother who took this pleasure away. The result is a confusing period in which love and hate are being directed simultaneously towards the mother. How he comes to adjust to these warring emotions will influence his later attitudes towards love and hate, for both of these feelings will be repeatedly aroused in later personal relationships. The maintenance of a warm mother-child bond is especially important during this time to tide him over this necessary stage of development, which represents his first movement away from complete dependence on the mother. Experience suggests that he will cope better with weaning and its resultant frustrations when it is made a gradual process of transition rather than occurring as an abrupt catastrophe.

Some mothers also have emotional problems of their own. If these lead her to be lacking in warmth towards him she will leave the child unable to trust and to display affection towards others. If she dominates him she will achieve submissive behaviour in him at the expense of growth in his own personality. If she overprotects him, not allowing him to meet and overcome the obstacles which must be conquered if one day he is to stand on his own two feet, she is likely to create prolonged immaturity in him and so-called "spoilt child" behaviour. If her attitude is inconsistent towards him, with unpredictable displays of affection and rejection, the child will be unable to develop a stable picture of people towards whom he may relate securely. (The topic of maternal rejection is dealt with more fully in Chapter 13, p. 292.)

Separation from mother at this stage may have serious results, even when the relationship has been a good one. It has been noted that babies between six and 12 months of age go into a state best described as **infantile depression** when parted for any substantial period from their mothers. They appear to be fearful and sad, and may withdraw from or even totally reject their environment. All activities may be slowed down and the child may sit or lie as if in a dazed state, making no attempt to contact people in the vicinity. **Bowlby** and his colleagues have shown that " some children in their personality development suffer grave damage and others lesser damage from a separation experience ". The practical recommendation is that " the separation of a young child from his mother figure is not to be undertaken without weighty reasons, and then only provided there is a suitable and stable substitute available to him ".[1] Separation does not have to involve physical distance to produce damage to the developing personality; " emotional distance " may be as harmful as actual physical absence.

Hand in hand with this development of emotions and relationships goes an increasing awareness of the limits of his own physical body and some dawning realisation of the existence of his own inner world of thought. Gradually he comes to recognise objects in his environment and to attach meaning and feelings to them. Watch a baby " find his toes " and see that he is learning that these distant " objects " are actually a part of his own body—they are him. At the same time he is learning to separate feelings coming from inside himself from those which arise outside him. Piaget has used the term **adualism** to describe

[1] Bowlby, J. (1958). *Brit. J. med. Psychol.* 31, 247.

the state of mind in infancy before the baby is able to recognise the difference between himself and the external world; gradually he matures from this stage to the point where he can recognise himself as an individual, distinct from his surroundings, and can test this individuality against the people and objects in the world about him.

Summarising these early months, the infant begins life in a state of total, helpless dependence upon his mother, from whom all his satisfactions come until the time of weaning marks the beginning of a new type of relationship with her. During this time he begins to progress from the state of adualism towards the recognition of himself as someone separate from the other objects in his environment. Emotions of love, anger and anxiety are experienced for the first time. Up to this point his developing personality structure has been almost entirely shaped by the adequacy, or inadequacy, of his relationship with his mother.

The infant is now coming to develop a recognition of the boundary of his body, the beginnings of a mental picture of himself known as the **body image;** the mother comes to be seen as a separate person and not as part of himself. But even when he is capable of recognising objects, these objects at first exist for him only while they are actually present and it is not until somewhere near the end of the first year that a clear memory image exists in the object's absence. Despite this, his distress when mother is absent and his satisfaction on her return indicate that he is able to register that *something* is missing. At the same time he recognises that the feelings and needs which he experiences are his own, coming from inside himself; only when he realises this can he begin to seek to control them. Muscular development allows progressive co-ordination and control, shown in sitting up, crawling and walking, indicating his increasing ability to make his body respond to his bidding. The gradual development of language provides a means of communicating his needs, wishes and feelings.

PSYCHIATRIC NURSING

FRUSTRATIONS AND REALITY

Now, while seeking to explore and to assert himself, he increasingly runs head on into frustration, ranging from the play-pen that limits his wanderings to parental judgements and restrictions on his behaviour. Gradually he finds himself expected to conform to parental attitudes and values. As an independent being, he would like to decide some things for

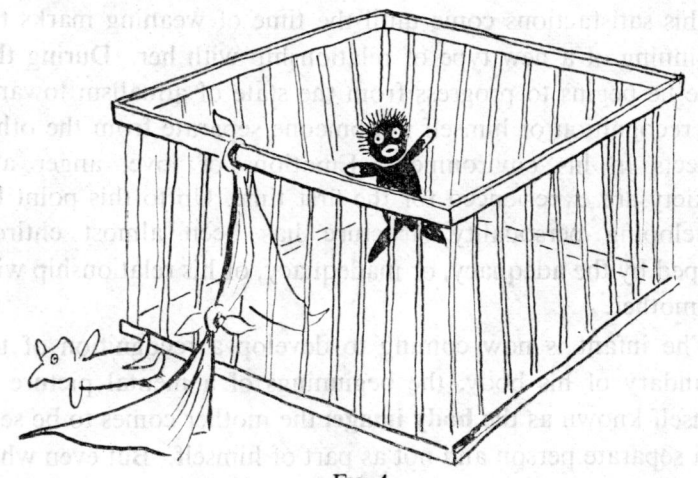

FIG. 4
The play-pen that limits his wanderings.

himself, but finds his decisions repeatedly opposed. This struggle, at its height from about 15 months to approximately three years of age, is highlighted in toilet-training, in which we find a dramatic example of the changing relationships between parent and child.

There are a number of reasons for this. After the weaning period the child becomes increasingly interested in his bodily activities and in time the oral phase is replaced by that stage of development in which he derives particular pleasure from excretory functions—the so-called **anal phase**. Defaecation is for the infant a pleasurable act and he shows an intense interest in his own faeces, largely because they are his first recognisable product, the first sign that there is something which he can do for himself and which nobody else can do for him. (Because these important faeces are deposited in the toilet, some children come to regard this as a rather important place and may feel therefore that it is an appropriate spot in which to put all the most valuable possessions of the household!) Remembering that the child's emotional life is still largely governed by the pleasure principle it is not surprising that he resists parental frustration of his wishes. Here the parents' feelings about the child are well shown; some are determined to mould the child to their own ideas, whilst others are content to allow him to develop at his own pace. (Some children may *appear* to be toilet-trained prior to 12 months of age, but this can only be due to the establishment of a simple reflex habit, as it is not until the age of 15 months that the child even begins to exercise voluntary control over his excretory functions.) With the realisation that he is the boss in this particular aspect of living the child may revolt against parental attempts to direct him. Some parents, anxious and determined to " make the child obey ", place him on the pot for an extended period, scold or rebuke him if he fails to perform, or pass into raptures at his most meagre contribution. It is not surprising that, when parents behave in this fashion, he quickly realises what a powerful weapon he possesses in his excretions. Accordingly he may use them to please his parents and to gain their praise, but if he is feeling angry with them he may also use them to show his hostility, resistance and independence.

How they react to this resistance will affect both the speed and certainty with which he gains personal control over his toilet functions. Usually somewhere during the course of the second year of life the child will normally reveal his readiness for toilet-training and wish to behave like his parents or older brothers and sisters; he is beginning to copy his elders and follow in their footsteps. Moreover, he is prepared to conform to some extent to their wishes in order to obtain their approval.

Parental, and particularly maternal, attitudes of patience, acceptance and tolerance will be more rewarding through this period than a rigid and restrictive training. By the same token, if parental feelings of dislike or disgust towards toilet functions are expressed in their behaviour, such feelings may be reinforced in the child and remain a part of his later personality structure. Such parental attitudes may result in later unusual interest in excretory functions or excessive shame concerning them and may produce a later personality characterised by over-organised patterns of living and by a preoccupation with excessive cleanliness and avoidance of dirt. The fact that excretory behaviour can be used to express complicated emotions, particularly anger, is very apparent in some of the bowel and urinary disturbances of childhood (p. 286) and may also be shown in the incontinent habits of some psychiatric patients (p. 443).

During this period, the child is in a conflict situation. He realises that to obtain the much desired love of his parents he is required, at least to some extent, to conform—but conforming conflicts with his wishes based on the pleasure principle. This is the time when the formerly placid child becomes rebellious and tends to do the opposite of what he is told. But in normal development conforming wins out—to a greater or lesser extent he modifies his own wishes, adapts to the demands made by the outside world, and is now said to have developed the capacity to live according to the **reality principle** (p. 83).

THE CHILD AND THE FAMILY

Gradually the child's possession of the mother is whittled away by various separation experiences. Yet, if he is the youngest child, he retains a favoured position in the family until he is dethroned by the arrival of a brother or sister. The intensity of his reaction to this event will be greater at 12 months than at five years of age—at the latter time the child has a certain ability to make up for this sense of displacement by using his own resources and his increased independence. But to some extent at any age, seeing the new arrival dominating the scene and possessing mother's time and attention leads to feelings of rejection, rivalry and aggression towards the intruder. This competitive jealousy for mother's love is known as **sibling rivalry** (sibling: brother or sister). Expressions such as " let's send him back, I'll be your baby " are indicative of this

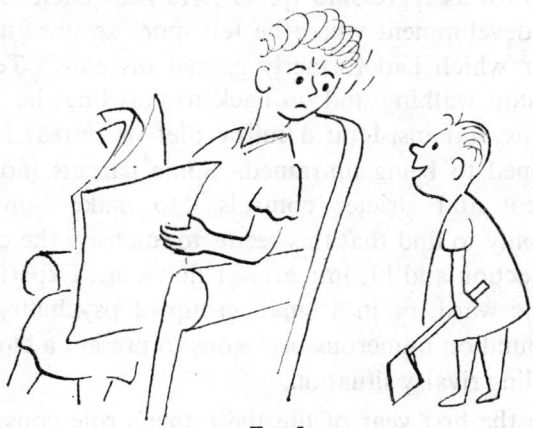

FIG. 5
" I think the baby has stopped breathing ".

feeling of jealousy, whilst aggression may appear either thinly veiled in comments such as, " Mummy, I think the baby has stopped breathing ", or in openly hostile attitudes and behaviour.

Within limits, such behaviour is normal and contributes to the experience of " growing up ". He has to learn to share, first his mother, later his possessions; how he finally adjusts to this will influence his behaviour in the later situations requiring sharing which will occur throughout his life. In normal circumstances he learns to modify his demands and needs so that he comes to benefit from the new family structure and from its opportunities for increased companionship. How he adapts will depend considerably on parental attitudes. Parents may support the child through this period by recognising his anxieties and by offering alternative pleasures for him. At the other extreme are those parents who exclusively centre the family's thought and attention on to the new arrival while the older child is reduced to the position of " second cab on the rank ". Particularly if insecure with mother even prior to the arrival of the new child, rivalry may be so intense that his only means of coping is by a return to immature behaviour, a technique known as **regression** (p. 99). He goes back to an earlier stage of development where he felt more secure and uses the behaviour which had formerly gained his ends. Temporarily he may stop walking and go back to crawling, he may reject solid foods and insist on a milky diet or retreat from being toilet-trained to being untrained. Some parents move in with punishment and stricter controls " to make him grow up again ", only to find that this seems to intensify the child's feeling of rejection and his immature behaviour. Experiences on a psychiatric ward, or in a small group of psychiatric patients, will be found on numerous occasions to present a close parallel to the sibling rivalry situation.

During the first year of life the father's role consists largely of supporting mother and providing her with a trouble-free environment in which she is able to relate comfortably to her baby. Later of course father's personality becomes increasingly reflected in the family experiences. From father the child's picture of males begins to develop and this picture he carries with him to some extent into adolescence and adulthood. But when father is seen to have a special kind of relationship with mother, not shared by any other member of the family, then a new factor creeps into the child's development.

FROM THREE TO SIX

At about four years of age a third stage of development ensues known as the **phallic stage** (phallus: male sexual organ). At this period there is an increasing interest in his own and other people's bodies and a growing recognition of the physical differences between people and, in particular, great curiosity about the anatomical differences between the sexes. To explain these differences the child forms theories which often appear fantastic to the adult mind. Initially he thinks of other people as being the same as himself; when the difference in anatomy is recognised it is thought of, not as a basic difference present from birth, but as the result of something that has happened either to the boy or the girl. Often one can observe a perfectly normal little boy who, on seeing an unclad girl, queries with obvious perplexity and sometimes recognisable anxiety " what has happened to her wee-wee?" His reaction clearly indicates that he thinks that her penis has been taken away and this leads him to the fear that if he does wrong he could be similarly punished. This anxiety is referred to as **castration anxiety.** In the young girl the recognition of difference often results in feelings of envy; this is expressed later in jealousy of the boy's games, his strength and even his clothes. In cases where development proceeds unfavourably for one or another reason, this pattern may persist into adulthood, leading to the woman who consciously or unconsciously is dissatisfied with her feminine role in life and who constantly envies and tries to rival the male in his own tasks. This behaviour, evidence of what is called **masculine protest,** is derived from the basic anxiety about sexual differences. Though many a little girl openly shows her feelings by asking, as a Christmas present, for " a bottom like my brother's ", only an unfortunate few fail to solve this problem in the course of development. Perception of the boy's penis can also lead the little girl to feel that she herself must in the past have been punished for wrong-doing by the removal of this organ.

At about the same time the child becomes increasingly possessive of the parent of the opposite sex and this attitude is accompanied by feelings of rivalry, aggression and resulting guilt towards the parent of the same sex as himself. This situation was termed by Freud the **Oedipus complex,** a crucial stage in development which, unsatisfactorily overcome, may have serious consequences for later personality development. There are essential differences between the reactions at this time of the little girl and the little boy, and these are best considered separately.

The Little Girl. The little girl shows increasing interest in her father and increasing love for him, expressed in her behaviour, imagination and play. In a home where she is permitted to express her feelings with reasonable frankness she may go through a stage of openly competing with mother for father's affections, calling him by his Christian name, racing mother to get what he wants and copying mother's behaviour towards him. Because basically she wishes to take mother's place with father this is a time of anger, anxiety and guilt; she fears her mother's retaliation and her father's rebuff. About this time she begins to develop household interests—through these she seeks to prove her ability to look after father as well as mother does but, as well as the component of rivalry, this behaviour also indicates the girl's movement towards an unwitting copying of her mother. She begins to see mother as the sort of person she would like to be and this is a good sign for the little girl's future, provided that the mother on whom she is modelling herself is a reasonably stable and feminine person. During this period she has to come to accept that she cannot have father for herself; she also has to face the painful truth about the parents' private relationship with each other, even though she will not fully understand it. Parental understanding, toleration, support and interest will all help her resolve her conflicts and adjust to these complicated emotions. But if the response to her behaviour is laughter or anger, disgust or withdrawal, then her love feelings will be disturbed and this may lead to later difficulties in establishing satisfactory relationships with the opposite sex. Many instances of spinsterhood, divorce, sexual frigidity and homosexuality may be traced to a failure to resolve the conflicts of this period. Moreover such a failure is of great significance for the later development of psychiatric illness (p. 148).

The Little Boy. During the same period the boy's feelings of love and desire for his mother increase; he wants her for himself and feels his father to be his rival. He may say out loud to his mother: " If Daddy died, *then* could I marry you, Mummy?" Yet he is afraid of father and fears what the latter might do to him on account of these wishes. Commonly he imagines that father may punish him by removing his male sexual organ—in fact some particularly foolish fathers may even directly threaten this as a punishment for sexual or other forms of misbehaviour. If all goes well he begins, through games, displays of strength, interest in mechanical toys and so on, to copy his father's behaviour and to show his wish to be like him; in time he accepts the way in which his father looks after and thinks about his mother. This promises well for his future and ensures the satisfactory development of masculine behaviour. Here again unsatisfactory parental behaviour and attitudes, or an inadequate example of masculinity in the household, may prevent the child resolving the conflicts of this period, with the result that he retreats from his male role.

This gradual taking over of certain aspects of the parents' behaviour so that it becomes a part of the child's personality is known as **identification.** Identifying with a normal parent of the same sex leads to the establishment in the child of behaviour appropriate to that sex and gives him the capacity to take a person of the opposite sex as the later object of his love. But a poorly adjusted and disturbed father, whom the boy uses as a model, can have long-lasting unfortunate effects on the child's later development. If circumstances are such in the family, due to death, divorce, or the domination of one parent by the other, that either boy or girl identifies more easily with the parent of the opposite sex, then serious disturbances may be the result.

To the puzzled adult, who remembers little or nothing of this in his own development, it must be said at this stage that even in the normal person the anxieties and conflicts of this time are so painful that they are automatically removed from consciousness by the defence mechanism known as **repression** (p. 94).

In fact all the anxieties of these early years of life are kept out of adult awareness, not simply because of the great time which has elapsed since their occurrence, but because of this mechanism of automatic forgetting which is described more fully in Chapter 5.

THE CHILD'S THINKING

Adults are usually inclined to over-estimate the child's capacities for thinking, often assuming it to be guided by the same type of logic which characterises the normal adult mind. But it is not until the eighth year that truly rational thinking appears, its achievement being dependent upon the transition from adualism previously referred to and on the development of full and adequate recognition of the self. Prior to this attainment the child sees himself as the natural centre of the world and all of his thinking is focussed around himself, a mode of thought termed **egocentric.** During these early years he is unaware that his mind exists as such and he has the belief that everything happens outside the mind. This is called **exteriorisation** and is the type of thinking which underlies the defence mechanism of projection (p. 100). Another component of the thinking of this early period is **animism;** the child endows everything, including inanimate objects, with life. Thus a cup on its side is described as " tired " because it is lying down, an empty bottle is " thirsty "—because he is alive, everything else is seen as possessing life. Even when he later recognises that all objects do not possess life, he still thinks of moving objects in this way —to him trains and cars are endowed with personalities of their own.

Yet another form of thinking observable before the development of adult logic is **magical thinking.** The child's early fears are often associated with this—for example, he sees his angry thoughts and wishes as being so powerful that they can cause direct harm to other people. If he has fantasies of destructiveness towards a parent and that parent should die or disappear, then the resulting sense of guilt may be very great. On the

THE DEVELOPMENT OF HUMAN BEHAVIOUR

other hand magical thinking may be used as a means of self-protection; thinking good thoughts may, in this primitive way, protect him from harm. Though this type of thinking is to a large extent left behind in childhood, traces of it are common in adults, particularly in those who still have many superstitions —who believe, for instance, that throwing salt over one's shoulder will ward off bad luck. It is also a striking feature of that type of psychiatric illness known as the obsessive-compulsive reaction (p. 189) and is also very similar to the type of thinking seen in some uncivilised native tribes.

Also at this stage the child divides the external world into " the good " and " the bad ". Whoever protects and pleases the child is good, is liked by the child and the child feels liked by him. Whoever frightens and hurts the child is bad, disliked and felt in turn to dislike the child. He has further difficulty in separating his imaginings from external reality—often the events of his imagination are so vivid and real to him that he may believe that these have actually happened. In these early years he may find it almost impossible to understand that his own nightmare was something not felt and shared by his parents. The internal fears of some immature adults may have to them a similar quality of reality; fearing her overdue husband dead, the neurotic wife may almost be able to " see " him lying mangled in a ditch.

Understanding children is impossible without recognition of these differences in their manner of thinking. It has been pointed out, for example, that a young child going to hospital, told she is to have an operation, may visualise that the surgical procedure to be carried out on her body will be the same sort of thing that she does to her dolls when she pulls them to pieces and puts them back together again. All these patterns of thinking become interwoven with the child's feelings, for any separation between the two is artificial. Some of his problems he solves in play and fantasy; through play he learns to master his environment and his anxieties and particularly to act out in a harmless way the aggressive feelings which he dare not discharge directly. These games provide therefore a safety mechanism, frequently employed by child psychiatrists in their treatment technique of play therapy (p. 296).

THE DEVELOPMENT OF CONSCIENCE

The so-called " voice " of conscience exerts a strong influence and control over the behaviour of adolescents and adults; it approves or disapproves of each of the individual's wishes, feelings and decisions. The previous remarks about the importance of the pleasure principle make it obvious that the child is certainly totally lacking in conscience at birth and during his early years, although the contrary view is still commonly held. It does not begin to operate as an effective agent until about the sixth year of life. Prior to this time children obviously show in many ways that they understand the difference between right and wrong—they are able at times to restrain destructive impulses towards other children and to curb the wish to steal another child's toy. This behaviour, however, only discloses his ability to conform to the demands and codes of conduct laid down by adults; he obeys authorities which are still external to him and conforms to their values in order to protect himself from punishment and loss of their love.

With the development of conscience these previously external standards now become a part of his own personality and act as an internal guide to his own behaviour, which now comes to be *felt* as right or wrong, with the result that he is able to experience shame and guilt.

Obviously the standards which he acquires are mainly those of his parents. By and large the children of parents who lack reasonable moral values will be left without an effective conscience, a situation which is commonly found in those adults who have a character neurosis of an antisocial type (p. 203). On the other hand, parents with excessively rigid and unyielding moral values can influence the child to build into himself a conscience which is too demanding and which leaves him permanently troubled by feelings of despair and moral inadequacy. Conscience, like many of the necessary things of life, may yet if too weak or too demanding mar the individual's capacity to function as an effective social unit.

THE SCHOOL-AGE CHILD

The period up to six years of age is a vital one for the child's ultimate development. By this time he has developed fairly stable patterns of behaviour and feeling; he has learnt ways of dealing with emotions such as love, jealousy and anger. Following these years of highly charged emotional development there is a relatively quiet period during which the child displays an increasing interest in, and movement towards, the world of people and things outside the immediate family situation. This is the time of intellectual growth and of movement towards social development. Egocentric thinking and impulsive behaviour have largely to be left behind; he is required to work out an adequate balance between his own needs and the customs and demands of his society, for his own benefit and that of the broader community.

Social development is directed by three factors. Firstly, his bodily structure may be of considerable importance, particularly if there is any marked physical abnormality—for example, gross interference with sight or hearing, a paralysis or a disfigurement. All these limit a person's capacity for social behaviour and may make more difficult the acquisition of the desired independence. Secondly, environmental factors may produce a long-lasting influence; family attitudes may encourage growth towards outside friendships and relative freedom or may actively suppress such advancement. Moreover the environment in his district may encourage the development of a good adjustment to society or may foster antisocial values. Thirdly, social relationships depend upon the emotional development of the child. His security (or lack of it) and his feelings about himself will all influence his ability to relate to other people, to trust them, to seek out new experiences and to form increasing contacts with a broadening social group.

Schooling is a major step towards breaking down the child's dependence on the family. It brings an increase in his range of personal contacts and introduces new authorities, new playmates and new experiences. These experiences can, in unfavourable circumstances, reawaken many of the anxieties, conflicts and emotions initially experienced by the child in relation to his own family. His behaviour at school bears the stamp of his own family situation; teachers may be feared for no particularly good reason if authority has been harsh in the home, excessive rivalry may develop with other pupils for the teacher's attention as a consequence of unsolved sibling rivalry in the family. Teachers can become the targets for emotions, particularly rebellious ones, originally arising in relation to the parents. Gradually school becomes a learning situation; the child tests out the extent to which he may express his feelings and assert his own individuality and yet still conform to the limits laid down by society. In time he learns that if he goes too far the others will " gang up " on him; little by little he comes to recognise that certain forms of behaviour will be followed by undesirable consequences. Many parallels exist here with the behaviour which will be noted when patients live together in a psychiatric ward.

Sport brings the need for co-operation with others and for the acceptance of leadership. Team games require the submerging of the child's needs into the team's needs and show him both the difficulties and the advantages of co-operation. In all these activities teachers will be playing the part of substitute parents; if they fill their role wisely, they may do a great deal towards modifying any unfavourable parental examples previously established in the child's mind.

Of course the primary purpose of schooling is to provide the child with a formal education. How successful this will be depends, not only on his basic intelligence, but on the emotional atmosphere of the classroom and the way in which he reacts to his teachers. Where healthy, positive attitudes towards learning are created then, in the absence of other handicaps, he will tend to learn readily in order to please his teacher and to maintain good relationships. The rate of intellectual growth and the way in which new experiences are built into the child's personality will however depend to some extent on the particular meaning the experience has for him in the light of his previous background and feelings. The small boy's father has perhaps sneered at "book learning", while his mother has actively encouraged it; for such a boy lessons may be suspect because they are unwittingly thought of as being feminine and "cissy". Thus he comes to see the world through his own particular pair of spectacles which have been shaped and tinted from the beginning by his early relationships. Some of what he sees and thinks about the people and the world around him will often be distorted, clouded or misunderstood because he is putting into these situations something of the picture he carries inside himself. In a state of emotional stress learning may be impossible and situations may be incompletely understood; he may be unable to take in knowledge due to anxiety and tension. That is to say, his emotional state may suppress the development and the best usage of his basic endowment.

During this period, from the time of resolution of the Oedipus complex at the age of six or seven up to the time of puberty at the age of 12 or thereabouts, the child has little interest in sex and tends to associate largely with children of the same sex as himself. Gradually at the age of 10 or 11 we begin to see the reappearance of ideas and behaviour connected with the earlier wishes and fears of childhood. There is an increase in bodily feelings and the commencement of protest against parental domination. All this becomes the prelude to the physical and emotional upheavals of adolescence.

THE YEARS OF ADOLESCENCE

Following on the period of relative calm just described, there comes the time of sudden physical development at **puberty**. The years following this are known as adolescence and are characterised by a number of physical changes which call for a variety of new adjustments. This time is pressure-packed with conflicts as the adolescent experiences further collisions between his own needs and the demands of his family and social environment.

There are four fundamental changes during the adolescent period:

1. Physical Growth. A relatively sudden change in the activity of the endocrine glands leads to rapid muscular development and striking alterations in the size and shape of the adolescent boy and girl. With these changes goes a heightened awareness of the body and its feelings. Whilst endeavouring to cope with these marked and rapid changes the adolescent often expresses himself in awkward, unattractive behaviour.

2. Sexual Growth. At puberty begins the development of what are known as the secondary sexual characteristics. In the boy his approach towards manhood is signified by the growth of pubic hair, enlargement of the testes, a broken voice, the tentative use of shaving equipment and an upsurge of sexual feelings often accompanied by nocturnal discharges of semen. For the girl the growth of pubic hair, the development of her breasts, the general rounding of her bodily outline and the appearance of menstruation are the signs of her advance towards womanhood. In both sexes the feelings and attitudes earlier developed towards sexual drives and thoughts will be reawakened during this time.

3. Intellectual Growth. Somewhere around the age of 16 the individual's intellectual capacity achieves its full bloom. Obviously all people do not have the same endowment; not quite so obviously, intelligence is not to be confused with knowledge and experience. Whilst intellectual capacity does not develop further after this age, there is usually a substantial increase in the range of available information which makes the individual better able to form judgements and to deal with his surroundings.

4. Social Growth. This emerges from the physical, sexual and intellectual changes which direct and stimulate increasing social relationships. This growth is the essential bridge which enables the individual to step over from the dependence of the child to the independence of the adult.

The Effects of These Changes on the Adolescent

The conflicts of adolescence can be understood as arising out of the changes just listed and their meaning for the individual. In brief, these changes influence the individual's feelings about himself and his body, his sexual role and identity, his interest patterns and job ambitions and his adjustment to his family and society.

Bodily Feelings. Adolescence brings an increased awareness of the bodily self. The adolescent frequently wears these changes like a new suit, which either embarrasses by its newness or which fails to fit its owner. His behaviour is therefore characterised by clumsy bodily movements, by awkwardness and self-consciousness, all of which can be reflected in his social contacts. There is usually an increased attention to personal detail and the adolescent's concern with hair, teeth, freckles and pimples is indicative of this increased self-awareness. This sensitivity about the self is accompanied by an increased sensitivity towards the people around him. Already on the defensive, the adolescent is over-critical of adult attitudes and his self-consciousness leads him to read personal meanings into statements where none were intended. This is often aggravated by comments from adults which indicate intolerance or amusement at his efforts. Faced with such beliefs he may retreat from or aggress at his real or imagined tormentors, or may reject their standards and what they represent. Any of these defences can have undesirable effects on his search for a secure identity for himself.

Sexual Role and Identity. In the boy his increasing sexual feelings will reawaken any anxieties associated with his earlier sexual feelings towards his mother, even though he may not be fully aware of these, and may reactivate the guilts and fears arising from his expectation of father's retaliation. The same Oedipal anxieties occur in the girl, as well as a concern about what is happening inside herself. If not adequately prepared for the event, or if harbouring frightening fantasies about sex, the first menstruation can be experienced as a severe psychological stress. A special aspect of bodily change is seen in some adolescent girls with hidden sexual anxieties who may be acutely embarrassed by breast development and may go to great lengths to avoid this being noticeable.

Increasing emotional demands may be directed towards the opposite sex parent and the denial of these demands may result in anger. Usually the adolescent turns to someone of his or her own age, both to express and to receive the love satisfactions desired. Temporarily, the boy may turn away from women and may find his love object in his own sex, for example, by having a strong attraction for the captain of the first football team; the girl may do likewise or, more seriously, carry her unsatisfied needs for her father into companionship or marriage with much older men. In early adolescence both boys and girls may develop one or more relationships which warrant the label homosexual, that is to say, they develop physical feelings towards a person of the same sex. It is by no means rare for such relationships to involve physical acts of a homosexual kind; Kinsey suggests that one-third of American males have had such experiences, but very few of these go on to develop an exclusively homosexual outlook. If homosexual practices have occurred only rarely it is probably unlikely that they will have any serious significance for the adolescent's future, though they may lead to a crushing sense of guilt in some instances. Later in adolescence the teenager's interests, if development proceeds normally, become exclusively heterosexual (that is, characterised by physical feelings towards a person of the opposite sex).

During this time a periodic awareness of sexual desires and

the occasional practice of masturbation (self-satisfaction of sexual need) are both essentially normal. But for some individuals these bring intense, often persistent and sometimes socially crippling emotional stress. If the child has been trained to regard sexual feeling and functions as sinful, or if the attitudes expressed in the family towards sexual matters have been coloured by overtones of disgust, then the emergence of the sexual drive may lead to intense guilt and depression. Many parents unfortunately are so anxious and confused by their own sexual conflicts that they instil into their children unnecessary fears and incorrect information. Often parental anxieties result in sexual education being carried out mainly in the form of " threats " of what might happen if they indulge in any form of sexual activity, so that the adolescent's already great difficulties are intensified. Anxieties of this type will frequently be connected with the many psychiatric symptoms which may develop during adolescence, in some cases only for a brief period, but all too frequently as the beginning of a major emotional disturbance. To escape the " evil " thoughts associated with sexual matters some individuals may withdraw substantially from social activity in order to isolate themselves from the opposite sex; others are forced to defend themselves by a wide variety of fears and rituals.

Western cultures formerly imposed a lengthy waiting period between the time of puberty and the time of marriage, when sexual needs could be satisfied in what was then the only socially approved way. The culture as a whole tended to frown on premarital sexual activity, even whilst acknowledging that it existed, though other societies permitted or encouraged sexual experimentation during adolescence. Even the most normal adolescent, carrying few anxieties concerning sexual matters from his earlier development, had to deal for some ten or more years with pressing biological needs and find a solution acceptable to his own conscience and to the conventions of his social group.

Conventions reflect the attitude of a culture and mirror its changes. In the last decade or so the so-called " sexual revolution " has had a marked effect on Western societies, readily evidenced in the standards of the culture as expressed in art and literature, in altered standards of censorship and in the behaviour of individuals, both adolescent and adult. In consequence there has been greater scope for direct sexual expression, in ways approved by the adolescent peer group, with much less feeling of guilt. Concurrently a good deal of this sexual energy is still discharged in not directly sexual ways through the mechanism of **sublimation.**

For some, however, it has been a disappointment to recognise that increased sexual freedom has not always led to freedom from personal unhappiness or even overt psychiatric illness. Changed social attitudes, unfortunately, do not in themselves provide much relief for those many individuals who retain major conflicts concerning sexual matters arising from childhood experience and relationships. For these people, adolescence and adult life may still precipitate considerable and sometimes disabling anxiety, guilt and distressing interference with their personal and social relationships.

INTERESTS, AMBITIONS AND JOBS

The ideal environment for the adolescent is one of security, stimulation and encouragement so that he may make the best use of his capacities and opportunities. Unfortunately, the development of his capacities will in some instances have been marred by past emotional experiences; instead of curiosity there is disinterest, with a lack of any eagerness to learn, a distaste for any intellectual pursuits and a reluctance to master a difficult task. An unfavourable environment in the home or suburb may channel all his intelligence into feats of memory concerning race results or the " top forty " on this week's hit parade.

How the more promising adolescent develops into an adult will depend upon the reaction he gets to his curiosity and enthusiasm. He has always been noted for more fervour than subtlety; often his opinions are wildly impractical, yet are the result of his inexperience and his desire to explore new fields. All too frequently these are squashed by adults whose short memories prevent them recalling their own adolescent days. If his ideas are consistently disregarded, he may see this as amounting to rejection of himself as a person; in consequence he may protect himself from such hurts by withholding his own ideas or by, in return, partially or completely rejecting adult values.

During this period he contemplates a career. Because work involves routines, discipline, a variety of relationships with other people and complex new experiences, it may be evaded, passively accepted or actively sought. On the one hand work may be seen as an undesired restriction on his leisure, on the other hand visualised as a means, desirable and in itself enjoyable, of obtaining long-term goals. When he leaves school the adolescent is taking a major step towards adulthood, for here he begins to "pay his own way" and to be responsible for himself; the fortunate one has guidance and encouragement from his parents at this time. The job he takes on becomes part of his identity and security, as well as a means of obtaining possessions and status in life; it may (but all too frequently does not) provide emotional satisfaction. In some people persistent resentment towards discipline and authority is reflected in their work habits, in unpunctuality, resistance to guidance and direction, in absenteeism and repeated job changes. Because individuals possess varying aptitudes these are usually measured prior to career selection (a process known as **Vocational Guidance**). In all too many instances parents are either disinterested or, perhaps even worse, have unrealistic ideas about what their child should be and guide him into a job for which he has no particular talent and in which he has no interest. Such a situation leads inevitably to tension and conflict.

RELATIONSHIP WITH PARENTS

During adolescence there is on the one hand the wish to be free, to make decisions, to explore, to throw off parental restraint, to make light of adult ideas, values and judgement, to ridicule all grown-ups and to be angry at their " stupidity ". On the other hand the adolescent is somewhat bewildered by the rapidity of his many changes and has a strong need, which he often does not recognise himself, for security, guidance, control, affection and a stable home background. At times he seeks to move out from his domestic environment to cope with the world outside and " sort himself out "; at other times, perhaps even the following day, he retreats back into the shelter and protection of dependence on his family. His moods may swing rapidly from love to hate; one day he seeks advice, the next day scornfully rejects it; sometimes he sees his parents as doing no wrong, at other times he has little regard for them. If all goes well the adolescent, out of this conflict, strengthens his feelings of individuality and independence and his parents come to be accepted as people in their own right, people whose ideas and values he largely accepts, but from whom he can differ in some instances without bitterness. But parents for their part may fail to understand his needs, either neglecting to provide sufficient support and direction or enforcing tight restrictions on his behaviour or, worst of all, swinging unpredictably between these two extremes. If his opportunities for development and self-expression are suppressed, or if there is little real affection and acceptance in his environment, then the result may be persistent dependence; alternatively, there may be a rejection of family influences and aggression through delinquent and antisocial behaviour.

RELATIONSHIPS WITH SOCIETY

During adolescence the individual is busily engaged in testing out his relationships with others, attempting to find for himself a social group in which he feels comfortable and which has standards acceptable to him. Unfortunately society, like some parents, may also demand on the one hand that he behave like an adult and accept adult values of self-assertion and independence while, on the other hand, expecting him to conform in every way and discouraging or disregarding his opinions and judgements. For a period, even in the most normal circumstances, the adolescent tends to react to this with a state of protest. To protect himself and to ensure that he belongs somewhere he bands together with his own kind; adolescents often form their own groups or " gangs ", with private membership badges (special clothes or hair-styles) and sometimes even constructing their own language as a barrier to outsiders who are regarded as " squares ". By these devices they assert their own values and support their insecurity by group membership. Obviously, the standards of the group to which the adolescent is drawn will play a significant part in determining whether he adopts healthy or unhealthy, social or antisocial, behaviour. Adults so often accentuate such gang behaviour, with its possible undesirable consequences, by showing open resentment towards this rising group of people which will ultimately replace them.

Another important factor is the adolescent's disillusionment Throughout childhood he is taught certain principles to guide his social behaviour; many of these principles stress love and respect for the life and property of mankind. In adolescence many of these guides to conduct crash as he surveys the domestic and international scenes and begins to note the jealousies and rivalries of some aspects of the business world and becomes aware of the increasing emphasis on military power. He comes to hear that the annual budget for health or education is less than the weekly budget for the development of scientific weapons of destruction. To the adolescent the adults have " made a mess of things ". Even in the family, he may all too frequently suffer serious disillusionment as he finds that the principles drummed into him by his father are not always strictly adhered to by his parents. Consequently adolescence is a period of perplexity. One sees the picture of a group of " angry young men " and women trying to establish a balance between their own values and those of adults—all this in a world where at the present time values are in any event rapidly changing.

SUMMARY OF ADOLESCENCE

The adolescent years are marked by rapid and numerous changes, by the pressures of physical development and by emotional turmoil. Despite the need for the adolescent to express and establish his own increasing individuality there is also continuous need for security, guidance and supportive direction. Emotionally this is still a period of impulsiveness, dominated by a search for a personal identity. The ways in which he reacts to these changes and the resulting emotions are considerably influenced by his early experiences. In turn, the type of response which the adolescent makes to the conflicts of this time will substantially affect his adjustment as an adult.

4
ADULT LIFE, MIDDLE AND OLD AGE

THE previous chapter showed that personality development is a continuous process which can be traced from infancy onwards. While the infant begins life needing immediate satisfaction for all his demands and is totally self-centred as well as completely dependent on others, the mature adult is required to be relatively independent and to accept responsibility for himself and his behaviour, in order to develop satisfactory living patterns with the other members of his society. By the time adult life is reached, childhood and adolescence have in one sense been left behind—yet the stored experiences and memories of these times live on in the individual's mind and persist in making themselves felt by influencing his reactions to later experience.

When does adulthood begin? Chronologically, socially and legally the individual becomes an adult in most Western communities at the age of 21, when he may traditionally be given " the key of the door " and is allowed to vote, to receive an adult wage and, in the eyes of the law, is no longer a minor. Psychologically speaking, however, some individuals may not be truly adult at this time; for some people maturity is late in coming, others throughout their lives may at times show behaviour characterised by immature, childish attitudes.

In Chapter 8 we consider the difficulties in defining exactly what we mean when we talk about a normal person. Certain general features can however be said to distinguish the mature adult, the adult who has left behind almost completely those forms of feeling and behaviour which would have been only appropriate at an earlier period of life. Such an adult has been able to merge his feelings and thoughts into a spontaneous, warm, expressive response to people which is rewarding to him and to others. Control of himself is not a major problem to

PSYCHIATRIC NURSING

him and he is largely able to foresee the consequences of his own behaviour and plan for a relatively long-term goal. He is secure in his own independence, yet able to acknowledge that in a complicated society we are all to some extent dependent on one another for both material and emotional satisfactions. He has some degree of understanding of himself, realistically acknowledging his own limitations and with plans for his future which are within his capacities. He is an integrated person, that is to say, the various "parts" of his personality all fit together—his drives and needs do not battle inside himself nor come into conflict with society.

THE ADULT YEARS

Work. Work is recognised by the adult to be an essential component of his continued independence and the means by which other needs and status are obtained. A job is also capable of providing personal satisfactions from the application of one's abilities and from the social relationships which develop in the work situation. Unsatisfactory preparation in adolescence, or conflicts at that time, may however have led to a work history characterised by change and instability, constant dissatisfaction and antagonism towards authority, even protest (directly or indirectly expressed) against having to earn one's own living. Chapter 7 will show how the competitions and rivalries, even the monotony and frustration, which may be experienced in a work situation can act as substantial stresses on immature individuals (p. 140).

Social Interests. By the time early adult life is reached most people have developed a fairly consistent pattern of social interests which does not undergo much change in the next 10 or 20 years. For many individuals, their contacts and responsibilities in clubs, in sporting groups or in charitable work form very important segments of their lives; satisfactions here can do much to compensate for difficulties and stresses in other areas. Hobbies also may provide a means of gratifying certain needs which otherwise would not secure a legitimate outlet in our society. Some individuals, however, throw themselves with such frenzy into social pursuits, sports or other activities that they are clearly seeking a compensation for dissatisfactions or feelings of inferiority aroused by conflicts inside themselves. Even a man's job, or a woman's household tasks, may become such an absorbing preoccupation as to indicate clearly the way in which such activities are being used as an escape from personal difficulties.

Adult Sexual Life. Real sexual maturity requires a level of emotional development which can only be based on a ready acceptance of one's own sexual role, together with positive feelings directed towards a love-object of the opposite sex. Anxieties, conflicts and guilts persisting from early childhood experiences and imaginings can retard or prevent such maturity and can be the prelude to later sexual and marital difficulties. All love feelings and relationships are coloured to some extent by earlier love feelings and needs which persist and unknowingly influence the attraction to a sex partner. Relationships, however exciting on the surface, can be healthy or unhealthy, depending on the extent to which the choice of the loved person is based on his or her real characteristics and on how much the individual's immature needs influence his desire. Unhealthy relationships, for example, are those where there is a great discrepancy in the ages of the two persons so that the older partner is clearly a parent substitute, or where effeminate men choose masculine women, or where the relationship is based on a need to dominate and control rather than to enjoy mutual tenderness.

Marriage. To be successful, this requires the merging and adaptation of two personalities in order that each shall attain mutual satisfaction. Initially marriage requires numerous adjustments to the loss or restriction of past freedoms and to new roles of dependence and responsibility. The sexual union of marriage should prove mutually satisfying but may liberate anxiety, anger or even disgust because of earlier conflicts concerning sex. In-law problems can also complicate the issue; various attitudes of liking or disliking, acceptance and rejection may have to be worked through and may involve rivalries (such as between a wife and her husband's mother) which may be real sources of tension and stress.

Pregnancy and Parenthood. The wife's first pregnancy should be a satisfying personal experience, adding to the husband's and wife's mutual capacity to love and share. On the other hand pregnancy may lead to reactions of anxiety and disappointment, even frank hostility, because it is seen as producing an ugly body or as restricting future personal liberty. Whilst every young mother has some degree of anxiety about pregnancy and confinement, many of the fears expressed during this period are quite irrational and stem from persisting fantasies about childbirth arising in the early years of life. These may derive from persisting Oedipal guilt or from anxieties about the " goodness " and " badness " of what is inside the body. The husband may also experience irrational over-concern about his wife and about what he has done to her because of anxieties remaining from his own development. If none of these unhealthy attitudes are marked, then during the pregnancy and confinement there will be a close and satisfying contact between the parents-to-be, the contentment derived through these experiences having a favourable effect on the birth process and on the mother's response at this time. If all goes well, the child will symbolise to both parents the product of their feelings towards each other and will further add to the emotional satisfactions derived from the marriage.

For some young mothers the interest attracted by the infant is resented, as are the demands which he makes upon her, because she herself wishes, by reason of her own immaturity, to remain the centre of attention. Likewise the mother's attention to the infant may cause similar jealousies in an immature father, who feels left out of the picture. For such a parent the arrival of the new baby may produce feelings of rivalry and anger, which may or may not be consciously recognised, perhaps

ADULT LIFE, MIDDLE AND OLD AGE

linked with early childhood experiences in which the birth of a younger sibling interfered with his own supply of love. Breast-feeding will produce in mothers emotional reactions ranging from natural satisfaction and pleasure to anxiety and even disgust, these feelings being developed out of her own earlier

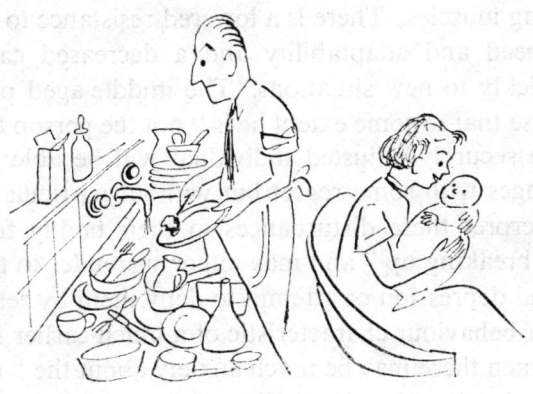

FIG. 6
Father feels out of the picture.

experiences of mothering when she was the child with her own mother. Unhealthy attitudes in the mother in turn affect the infant, who is surprisingly sensitive to changes in her mood; the presence of marked tension can be communicated to the child and lay the foundation for personality difficulties in him. In short, many of the problems which we looked at in the previous chapter from the child's point of view can now more clearly be seen to reflect the conflicts of the significant adults involved; we see how immaturities in the personalities of the parents create or magnify difficulties in the process of child-rearing. Whether a child is loved and supported and accepted as an individual, or whether he is dominated or over-protected, all these pieces of parental behaviour are a product of the parents' own experiences during the process of their development and indicate the degree of stability which they have reached in adult life.

THE YEARS OF MIDDLE AGE

Middle age is that period of life occurring between 40 and 65 years of age and is a time which calls for a series of further adjustments to certain characteristic changes.

Decline of Physical Capacities. In both sexes there are changes in appearance noticeable in wrinkles, skin blemishes and sagging muscles. There is a lowered resistance to fatigue, a loss of speed and adaptability and a decreased capacity to adjust quickly to new situations. The middle-aged person has to recognise that to some extent he is " not the person he used to be ". The securely adjusted individual will be able to accept these changes with some regret but without particular anxiety; others interpret these disturbances in their bodily feelings as signs of " breaking up " and may either surrender to them with despair and depression or attempt to deny them by returning to patterns of behaviour characteristic of a much earlier time.

For women there may be much anxiety about the " change of life ", that is, the cessation of menstruation (the menopause) and the loss of child-bearing capacities. The woman who has been secure in her sexual role and who has been fortunate enough to have gained real fulfilment as a female will not find these changes of crucial significance. For others, over-concerned about their bodily appearance and previously denied for whatever reason full satisfaction as a female, their declining attractiveness and an awareness of having missed opportunities which have now gone for ever may lead to a variety of distressing symptoms. In the latter group the menopausal period is frequently accompanied by hot flushes and sweating and unpleasant emotional reactions such as extreme fatigue, headaches, irritability and insomnia. In the male, the decline in potency and virility which usually begins at this time can also be a severe stress, especially for the man who has derived excessive satisfaction from his own sexual powers.

Relationships with Children. Middle age is usually the period during which the structure of the family alters as adolescent children gradually acquire independence. Parents' reactions to these changes vary from happy acceptance of their children's courtship and marriage to jealousy and resentment about the breaking away of their offspring from parental ties. Parents who feel they are " going over the hill " may be jealous of the adolescent's emerging capacities and new experiences, often without being really aware of this jealousy. The insecure middle-aged woman may be seriously threatened, though perhaps without admitting it to herself, by the good looks and sex-appeal of her teenage daughter; the insecure father can be

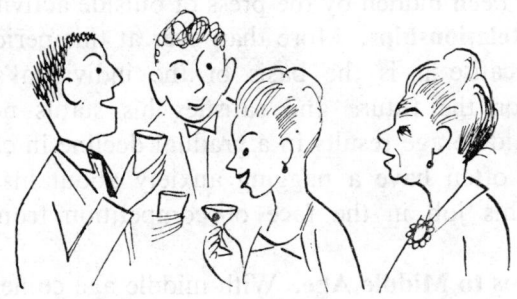

Fig. 7
Threatened by the sex appeal of her teenage daughter.

disheartened and secretly resentful when his son beats him soundly on the golf-course. Some parents, threatened in these or other ways, are unwittingly reluctant to allow their children to become independent adults and seek to maintain their control over them. More mature parents, on the other hand, find satisfaction and reward in the marriage of their children to suitable mates and the consequent production of grandchildren on whom they can dote.

Relationships towards Ageing Parents. Many middle-aged persons experience problems centred around their elderly parents, towards whom they may feel responsible, rejecting, guilty or on whom they are still dependent. The death of parents is common at this time and for some the resulting separation experience will reawaken earlier anxiety about separation, as well as guilty feelings because of previous hostilities towards them.

Relationships of Husband and Wife towards Each Other. Because of the changes in the family structure and the lessening of responsibility for others, there will be increased opportunities for new and different interests which the man and wife can share. Usually spending rather less time in sports and social pursuits, they have more time for each other and can build from this a new and satisfying unity. On the other hand, the enforced closeness brought about by the above factors can intensify frustrations and resentments between them which had previously been hidden by the press of outside activities.

Work Relationships. More than ever at this period work is valued because it is the basis of the individual's financial security for the future and satisfies his status needs. But because middle age results in a gradual decline in capacities a man may often have a nagging anxiety about his ability to maintain his job in the face of competition from younger people.

Reactions to Middle Age. With middle age comes a certain rigidity of personality as a result of which individual characteristics become more permanent. There is a reluctance to accept change and the usual and familiar tend to be preferred. These characteristics may make flexible and healthy adjustments to the stresses just described particularly difficult and it is not uncommon for a wide variety of defensive reactions to be brought into play at this time. Compensation may be attempted for the loss of youthful appearance by love affairs in an effort to prove one's attractiveness. Tension and anxiety may bring out for the first time a tendency towards excessive alcohol consumption or may lead to minor forms of drug addiction. Very commonly, as will be seen later (p. 246), moods of depression arise during this period which may in some instances go on to major depressive illnesses.

THE YEARS OF OLD AGE

Because of greater medical knowledge and more effective treatments for a wide variety of illnesses, there has been in

Western societies a gradual and persistent extension of the human life span which has led to a substantial increase in the number of old people in our culture. This situation has brought its own complications, not only because more accommodation is required in psychiatric hospitals for patients showing the mental disorders of old age, but also because of the great numbers of old people who have no specific need for hospital care, yet who are nevertheless social problems by reason of their loneliness and the general disinterest of the community.

Decline in Physical Capacities. Virtually every organ and system of the body tends to function less efficiently in old age. There is a loss of strength and energy, dexterity is reduced, digestive upsets are frequent and there is a gradual deterioration of the sense organs leading to difficulties in vision and hearing. Physical illnesses such as angina pectoris, arthritis, gynaecological disorders and prostate trouble are particularly common at this time and may increase the disability of the old person. As he becomes increasingly aware of these handicaps, some degree of threat is inevitable.

Decline in Intellectual Capacities. In old age there is a decline in the person's capacity to attend and to concentrate; memory is interfered with, he retains new information poorly and in particular is unable to cope with problems involving new experiences. He is therefore slower to pick up new ideas, his attention is harder to sustain and he has greater difficulty in grasping a situation in its entirety and is inclined to react to only a part of it. He is less able to switch from one idea to another—hence his difficulty in following a complicated conversation. Although emotional factors also play an important part, this decline in intellectual capacity is partly responsible for the misunderstandings and misinterpretations which the elderly sometimes attach to the events about them. Also, because of his intellectual and physical decline, there is a decrease in the old person's range of interests. This is accompanied by an increasing absorption in himself and he is apt to recall and relive many times the events of yesteryear—frequently conveniently rearranged to provide him with personal satisfactions. This tendency is exaggerated in our type of society where the old person is, generally speaking, of low status, unlike certain other cultures where the elders are still the wise men whose views are respected by all.

Retirement. Sudden cessation of work usually brings some sense of loss and for many is the forerunner of economic uncertainty. The sudden change in routine may produce feelings of insecurity and bewilderment and lead in some people to the

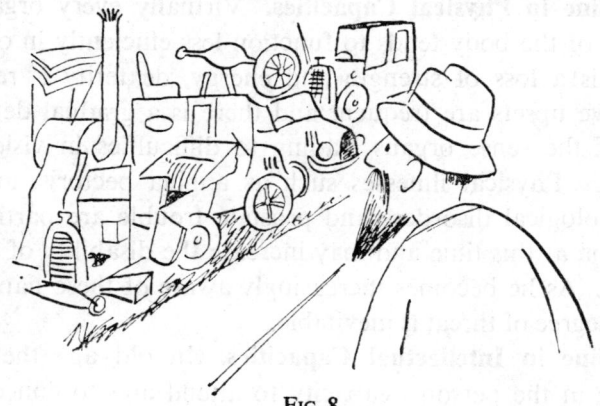

FIG. 8
The belief that they are " on the scrap-heap ".

belief that they are " on the scrap-heap ". The wise and welladjusted person has planned ahead for this day and has already other interests and hobbies with which to fill the gap. Such people may lead a contented and even productive old age, whereas those who react to retirement by passive surrender and who develop the belief that they have outlived their usefulness generally do not live to draw their retirement cheques for very long.

Relationship with the Family. Older people tend to become progressively more dependent on and more demanding of their children for satisfaction and security. The children, by now well and truly grown up, will react to the parents' needs and attitudes with behaviour which ranges from active acceptance to annoyance, embarrassment, guilt or rejection. If all goes well, the relationships between people and their aged parents may provide the latter with stimulation, encouragement and the knowledge that they are valued; in less favourable circumstances, their feelings of uselessness may be intensified to the point where they colour all their social relationships and lead to a general sense of isolation and loneliness. These feelings of loneliness, which are the scourge of old age, may lead the individual into a further retreat into himself, even while he is longing for some situation in which he could feel wanted and respected. With loneliness there frequently comes a decrease in social standards and self-respect; if the person lives alone and is virtually isolated from his surroundings it is often difficult to decide at first whether personality changes are due to senile deterioration in his brain or simply to a deprivation of social stimulation.

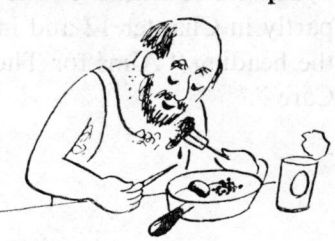

FIG. 9
A decrease in social standards and self-respect.

Reactions to Old Age. In many ways the emotional reactions of the aged are very similar to those of the child, in that their behaviour becomes self-centred and less inhibited. It is no accident that an old person is frequently described as being " in his second childhood ", because he commonly reacts to inconveniences and frustrations with outbursts of emotion which were not typical of him in adult life. Any type of extreme emotion—anger, suspiciousness, quarrelsomeness, tears and overwhelming gratitude—all may be part of the responses of the aged. These childish ways of behaving are often defensive, being intended to gain for them the same satisfactions that such behaviour received at an earlier time. As will be seen later (p. 261), much of the troublesomeness of the aged is a reaction, not just to deterioration in the brain cells, but to personal and social difficulties experienced in this period of decline. Hospitalisation, though ideally it should be otherwise, all too frequently can be an added stress and destructive of the old person's adjustment by helping to remove further his identity, independence and self-respect.

The nurse's aims in the care of old people are considered partly in Chapter 12 and in further detail in Chapter 22 under the heading " Aims for Those Who Need Long-Term Hospital Care ".

5

THE DYNAMICS OF HUMAN BEHAVIOUR

AT the commencement of Chapter 3 various examples were quoted to show that human behaviour was not, under any circumstances, a meaningless, chance phenomenon but could be explained in terms of the individual's past experience. If behaviour has meaning, then this meaning can only be understood if one is able to perceive some of the various " forces " which act on the individual at each moment of his life. Because these forces are in some respects constantly changing, then human behaviour is never a static or stationary thing, but is always being modified by these forces in what is referred to as a " dynamic " way. The study of the dynamics of behaviour, then, is the study of all those forces, both inside himself and outside himself, which have acted on the individual during his development, together with those which are acting on him at the point in time when his behaviour is being studied.

Broadly speaking, these forces can be classified into two large groups—those which are the result of his needs and drives and which arise within him; secondly, those which are the result of the various pressures brought to bear on him by the environment in which he lives. All human behaviour, normal or abnormal, is capable of being understood as a result of the interaction between these basic needs and the influences of the environment.

Initially, as was suggested in Chapter 3, these basic needs strive only for their own immediate satisfaction (p. 35); there can be no doubt that the development of more noble and dignified motives in a human being is the result of modification of these needs by the various experiences and frustrations of his life and the type of education which he experiences in home and school. Successful personality growth requires that these drives be " tamed "—in other words, that the individual learns to seek his satisfactions within the framework of his society. Ultimately the normal human being has to reach a satisfactory compromise between his own needs and the requirements of the society in which he lives; it is probable that some types of emotional disorder are more prevalent in Western civilisations because of the complicated nature of the demands which are imposed by such a civilisation on its members, demands which are quite different and much more exacting than those imposed by many primitive native tribes. The needs of human beings show less variation than do the societies, or the family groups, into which individuals are born, but even the strength of various needs may vary from one person to another, even within the one family, because a different hereditary mixture has been acquired from the parents. An environment which is quite congenial to a child who conspicuously lacks self-assertiveness may be an extremely trying one for another child who has a great need to master and control the people around him.

UNCONSCIOUS MENTAL LIFE

We owe mainly to Sigmund Freud (p. 10) the notion that many important features of each individual personality are, as it were, hidden below the surface, outside the range of that person's ordinary awareness. Before this idea was fully grasped much human behaviour, particularly abnormal behaviour, seemed to be meaningless because a surface study of the individual, however elaborate, did not make any real sense out of the observations. It is not easy to accept that we do not in fact know ourselves as well as we would like to think—to face up to the fact that inside each one of us there are drives, anxieties, guilts and memories of which we are not aware. The whole concept of unconscious motivation therefore met with a great deal of resistance in the early part of this century, despite the large amount of evidence which can be brought together to support the idea.

There are **three major pieces of evidence** for the existence of unconscious motives in human behaviour:

Dreams. These take place at a time when the dreamer is certainly not conscious and has no awareness in the ordinary sense. It is easy to dismiss them as being nonsense, because so many dreams do present themselves in an extraordinarily absurd light, but the researches of Freud and the later psychoanalysts show that dreams in fact do have a considerable meaning in the mental life of the individual. Careful research has established that the healthy adult experiences four or five episodes of dreaming each night, totalling between 15 and 25 *per cent* of his sleeping time, during which periods his EEG (p. 278) shows a very different pattern from the pattern existing during non-dreaming sleep; rapid eye movements are characteristic of this phase, which is sometimes therefore known as REM sleep. Contrary to popular opinion, one does not have a long dream in a flash, and the dream can be shown to occupy about as much time as watching the same events in waking life. What we remember of the dream on waking up in the morning is known as the **manifest content** and this, however rubbishy it might appear, can be found by psychiatrists to be derived from more basic wishes and drives which are the stimulus to the dream and form the **latent content.** What has happened is that certain of the individual's wishes, which would be unacceptable for him to acknowledge as part of himself in the waking state and are therefore kept out of consciousness, try to express themselves during sleep, though even here, because of their unacceptable nature, they emerge only in a distorted and heavily disguised form. This disguise is less obvious in the simple dreams of children, where the underlying wish can often be seen very easily; the child who is prevented by illness from going to a birthday party may dream a happy dream about the party the night before.

It is not any part of the nurse's task to become involved in an attempt to interpret the dreams of her patients; she may at times in case conferences hear how the understanding of a dream assists the psychiatrist in his task of unravelling the patient's problems, but the subject is raised here only to produce evidence for the existence of an unconscious level of mental activity.

Slips and Errors in Everyday Life. It was also Freud who drew attention to the fact that many of the so-called accidental slips which we all make in everyday life are not in fact " accidents " at all, but represent the result of a clash between a conscious intention and an unconscious wish. The nurse, if she has the ability to look at some of her own motives, may test this out for herself; she may easily find, for example, that when she seemingly forgets an object whilst on a visit and therefore has to return to the place to collect it, she has secretly wished to see a certain person again. When she completely forgets the name of a person whom she knows quite well, she may find that her feelings towards this person are not characterised by pure friendliness, as she had previously believed in her conscious mind. Deep down, many of us know that the apparently accidental slip may tell us much more about a person's real intentions than his conscious utterances; a girl who finds that her boy-friend has forgotten to call for her at an appointed time will naturally be angry with him, and rightly so, because her feminine intuition tells her that his feelings for her cannot be as genuine as he makes out. Another example can be taken from the Armed Services; a soldier who forgets to turn up for a certain duty will receive no sympathy from his superior officer and his offence will be regarded with the same seriousness as if he had openly admitted a reluctance to be present. When one forgets to carry out instructions of any kind, only a little self-examination may be required to realise that the act of forgetting may result from some degree of hidden antagonism to the person giving the instructions or to the instructions themselves.

Symptoms of Psychiatric Illness. The more abnormal a patient's behaviour becomes, the more difficult it is to understand what is happening in superficial, descriptive terms. A patient may present with a disabling fear, which he himself realises to be quite absurd, but which nevertheless is strong enough to paralyse some or nearly all of his activities. The more one scrutinises this fear, known as a **phobia,** the more illogical does the situation seem. A woman expresses a strong fear of going out of the house alone; she knows that there is nothing logically to fear in the city streets, but is quite unable to convince herself, or to let herself be convinced by others, until deeper anxieties are taken into account. During a perhaps lengthy process of treatment she comes to realise that this surface fear serves only to camouflage a deeper, previously unconscious dread—namely, that she does not have adequate control over her sexual impulses and that, if she goes out alone, she may not be able to turn away from a stranger who makes a pass at her. She is usually a woman who in her conscious life has little or no awareness of sexual feeling at all; yet, in the deeper levels of her mind, her sexual strivings are real and frightening to her.

CONSCIOUS, PRECONSCIOUS AND UNCONSCIOUS

In fact we recognise three varieties of mental activity. The first of these is labelled **conscious,** and refers to all those aspects of mental life which are ordinarily within our awareness. The second variety is known as **preconscious,** and describes the quite large mass of information which is stored in the mind of every individual, not constantly at the level of awareness but able to be brought up to awareness should the need arise. One may encounter in the street, for example, a person not seen and barely thought about since school-days several years before, yet in a flash be able to remember her name and several details about her. Many of the facts which the nurse acquires during her training are stored at this preconscious level, being readily available (one hopes) to her conscious mind when they are required by the demands of a particular nursing situation, or of an examination.

The deepest layer of mental life is that described as

unconscious. Why certain mental processes remain unconscious can only be understood by a realisation of the fact that, in the process of becoming civilised, the ordinary human being finds that many of his basic wishes are not acceptable either to society or to the conscience which he has developed as a result of the training given to him in his family. They are therefore kept out of awareness by a mental process called **censorship,** which maintains his own peace of mind and keeps his image of himself undisturbed. The unconscious also contains various unpleasant memories, free access to which would cause the individual to relive painful experiences.

ID, EGO AND SUPEREGO

We have seen that each individual begins life with a collection of basic needs which clamour for satisfaction quite regardless of the views of the world about him. The infant is hungry and wants food; he wants it regardless of whether his mother is tired, busy or occupied with other children and, if his need is not satisfied, he creates a disturbance until it is. All the primitive needs, taken together, constitute what is known as the **id.** This component of personality is primitive, greedy and quite lacking in social graces; it takes no account of the ordinary processes of adult logic and acts with no thought for the well-being of others. Motivated entirely by self-interest, it functions in accordance with what has previously been described as the **pleasure principle** (p. 35).

Sooner or later, with the further development of the central nervous system, the baby starts to realise that there exists an external world and that, however much he might like to do so, he cannot remain entirely selfish in his behaviour if he is going to come to terms with this world and obtain the most satisfaction from it. He gradually comes to learn that, even though he may be hungry, his needs will be more agreeably satisfied if he controls his desire to scream for food and waits until mother is ready to provide it. He is starting to adapt himself to reality; he is able to use some form of judgement to sum up the various aspects of a situation. He is developing the capacity to postpone the need for immediate gratification of his every whim. This more mature layer of his personality is known as the **ego**. More and more, using ego functions, he leaves behind behaviour governed purely by the pleasure principle and is now said to be acting in accordance with what has previously been described as the **reality principle** (p. 44). The development of the ego also gives him a sense of his own personal identity and means that he has fully mastered the distinction between what is himself and what is not himself (p. 41). In an unfavourable environment, particularly when a stable mother or mother-substitute is not available to help him in this difficult task of adapting himself to the hard cruel world about him, then inadequate ego functions may develop, or may develop in such a way as to break down under subsequent stress. It will later be seen that some of the symptoms of psychiatric illness can be explained in terms of inadequately developed, more easily broken down, ego functions.

But the growing child is still, even at this stage, intent only on his own satisfaction, even though with the development of the reality principle he can set about the task of achieving this satisfaction in a more sensible way. Before ego functions operate he can smash a glass purely for the joy of hearing the sound which it makes and seeing the pretty fragments. When ego function is established the normal child will no longer break glasses (at least not deliberately or unless he is uncontrollably angry), but he refrains from doing so, not because he feels it is wrong to break glass, but because his mother's previous reactions have convinced him that she disapproves of this behaviour and will punish him if it is repeated.

Ideas of rightness and wrongness, far from being born with the individual, are developed in him as a result of his experiences in the family group; restrictions on his behaviour which originally only operated when his parents were present to see that they were enforced gradually become effective in the parents' absence and he thus develops his own morality (p. 52). This further development of personality, known as the **superego**, really has two components. On the one hand he develops a system of internal checks on his own behaviour, refraining from carrying out certain acts, not just because his parents would disapprove, but because he himself would disapprove of them. On the other hand, the development of the superego leads him to form some idea of what he wishes to be like and he acquires an internal standard of conduct, derived from his parents' standards but becoming finally separate from them, on which he attempts to model his own behaviour. It should be noted that " superego " is a term of wider meaning than " conscience "; the latter refers only to conscious attitudes, whereas an adequately functioning superego quite automatically prevents us from carrying out certain acts, even though we are not aware that wishes have been presented to and rejected by our internal morality.

It is difficult when using these terms to avoid the idea that the id, the ego and the superego are literally parts of the brain, objective things which have an existence of their own. On the contrary these are simply convenient ways of describing certain functions of our personalities—a sort of shorthand which enables us, instead of saying " this young man seems to have a good capacity to adjust himself to the realities of life and to tolerate difficulties and frustrations ", to say " this young man appears to have adequate and stable ego functions ". The practical usefulness of these ideas will be more apparent in later chapters.

ANXIETY

However adequately the individual develops the capacity to live in harmony with the reality principle and with his conscience, he is still motivated by the desire to avoid painful experiences and wants as far as possible to maintain a state of internal contentment. This is obviously true at the physical level—any normal person draws away from a situation liable to cause physical discomfort and leaps up instinctively should he sit down on a drawing-pin. Similar principles apply to psychological life; the individual does not wish to undergo unpleasant experiences such as are associated with feeling anxious or guilty and tries if he can to avoid situations which might produce these unpleasant emotions. To avoid anxiety, or to master anxiety should circumstances cause it to be felt, is a constant motivating force in human behaviour.

What is anxiety? Like most emotional states, it is easy to recognise the feeling in oneself but hard to describe it in words. Though it may be accompanied by certain bodily changes such as a racing heart or sweaty palms, everyone would agree that it is something more than these purely physical sensations. A useful definition is that it is *a state of painful internal tension associated with apprehension*. It can be usefully understood as a danger signal, a state of feeling which is set up to warn the individual that some disaster may be impending. It occurs whenever the individual is threatened, whatever the nature of this threat and whatever its origin.

Much of the anxiety experienced during life is brought about by the occurrence of circumstances over which the individual feels he has no control, or by the threat of such situations developing. Probably the earliest anxiety is experienced shortly after the beginning of life—a sad blow to the poets, who have always tried to persuade us that infancy and childhood were times free from trouble and strife. Only a superhuman mother, possessed of the capacity to satisfy all her baby's wishes as soon as he expresses them, could prevent in him the unpleasantness of having nasty, painful feelings of hunger inside himself which he, unaided, is unable to relieve. This is a threat aroused in the child from within himself. Gradually, provided that he receives adequate mothering, he becomes aware that mother is capable of doing things which take away these unpleasant feelings. As he can at this stage only master distressing sensations, whether they come from inside himself or from outside himself, with constant adult help, then his degree of contentment will depend upon the amount and constancy of love and protectiveness shown to him. The presence of this loving environment is necessary for him to develop self-esteem and security and to provide him with the repeated reassurance that nasty feelings can be taken away.

Because the infant is so dependent upon adults, then if love is lacking in his environment, or if love is for any reason suddenly withdrawn, he loses, wholly or in part, his protection against unpleasantness, and he feels helpless and anxious. This situation is referred to as **anxiety aroused by loss of love**. Throughout his early years, he behaves in such a way as to show us clearly how much he needs the sense of being loved to provide him with security; he will give up many pleasures, endure many frustrations, control his instincts, all for the sake of being loved. Children are only teachable at all, in the home or in school, because they wish to gain the loving approval of the important adults in their lives. While they are very young indeed any situation which interferes with their supply of love, or looks like doing so, will make them anxious. But if the child receives an adequate, continuous amount of loving protection, then progressively he is more able to stand on his own feet, to develop his own inner sense of security and does not require that others should constantly show they love him in order for him to feel worthwhile. For the child denied this experience, many situations in later life may make him anxious because, automatically and usually unconsciously, they are a reminder of this early childhood threat of loss of love. Perhaps in childhood this danger was made very real to him by an unwise mother who said repeatedly " if you go on like that, Mummy won't love you any more ". Such a child, reacting with anxiety to this threat, can well become the adult who responds with great distress if significant people in his life withdraw, or look like withdrawing, their love from him. This is the type of person who reacts with overwhelming anxiety and perhaps frank psychiatric illness to a broken engagement, or to the death of a marriage partner who had shown great protectiveness towards him. This need for love, stemming from uncertainty and insecurity about the love received in childhood, may also lead the individual into a constant, though unconscious, search for proof that the world loves him.

It has already been said that the basis of this sort of anxiety lies in the child's early experience of being unable to master and satisfy his own feelings. For all sorts of reasons his environment may be such as to lead him to believe that his own internal impulses are dangerous and frightening things. During the toilet-training period he may be handled in such a way as to develop the idea that control over his own impulses is important above all other things in the world. If he becomes angry and mother reacts by saying " I'll go away and leave you if you behave like that ", he may become terrified of the strength and possible results of his aggressive wishes. If he shows sexual interest and is scolded for this, then he may develop a similar fear about the dangerous nature of his sexual drive. He thus can come to develop a series of rigid controls over all his instincts and feelings, so that he becomes almost a complete stranger to his real emotions. Such a person, feeling his own instincts to be dangerous, will react with anxiety later in life if situations arise which stir up these forbidden, frightening feelings. This is what is known as **anxiety aroused by one's own instincts** and many of the stressful situations which precipitate psychiatric illness do so in large measure because of the underlying instincts and emotions which they stir up. The normal adult does not fear his own impulses, but for the sort of person described here many situations in life create anxiety because they seem likely to lead to loss of control of oneself, especially loss of control of sexual or aggressive feelings.

A third basic anxiety-producing situation which arises in childhood develops out of the recognition of the anatomical differences between the sexes and is known as **castration anxiety** (p. 47). This form of anxiety, present in both sexes though showing different manifestations in each, normally subsides to an insignificant level in those children who are able to model themselves upon a healthy parent or parent-substitute of the same sex. But many less fortunate individuals grow up into adolescence and adult life retaining a substantial amount of hidden anxiety concerning sexual differences. One of the most obvious examples can be found in a man who becomes a homosexual, avoiding sexual contact with women because, in the unconscious segment of his mind, he still as an adult does not want to be brought face to face with the realisation that the anatomical difference between the sexes really exists. Much more commonly, psychiatric patients who show no obvious evidence of sexual peculiarity can be shown to have hidden castration anxiety as one factor contributing towards their illness.

These three basic situations which arouse anxiety in childhood remain as the chief sources of anxiety in later life, even in circumstances which superficially appear to have no connection with them. In an adolescent boy who develops a psychiatric illness, for example, the sources of his anxiety may be able to be traced back to one, two or all three of these basic situations. He may want to advance to independence, yet fear that breaking away from his parents may lead them to show less love towards him and thus create conflict essentially based on anxiety due to loss of love. He may feel the stirring of sexual desires within him yet these may arouse, not only anxiety associated with awareness of his own instincts, but also a new version of the castration anxiety felt as a small child when sexual wishes seemed likely to be followed by punishment directed towards his genital organs.

We can summarise the causes of anxiety arising throughout life in another way, which does not clash with the explanations just given but which states them in a different form. Anxiety can in this scheme be classified into three main types:
1. Anxiety which arises due to awareness of pressure of the instincts from the id, which has been called **neurotic anxiety**.
2. Anxiety which arises due to real threats to the individual from the external world, known as **reality anxiety**.

3. Anxiety which arises after the third major component of personality has been formed and the individual fears offending his own superego, the so-called **moral anxiety**, usually known as **guilt.**

As has been said previously, a mature individual lives in such a way as to bring about a reasonable compromise between these three great forces—his instincts, his moral standards and the demands made by society. Anxiety is the signal which warns him that all is not well in his adjustment to any one or all three of these pressures.

The objection may well be raised by the nurse at this point—" this talk about anxiety is all very fine, but I personally only feel anxious on quite rare and special occasions and I cannot see that its importance is nearly as great as you are trying to suggest ". This is an understandable comment, but one which overlooks one vital aspect of the anxiety problem. Due to the inevitable occurrence of anxiety in childhood, and because anxiety is a painful experience which everyone tries to avoid, there become developed within the personality a series of **defences against anxiety,** set up during the early years of life and becoming automatic features of every individual's behaviour. Should a situation arise which is perceived as likely to lead to anxiety, these defences automatically, and quite unconsciously, swing into action to deal with the threatening circumstances. The nature of these defences, and the way in which they are employed, produce many of the distinctive characteristics of the personality; furthermore, the type of defence which is used plays a significant part in determining whether stress later in life is likely to lead to psychiatric breakdown or not and, if it does, plays a major role in determining the form of the illness. Because these defences are a function of that part of the mental apparatus known as the ego, they are referred to as ego defences.

EGO DEFENCES

It has been said in the previous paragraph that the defences which the individual uses to protect himself against anxiety are automatic and unconscious. Before these are considered, however, we should look briefly at two conscious and deliberate types of action which the person may undertake in an effort to avoid mental discomfort. The first of these is **suppression,** a consciously recognised process by which the individual, aware of a thought, drive, feeling or memory which is experienced as frightening or unpleasant, endeavours to " forget " and put out of his conscious mind this troublesome part of his personality. Most people can probably remember saying at some time " I won't think about it, I won't let it worry me, I will push it out of my mind ". The child who has stolen and feels guilty, the adult who is aware of a dangerous temptation, the mother who becomes conscious of destructive feelings towards her children —all these and many other persons may seek to ease their distress by " trying to forget ", or by involving themselves in continuous activity so that they will have " no time to think about it ". This consciously attempted defence may provide brief periods of relief, but most people also know from their own experience that in the long run it is usually an unsuccessful manoeuvre, often leading to even greater tension when the conflict is found to persist.

Deliberate **intellectual control** is another way in which a person may attempt consciously to regulate his behaviour and to deal with his emotional reactions. Distressed by a feeling which is out of proportion to an apparently trivial hurt, the individual may say to himself " I must stop feeling this way because it is so silly, it just isn't logical to go on like this ". However, because so much behaviour is prompted by motives which are unrecognised, it is difficult and often impossible to provide effective control by conscious, logical thought processes over impulses and wishes and feelings which are, by their very nature, beyond the reach of such control. This is perhaps the hardest single fact which the ordinary person has to grasp about psychology and psychiatry—this notion that we are not as logical as we like to think we are, that forces inside ourselves compel us at times to act and feel in certain ways, despite the fact that we know with our intellectual functions that such ways are not rational. We have also to face the fact that many of the major decisions in our lives are made because of emotional needs which we have not recognised and are not simply the result of brilliant, logical reasoning as we would like to believe. This is not to say that conscious controls do not in many instances contribute significantly to a person's adjustment, but they are only effective in the presence of a well-organised and strong ego which permits some realistic understanding of oneself. Patients with many types of psychiatric illness quickly realise that all the intellectual controls in the world do not help them to reason themselves out of particular fears, obsessions or depressed moods. At the other extreme, some people do in fact regulate their lives with these conscious, deliberate controls up to the point where their whole personality is cramped, lacking the capacity for spontaneous reaction and robbed of any genuine emotional expression.

The preceding two paragraphs refer, as has been stated, to defence systems consciously organised in an effort to protect the individual. The remainder of this chapter deals with those defence mechanisms which are brought into play unconsciously and automatically, built into the personality during the early years of childhood. Although the use of the term " defence " may suggest that we are talking about something which is always abnormal or pathological, it should be emphasised that the concept certainly includes methods of handling anxiety, sometimes referred to as **coping devices**, which are completely compatible with healthy personality adjustment.

Sublimation

Earlier in this chapter it was pointed out that every human being begins life with drives and resulting emotions which in their natural state are primitive, often antisocial, unacceptable to society and, once his conscience and ideals have developed, often unacceptable to the individual himself. Civilised society does not allow some of these drives to be discharged at all—for example, it is not at any time permissible, except during the special circumstances of war, for one individual to kill another. Other drives are only permitted to be released in our society under special circumstances—sexual impulses, for example, are only supposed to be gratified in certain socially approved ways. If the person is not to go through life as a seething mass of bottled up instincts, then some way must be found to discharge the tensions which result from these forces, and the process by which the energy arising from these drives is directed into socially acceptable channels is known as sublimation. Its essential characteristic is that *the drives do find an outlet,* and in this respect sublimation is a coping device rather than a pathological defence; from this point of view it can be contrasted with all the mechanisms described subsequently. It is a mechanism that has contributed extensively to the development of the arts, the sciences and to all areas of creative activity. Composers, authors, poets, painters, engineers and artisans have often through sublimation channelled energy from their primitive drives into new creations which have enriched our lives. It is a mechanism which also has many uses of a less conspicuous nature; the adolescent uses sublimation to express in disguised form his sexual strivings and in his sporting activities he sublimates his aggressive impulses into socially acceptable behaviour. Likewise the spinster, unable to express her sexuality and creativeness in marriage and child-birth, may sublimate these needs in gardening, in the breeding of cats or in charitable work with children. The list of examples could be endless ... for sublimation is all around us.

Because of its unconscious, automatic nature, it is unusual for the individual to recognise that various forms of socially approved behaviour which are giving him considerable satisfaction are stemming from his primitive and often antisocial strivings. Some people do in fact still strenuously resist this idea, wanting to believe that man is by nature a noble, idealistic person. The explorer, the school-teacher, the doctor and even the nurse are unlikely to have much conscious recognition of the extent to which sublimation has determined their interest in their chosen field.

Sublimation can be regarded as a healthy coping device, an effective safety-valve through which the individual constructively discharges the energies arising from his conflicts and frustrations; it contributes substantially to normal personality development and to the attainment of social maturity. If the family and social environment is not such as to permit successful sublimations, or if the extent of the hidden drives is too great to permit their total management in this way, then the individual is forced to use less healthy methods in a search for relief from tension; these are now described.

Denial

The primary and fundamental defence mechanism is denial; its origins are to be found in the primitive, magical and illogical thinking of the young child (p. 50). This is the mechanism which permits drives, thoughts and feelings which would be unacceptable to the conscious mind to be disowned by the simple procedure of refusing to acknowledge their existence. The individual is freed from conscious concern about such feelings because to him " they do not exist "; reality is reshaped so that it is no longer unpleasant. It must be stressed that the word denial, when used in psychiatry, refers to this unconscious defence and does not include conscious activities such as straightforward lying or " putting on an act ".

Like many aspects of mental function, denial is normal and understandable in early childhood but indicative of serious immaturity when it is found in adult life. A quite normal small boy, whose eyes are heavy with sleep, can yet shout angrily " Mummy, I am *not* tired ". At the other end of the scale is the unmarried psychiatric patient, clearly eight months' pregnant, who asserts that her swollen abdomen is " all due to wind " and that the movements of the foetus are " butterflies in the stomach "; this latter usage is clearly indicative of a major break with reality and is diagnostic of a psychotic reaction (p. 158). One type of denial which is often not recognised as such by the nurse is displayed by the patient whose mood is excessively cheerful, showing the psychiatric symptom known as **euphoria** (p. 122). Here the person is in effect saying " I am not distressed by this situation, I am not worried, everything is wonderful, just see how happy I look ". It can be seen how denial of this kind is a primitive, unhealthy and dangerous way of defending against reality.

Repression

This is one of the most commonly used mechanisms to deal with impulses and emotions which are too hot for the individual to handle and accept and which therefore threaten his ability to live with himself and with others. The term denotes that process whereby disturbing impulses and thoughts are removed from conscious awareness and buried in the unconscious segment of mental life, where they are not open to direct recollection and conscious examination. Unlike suppression this is an automatic, involuntary, unconscious process. By removing from awareness those aspects of himself which are not acceptable to his conscious mind, the individual seeks to avoid the unbearable and possibly disruptive anxieties which would be associated with their recognition. For the time being such a problem is " out of sight "—but it is not " out of mind ", for the drives dealt with by repression still persist as dynamic, active forces inside the individual and continue to influence his behaviour and personality development. This repressed material may appear in personality traits, in interests, hobbies and choice of jobs, in attitudes towards independence, authority, marriage and responsibility, or can be expressed in disguised ways in the symptoms of psychiatric patients.

Repression is a mechanism which figures prominently in all our lives by hiding from us much of our own past. Used in moderation it will help the individual cope with the demands and requirements of his society, and may contribute to the quality of his adjustment to his surroundings. Excessive use of repression, however, produces an individual who has no awareness of a large part of his true self, and a part, as has been previously stated, which may still strive for expression and satisfaction. For some people, whose life experiences have left them with an excessive overdraft of unsatisfied strivings and emotions, repression may not in itself be a permanently effective protection from anxiety, certain circumstances later in life leading to the breakdown of repression and the substitution of other even less satisfactory defence mechanisms. The fact that repressed material still plays an active role in the individual's life, even though he is unaware of it, is clearly shown in each of the three pieces of evidence detailed earlier in this chapter for the existence of unconscious mental life. Furthermore, during the repeated interviews which some psychiatric patients have with a psychiatrist, a great deal of previously repressed material is often brought up into the individual's conscious awareness.

Reaction Formation

This can be regarded as a more permanent and in some ways more effective type of repression, in which the individual unconsciously deals with his forbidden desires by behaving in ways which are the very opposite of these hidden aspects of his personality. It is as though he says " I do not desire something which is unacceptable; on the contrary, I intensely desire the very opposite ". The impulses and desires involved are mainly of a hostile and sexual nature.

Many character traits are reaction formations against such forbidden desires, and aspects of a person's character formed in this way tend to appear in an exaggerated form. The very submissive person may be disguising by his submissiveness his unconscious destructive wishes; the constantly aggressive person may hide in this way his inner insecurity, dependence and uncertainty; the individual who is always excessively loving and forgiving may be thus managing to disguise his hate; the extremely prudish and narrow-minded person may through these attitudes be defending against the recognition of strong sexual impulses. It must be repeated that these are unconscious disguises which are organised to fool, not only the external world, but the individual himself. Many aspects of behaviour therefore have a deeper significance which is exactly the opposite of that which appears on the surface; for example, extreme over-concern about a certain person's health may be a defence by reaction formation against the recognition of unconscious wishes for this person's death. This last type of behaviour, which is far from uncommon in our society, may have a double motivation at an unconscious level—on the one hand, the uncomplaining devotion of an unmarried adult to an elderly parent being in some instances a reaction formation against death wishes directed towards the parent and, in addition, this devotion serving to allay a feeling of guilt and representing an attempt to " make up for " the fantasied destructive wishes.

Even more so than repression, reaction formation makes the individual a stranger to his own inner self; a person full of hostile, destructive wishes may in this way be able to say to himself " obviously I am not an angry person, on the contrary I am an extremely good, kind, loving person ". But reaction formations, like repressions, may break down; sometimes this breakdown is a very temporary process—an individual always thought of as meek and mild shows a sudden flash of murderous rage and we are all inclined to say " well, that *was* a surprise, I didn't think she was like *that*!" In psychiatric illnesses the breakdown of reaction formations can be more long-lasting; for example, the excessively prudish person can find his mind filled with obscene and perhaps blasphemous thoughts. It is also striking that reaction formations may to some extent disintegrate during dreams, so that a seemingly timid person comes to have nightmares full of blood and destruction.

Like repression, however, reaction formation can be a useful defence against anxiety, used by many people without ill-effect provided that this use is kept within reasonable limits.

Displacement

This mechanism may be used to deal with conflicts when repression has failed or when new circumstances seem likely to lead to the re-emergence of unacceptable wishes. It reduces anxiety by displacing or transferring frightening feelings from one very dangerous object or situation to a substitute, more socially acceptable object or situation. The substitute situation, one which does not frighten a normal person (or at least not to anything like the same extent), now becomes invested with a great deal of anxiety for the individual concerned, for reasons which he fails to understand and which are not obvious to an observer on superficial scrutiny. This is the defence mechanism behind the formation of a **phobia** (p. 81 and p. 119). A woman may have a completely unjustified and irrational fear that she has cancer, the cancerous growth standing for all the mental badness and rottenness which at one level of her thinking she feels to be inside herself but which she is unable to allow herself to recognise; the anxiety attaching to this unacceptable idea is transferred to a more socially acceptable, even though in this case still very distressing idea. She is thus able through displacement to continue to keep out of awareness frightening feelings about herself, even though she is still anxious and may in fact be socially crippled by her fears. (Displacement and the formation of phobias are further considered in Chapter 9, p. 187).

Conversion

This is a further defence mechanism by means of which the individual attempts to avoid facing painful truths about himself which seem likely to escape from repression. The unconscious conflict becomes represented by a bodily symptom, with the result that some function normally carried out by the central (voluntary) nervous system is paralysed or distorted. The symptom is one which will protect the individual, although he does not consciously recognise this fact, and the nature of his disability gives us a clue as to the unconscious conflict against which conversion is being used as a defence mechanism. Though he consciously protests against the inconvenience of his affliction, it is often very difficult to shift and clearly gives him some unrecognised emotional satisfactions, not the least of which being that he is able because of its existence to avoid facing up to a situation which would provoke anxiety. The young woman afraid of her sexual feelings may develop paralysed legs or a spasm of the muscles surrounding her vagina, both these symptoms effectively defending her against sexual relationships; the student afraid of examination failure may develop a paralysed hand which prevents him from writing; the adult male afraid of his aggressive impulses may develop a weakness of his arm which prevents him from lashing out. Even blindness, deafness and lack of speech may be brought about by this mechanism, in each instance to protect the individual from unconscious anxieties. (Conversion is further considered in Chapter 9, p. 184.)

Dissociation

This is the defence mechanism by which a portion of the personality which cannot be tolerated or accepted by the individual's conscious self is split off from his awareness. In some instances part of his personality is completely " blacked out "; more rarely this part continues to function in a seemingly automatic way, side by side with, or alternating with, the individual's more usual characteristics. In some instances dissociation is closely related to repression, as in those not uncommon patients who state that they have no memory at all of their life before the age of 12 or even later, clearly because they wish to protect themselves from acknowledging the anxieties which originated from their experiences prior to that time. Other patients are able to dissociate their feelings from the rest of their personality and therefore can face very painful situations without any emotional response at all. (This is sometimes described as a separate mechanism, known as **isolation**.) Obviously in this instance their feelings have to be kept out of awareness because it is suspected that they would be of quite disruptive, even catastrophic, intensity if they were allowed to come to the surface. (The subject of dissociation and the psychiatric symptoms which may result from it are dealt with more fully in Chapter 9, p. 181.)

Rationalisation

We have established that much of a person's behaviour is determined by unconscious rather than by conscious motivating forces, yet in order to preserve our self-esteem we all to some extent try to justify our doings by a mental process known as rationalisation. Through this defence mechanism we are able to construct rational and logical reasons to "explain" our actions, reasons which may have little or no connection with the true underlying motives which are outside our awareness; in so doing we tend to select reasons which sound desirable and even noble and to reject reasons which would involve the recognition of socially unacceptable parts of ourselves. This "explanation" is not to be confused with a lie, which is recognised by the teller himself as a falsehood. A rationalisation is believed by the person who constructs it because it serves as a defence against the acknowledgement of deep anxieties and conflicts; any attempt to discredit his own account of his motives will usually provoke in him a strong emotional reaction. Too great a use of rationalisation clearly creates a quite dangerous lack of awareness about one's own true motives and desires.

Regression

Through this defence mechanism the individual confronted with a stressful situation reverts to an earlier level of development and to less mature modes of behaviour. It is as though the person says to himself "this situation is too much for me to cope with, therefore I will go back to the ways in which I used to behave, which were successful then and which gave me the satisfactions I wanted ". The most easily understood example of this technique is found in the regressive behaviour which is often used in an attempt to cope with sibling rivalry and which has been previously described in detail (p. 46). But all of us possess within ourselves traces of our earlier personality organisations and we can all, under severe stress, behave in ways less mature and more childish than those which we normally use. In otherwise apparently stable people, sickness and hospitalisation (because of the threat which these present to the individual) often produce evidence of regressed behaviour; anxious and frightened persons in such a situation may regress to a quite child-like demanding dependence (p. 390).

In its major forms regression is a disruptive and highly abnormal defence mechanism. At its most intense, as is encountered in many patients with schizophrenic reactions (Chapter 11), the person behaves in ways which indicate that at least large parts of his personality have returned to the early oral developmental level of the infant.

Projection

This is the mechanism by which the individual unconsciously disowns the unacceptable parts of himself and attributes them to other people or objects. It is in some ways like displacement though, in its major forms, it involves a distortion of reality, which displacement does not. In its simple manifestations it is demonstrated in the attitude of " the bad workman who blames his tools " rather than admit his own inefficiency or carelessness. Much more seriously, it is involved in the development of **delusions** (p. 112) and **hallucinations** (p. 117), in which the patient believes that certain things are happening to him which are not in fact true but which he experiences as the result of projecting (which means " throwing out ") a part of himself. The man who has never dared to face a deeply repressed homosexual component in his personality may later in life develop the completely false belief that people in the street, or other patients in hospital, are making homosexual suggestions to him whereas in fact, if all his own deeper wishes were to be revealed, the exact opposite would be found to be the truth. Many people who believe that they are hated and persecuted by others are in fact projecting on to their persecutors their own destructive wishes. Likewise a married man, unable to accept the guilt of his own infidelity or his own promiscuous wishes, unconsciously uses projection to change his attitude from " I would like to be unfaithful to my wife " to " I am sure my wife has been unfaithful to me ". The threatening " voices " which the psychiatric patient at times hears are often accusing him of practices which he has in fact carried out, the memory of which he has repressed, or of practices in which at the unconscious level he would like to indulge.

Introjection

Projection described the process of " throwing " unwanted attributes of oneself out of one's own personality; introjection describes the reverse process through which outside things are taken into oneself. In early life introjection is not in itself abnormal—in fact it is the forerunner and underlying basis of **identification** (p. 49), by which a child takes into himself the qualities of another person, in the way that a small boy takes over some of the attributes of his father. This mechanism often has an oral component; the very young child feels that goodness and badness inside himself may be created by the swallowing of " good " and " bad " things. This is more clear in primitive peoples—for example, in those African natives who, wishing to acquire the courage of a lion, eat his heart in the belief that this will achieve it for them. In our own society attraction for a woman and the desire to possess her may be expressed by a man in the phrase " she's good enough to eat."

Mature adults do not normally maintain relationships with other people by using introjection to any significant extent. However, introjection may have potentially dangerous consequences when it is used, either by child or adult, in an attempt to master the anxiety created by the loss or disappearance of a loved person. Consider a woman whose husband has died suddenly at a relatively young age; even when her relationship with him had been a reasonably satisfactory one, her grief will almost certainly contain an admixture of anger, however irrational this might be considered, because he has left her alone without warning and has caused her to fend for herself and the children, perhaps without adequate resources. But alongside her anger her loving feelings for him persist, and in order to defend against the complete loss of him from her life she may take into herself (introject) certain aspects of him— it is common, for example, for her to find herself for a period unwittingly copying some of his mannerisms. Two possibly serious consequences may follow. On the one hand, certain unhealthy aspects of his character or behaviour may have been introjected—she may for instance develop the chest pains which occurred during his last illness, or she may find herself drinking to excess as he did. Even more seriously, she may turn back against herself much of the anger she feels towards him, not only because she dares not admit to herself the extent of her rage, but because in terms of mental life some part of him is actually inside her. Many depressed moods are explainable in terms of this self-direction of anger which more appropriately, but perhaps more dangerously, should be directed outwards. Moreover, in many instances of **suicide** the individual is really trying to destroy only the introjected mental image of a partially hated person, but in the process he destroys himself as well.

CONCLUSION

Starting off life as a raw bundle of primitive instincts, the individual during the process of growth has to learn to tame these in order to achieve greater satisfactions for himself, to keep at peace with his own conscience and to avoid infringing the rules and conventions of the society in which he lives.

Because our present society is highly civilised, this process of taming is an extremely complicated one and may go wrong at numerous points. It would be easier if one could bury unwanted aspects of oneself and thereby remove their capacity to do harm, but this chapter has stressed that such is not the case and that many surprising and antisocial desires do in fact live on in the unconscious level of mental life. Because of the relative lack of opportunity in our society for the direct gratification of instincts, many and varied defence mechanisms are built into the personality, by means of which the individual attempts to delay or prevent instinct discharge or to arrange for such discharge in ways which will harm neither himself nor his surroundings. The more he uses the unhealthy types of defence mechanism just described, the more will he be a stranger to himself and the greater vulnerability will he have to the later development of psychiatric illness.

6

PSYCHIATRIC SYMPTOMS AND SIGNS

WHEN the nurse first meets psychiatric patients on the wards, and even more so when she encounters them in the outpatient or community clinic, she may be surprised to realise that in so many instances their appearance, conduct and conversation do not at first sight differ very greatly from that of the average person. Many of these patients on closer study will retain their outward appearance of normality, but are found to complain of peculiar bodily sensations or to describe in detail a particular fear or a state of intense inward misery. Within the psychiatric hospital she will certainly encounter some who are extremely quiet and withdrawn, others who are periodically violent and destructive, others again who carry on peculiar actions or huddle in strange postures. Some appear to talk sensibly apart from clinging to certain isolated and obviously incorrect beliefs, whilst a few chatter incoherently and almost incessantly. Some patients do not talk at all and may hardly move from one hour to the next. Others may deny completely that they are sick, or may be too confused to give any account of themselves at all.

If she is to make some sense out of all this unfamiliar material, she must first learn the correct ways of describing and recording what she sees and hears. Though everything that a psychiatric patient says or does could, if necessary, be reported without using technical terms, such reports would be in most instances extremely long-winded and confusing, and it is therefore essential for her to be familiar with the usual labels applied to the various abnormalities in the patient's thinking, feeling and behaviour. These abnormalities, like deviations from the normal in other branches of medicine, will be in the form of either **symptoms** or **signs;** symptoms are those complaints of the patient which are entirely personal and subjective, whereas signs are objective facts which can be noted by an outside observer. A complaint of pain, for example, is a symptom, but if at the time of his complaint the patient is rolling around in his bed in distress then he is also showing signs of his painful experience.

An individual symptom or sign, taken by itself, means very little, either in psychiatry or in medicine generally. In medical nursing, for example, the patient may be noted to be coughing; this fact will suggest the general region of the body affected, but the disease process may be involving one of several systems and the presence of a cough gives no clue at all as to the nature of the disease nor its cause. If, however, the cough is found in association with other symptoms and signs such as pain in the chest and fever, we begin to get a more accurate idea of what might be behind the patient's illness. The same is true in psychiatry; the nurse must first learn to recognise and describe individual abnormalities, and then will later see that certain of these symptoms and signs tend to occur in particular combinations characteristic of the various forms of psychiatric illness.

The material of this present chapter is set out under various major headings with which the nurse should gain an early and thorough familiarity. These will provide her with a scheme into which she can organise all the various observations she makes in her day-to-day contacts and conversation with individual patients, and she will be more certain that she has not overlooked significant aspects of their illnesses. Such a plan should also assist her at the time of her nursing examinations, as it will enable her to review with greater certainty of completeness the major features of any particular psychiatric disorder.

GENERAL APPEARANCE

Certain psychiatric patients (though less commonly than is popularly thought) display easily observed outward signs of their illness which should arouse the nurse's immediate interest, and which may in some instances at once provide important clues as to the nature of their disorder.

Facial Expression. This is chiefly of significance as an indication of the patient's mood, and on some occasions may be more reliable than his own report on the state of his feelings—he may claim to be cheerful and free from worry, but one look at his face may show this to be quite untrue. Feelings of depression, fear, anxiety or hostility are usually clearly shown by the facial expression and contrast strikingly with the blank, vacant gaze which is seen in some cases of advanced psychiatric illness. Anxiety or fear may also be indicated by beads of perspiration on the forehead and lips in times of stress.

In some mentally retarded patients, notably in Down's syndrome (p. 303), the facial appearance is highly characterstic.

Posture. Abnormal postures of the body may result from various diseases of the central nervous system or of the bones, muscles or joints. They may however be observed in some psychiatric patients in the absence of physical disease. The grossly depressed patient may slump in a huddled position, sometimes for hours on end if undisturbed. Other patients, notably those suffering from schizophrenic illnesses (p. 223), may adopt strange postures which they are capable of maintaining for long periods, this sign being known as **catatonia**. The patient's limbs may remain for some time in any position in which they are placed, even a highly unusual or uncomfortable one, and this state is referred to as **waxy flexibility**. These abnormalities of posture are based on a disturbance in the tone of the muscles.

Mannerisms. Many people show repeated small movements of an habitual kind—they may have unusual ways of smoking a cigarette, certain typical gestures of the hands, a characteristic way of raising their eyebrows, and so on. These are known as mannerisms and are not in themselves abnormal. In some varieties of psychiatric illness, however, such movements may be extremely peculiar in their form, sometimes giving the patient a quite grotesque appearance; the face may be repeatedly pulled into strange shapes or some part of the body incessantly and violently scratched.

Dress. Though normal people vary very widely in their ideas of what constitutes an appropriate style of dress, occasionally one sees patients whose mode of attire is so utterly freakish as to indicate immediately that they are mentally sick. Particularly in the long-stay wards of mental hospitals there will be met at times patients who choose to wear clothes of an absurdly out of date style or in an eccentric and hideous mixture of colours; one such male patient wore at all times a purple tie about four inches long, which had originally been a book-mark and which he claimed had a special religious significance for him.

Hygiene. Clues to the personality and illness of the patient will occasionally be picked up by noting the amount of time and attention he devotes to the care of his body. If this is unusually great such behaviour is said to show evidence of **narcissism,** that is, excessive love of self, a disturbance of character structure which is not infrequent in some immature personalities. On the other hand, some patients will show a progressive falling off in their standard of hygiene and a lack of concern for normal cleanliness and neatness; this is particularly common in the mental disorders of old age, or in other conditions where there is physical damage of any kind to the brain, but may be noted in any advanced psychiatric illness.

The nurse should be generally alert for any other specially noticeable features of the patient's physical appearance, whether or not they appear to have any connection with his mental state. If he looks markedly older or younger than his age, if he is conspicuously underweight, or if there are particular bodily deformities—all these things should be noted and may prove to be of assistance in diagnosis and management. The fact that a patient is heavily tattooed may, for example, provide some clue as to the nature of his personality; the actual content of the tattooed pictures, if they can be tactfully observed, may in some instances give an even clearer understanding of his emotional life and problems.

ACTIVITY AND BEHAVIOUR

The general level of activity in psychiatric patients may vary widely in both directions from the average.

Overactivity. This ranges from mild restlessness and an inability to sit still or relax up to the ceaseless, almost frantic activity of some seriously ill patients, most notably those suffering from an acute manic reaction (p. 242), whose restlessness may be of such an extent that they can find no time to eat and sleep. In these extreme cases nothing constructive is achieved, as one task is dropped almost as soon as it has been started and a new one commenced. Brief phases of violent and destructive activity may occur in schizophrenic or epileptic patients.

Underactivity. A general slowing down of activity level and of bodily functions is known as **retardation**. When this is severe and progressive the patient may finally reach a stage where he is completely motionless, a condition known as **stupor;** he is fully conscious but remains in the one position for hours at a time. This type of stupor may occur both in severe depressions and in some schizophrenic reactions; stupor of a somewhat different variety may occur in organic illnesses (p. 255). Retardation in its proper sense needs to be distinguished from the feelings of chronic fatigue, heaviness and inertia of which many neurotic patients complain; the latter can talk normally, often volubly, about their condition, whereas in true retardation speech functions are also slowed down and even simple conversation may be a painful effort for the patient.

Special Patterns of Activity are of importance in some cases. Some patients with schizophrenic illnesses repeat the same pattern of movements unceasingly, a sign known as **stereotypy;** the movements may involve the head or arms, or may consist of an unvarying walk around the same pathway in his ward. Also in schizophrenic reactions patients' behaviour may show gross abnormality in relation to what is asked of them; they may consistently do the opposite of what they are told (**negativism**), conversely they may copy with blind obedience any action they see carried out (**echopraxia**). (The other "echo" symptom is **echolalia,** in which patients consistently repeat any statement made to them.) At times their activity shows evidence of **ambivalence,** that is, a movement in one direction is immediately countered by a movement in the opposite direction; the patient's hand may, for example, go up to his mouth with an article of food but be withdrawn at the last moment, the cycle being repeated over and over again until sometimes, as if paralysed by two opposite desires, his arm remains for a considerable period in mid-air. (Such a conflict may lie behind the development of catatonia, described in the previous section.) Similar conflicting tendencies may make their appearance in his manner of walking, although abnormalities of gait will more commonly be found in conversion reactions (p. 184) and in many organic diseases of the nervous system.

The disturbances of activity known as **compulsions** are of a different kind altogether. Here the patient feels compelled to carry out a certain pattern of behaviour, while knowing full well that it is absurd and logically unnecessary, yet finding no peace until he has completed it. The piece of behaviour may be quite simple, such as getting out of bed to check once again if the front door is locked, even though the logical part of the mind knows with certainty that this has already been done; such happenings may occur occasionally in otherwise quite normal people. But in cases seeking treatment the required ritual may be exceedingly complex and time-consuming; repeated washing of the hands is probably the most frequent compulsion of this type. If the compulsion is resisted by the patient he suffers from unbearable tension, yet completion of the act is followed shortly afterwards by the further development of anxiety so that the behaviour requires almost constant repetition. Compulsions are invariably found in association with obsessions, described in the next section.

Though not symptoms or signs in the usual sense, many other features of the patient's behaviour may prove of assistance to the nurse in her task of understanding him. A detailed list of these aspects is given in the table in Chapter 20 (p. 419).

SPEECH

Disturbances in Rate of Speech. The rate of speech usually parallels fairly closely the general rate of activity. In states of excitement and overactivity the rate is accelerated; in mild cases this is referred to as **pressure of talk,** when more severe it is termed **flight of ideas.** The patient's thoughts move so rapidly that his words come tumbling from him at great speed; he makes such lightning changes from one topic to another that it may be difficult or impossible to understand him fully. He may follow one word with another which bears a superficial resemblance to it, for example, one patient said " my life is going with a bang—bang, bang, hang—you'll hang if you don't watch out "; this is described as a **clang association.** He may attempt to converse by means of poor poetry or may make feeble jokes and puns.

As with motor activity, slowing of speech is known as **retardation.** It is clearly an effort for the patient to talk, and he may state that he has no thoughts or that they come to him extremely slowly. In severe cases he may not talk at all, this being known as **mutism.** Not all silence, however, is due to retardation, as a patient may be prevented from speaking by feelings of marked anxiety, fear or hostility, yet have many thoughts racing in his mind. Occasional neurotic patients using the mechanism of conversion (p. 97) may be unable to speak for yet another reason, namely that they have a paralysis of function of the vocal cords—the sign known as **aphonia.** This further has to be distinguished from the condition of **aphasia** in which, due to organic damage to the speech centre in the brain such as may follow a " stroke ", the patient is unable to find the correct words in which to express his thoughts.

A somewhat different form of disturbance in rate is known as **blocking;** here the patient's thoughts and speech are proceeding at an essentially average rate, but are very suddenly and completely interrupted, perhaps even in the middle of a sentence. The gap may last for several seconds, even up to a minute, after which the patient resumes speaking, either where he left off or on a completely new topic. Blocking is often a part of the thought disorder found in schizophrenic reactions.

Disturbances in Form of Speech. Normal speech is understandable to another person of the same race and approximate standard of education because it consists of various words and ideas which follow one another in a sequence which we have learned to regard as logical. Normal communication between people is thus based on the fact that we all tend to link up ideas in our minds in basically the same sort of way, even though the ideas themselves may be very different; this process of thought linkage is known as the **association of ideas.** If one idea follows another without the usual type of logical connection existing between the two, then speech becomes progressively more difficult to understand; the patient begins to use ordinary words in such extraordinary combinations that his meaning may not be able to be grasped. He tries to express an idea, but talks around it and past it so that its point is obscure; he uses vague concepts which are difficult to pin down. All this is known as **thought disorder,** and is a striking feature of schizophrenic reactions. In extreme cases the patient develops **incoherence,** in which no glimmer of sense can be extracted from his speech; he may repeat the one word or phrase over and over again **(verbigeration)** or may use isolated, disconnected words mixed up in a hopeless jumble (a "**word salad**"). At times, in an effort to express the complex and confused thoughts with which a schizophrenic patient struggles, he may employ completely new words **(neologisms)**; one such patient described as "oversolarest" the process by which she believed men were arousing sexual feelings in her from many miles away.

Two other less important alterations must be mentioned **Circumstantiality** is that form of speech in which, without showing the basic disturbance of logical association seen in schizophrenic thought disorder, the patient rambles on and on in an effort to make some particular point but keeps being distracted by all sorts of side issues, overloading his story with many irrelevant and usually tedious details. (This is the person who keeps saying to his listeners " Oh yes, now where *was* I?") It may be shown by many normal people, especially those of dull intelligence or of advanced years; in psychiatric cases it is most readily observed in the mentally retarded and in patients with organic brain disease. In these latter patients there may also be observed a tendency to **perseveration,** that is, the abnormally persistent repetition of a single theme, even a single word, to which somehow the patient always manages to return in his conversation—here again this sort of tendency is not unknown, though to a lesser extent, in the typical party bore.

Disturbances in the Content of Speech. Under this heading one is looking for evidence of the various abnormal ideas with which a psychiatric patient may be preoccupied. These may in some instances be revealed very clearly during the first contact with him, but may on the other hand be carefully hidden and not recognised by the nurse until she has come to know him fairly well and has obtained his trust.

DELUSIONS. A delusion is a false belief, not shared by persons of the same race, age and standard of education, which cannot be altered by logical argument. The importance of " race, age and education " can be shown by the following examples: a belief that thunder represents the anger of the Gods might be normal if held by a member of a primitive African tribe, but would be delusional if held in a Western civilised community; a child's belief in fairies could not be called delusional, but would be labelled as such in an adult; the conviction that constipation is causing the accumulation of toxic substances in the blood stream would have a greatly different significance according to whether the individual had a primary school or University level education.

As delusions are by definition false and fixed ideas they can only be held by patients who are in some way able to distort reality. They are not therefore ever seen in neurotic patients, but only in personalities with the type of ego development which permits them to use the mechanism of **projection** (p. 100), the ego defence which lies behind all delusions. They are often, but not necessarily, found in association with hallucinations, and may occur in any type of psychotic reaction. They can be fleeting and vague, when they are known as **unsystematised delusions,** or may be built up into a complex, elaborate and more fixed structure of **systematised delusions;** the latter tend to be of more serious significance. The various types of delusion which can be described are:

Persecutory Delusions. The patient believes that certain happenings in his environment indicate the existence of some type of plot against him. Commonly, he believes himself to be the victim of some powerful organisation such as the police, the Communists, the Roman Catholic Church or the Masons and produces the most absurd " evidence " to justify his claim. Often his delusions are a further development of what are termed **ideas of reference,** ideas held by the patient that casual remarks or actions of people he meets are intended to have some special significance for him. For example, in the space of an hour a man passes in the street two complete strangers wearing red ties; he at first believes that this chance happening is intended to have some special meaning for him, and later elaborates the delusional belief that he is being followed by Communist agents. Various happenings may lead him to develop the idea that his body, his thoughts and his feelings are all in fact controlled by Communists, such beliefs of influence by others being known as **passivity feelings.**

Delusions of Guilt. Patients holding such beliefs state, without convincing evidence, that they have committed great wickedness in their past lives, often giving this a frankly sexual meaning. They may talk of having committed " the unpardonable sin " without ever being able to say precisely what this has involved. At times there is some slight basis in fact for the feeling of guilt and it is only its extreme severity and its sudden appearance many years after the event in question which indicates its abnormality; for example, a woman aged 60 developed out of the blue extreme remorse concerning an abortion which she had induced 30 years before but which had not significantly troubled her in the intervening period. A middle-aged man may suddenly develop intense guilt over the theft of a few pence from his mother in his childhood. In extreme cases these patients, who are almost invariably intensely depressed, may believe that they have caused enormous harm to others by their misdeeds and may refuse to agree that they are sick, insisting that they are being punished by God for their wickedness.

Nihilistic Delusions. The word " nihilistic " comes from the Latin " nihil ", meaning " nothing ", so that literally the phrase " nihilistic delusions " means " delusions of nothingness ". Such ideas may involve the patient's view of the whole world, which he believes to have been destroyed, or he may be convinced that a similar fate has befallen one or more of his relatives. In other instances such delusions refer to his own person; he may state that he is dead, or that certain parts of his body (commonly his brain, heart or intestines) have died or ceased to function, or that he has lost all his money or worldly goods. These symptoms are seen principally in severe depressive illnesses, less commonly in schizophrenic reactions.

Delusions of Bodily Disease. These delusions, sometimes known as **hypochondriacal delusions,** are those in which the patient holds a fixed conviction concerning the presence of disease or abnormality in some part of his own body. They differ from the excessive bodily concern shown by many neurotic patients in that, in the former instance, ideas are held which are clearly not compatible with reality. One young woman, for example, stated firmly that she was unable to swallow properly because her food, after passing her throat, deviated to the left of the midline and finished up in the bottom of her left breast. Patients may state, without any supporting evidence, that they are afflicted by cancer, venereal disease, brain tumour or tuberculosis. (Note that other patients may have a phobia, rather than a delusion, concerning these same diseases; phobias are discussed later in this chapter.) Such delusional complaints are almost confined to schizophrenic and depressive illnesses.

Delusions of Grandeur. These are firmly held ideas of great power, wealth and influence expressed most typically by patients with acute manic reactions, but also seen in some schizophrenic and organic psychotic disorders. The patient may believe that he is a King or Emperor, or that he is God or Jesus Christ; female patients may have a conviction of being the only true Virgin Mary. Other women develop the delusion that they are a source of sexual attraction to all men, and claim to have talents and beauty which remain sadly unsupported by the available evidence.

OVERVALUED IDEAS. Some patients devote an excessive degree of mental attention to some particular aspect of their life, appearance or personality, an aspect which has a definite factual basis but towards which they are directing an amount of concern which is clearly quite out of proportion. An example is that of a young male patient who had a very slightly disfiguring operation scar on his forearm which caused him extreme mental anguish, the extent of which was such that he felt obliged to leave his job as a fire-brigade officer because in a short-sleeved summer uniform the scar was clearly visible. The hidden reason behind his preoccupation was that the scar had resulted from the surgical removal of an old tattoo of a naked woman, the original acquisition of which had caused him great unconscious shame. Such a patient is not in the strict sense of the term distorting reality, but it is not uncommon for a symptom of this type to develop gradually into a definite delusion.

OBSESSIONS. These are also fixed or recurring thoughts in the patient's mind, but with one highly important difference from the abnormal ideas previously discussed—the patient himself recognises them to be abnormal. Despite this, however, the ideas recur over and over again in his thinking, often causing considerable mental distress because of their apparent purposelessness and their persistence and because they often seem to the patient to be completely out of keeping with what he considers to be his true self. One intensely religious young woman, to whom the conscious contemplation of the idea of divorce would have been horrifying, found her mind incessantly occupied with the thought "Christian involved in divorce case", an idea which, like all obsessions, could not be dismissed despite desperate efforts to banish it from her thinking. Such obsessional thoughts are frequently found in association with compulsions (p. 109).

It should be noted that the correct psychiatric meaning of the term "obsession" is quite different from its popular usage; the essential element in the definition is the patient's own awareness of his peculiarity. It is therefore usually quite incorrect to talk of a young man being "obsessed" with religion, or with some woman, or with his racial background, as in the majority of such instances the particular preoccupation is not seen by the person as foreign to his personality and is thus much closer in nature to an overvalued idea.

The difference between an obsession, an overvalued idea and a delusion, three terms which are often confusing to the nurse, may be illustrated as follows:

(i) A young woman has a slightly excessive growth of facial hair; while realising full well the absurdity of the idea, she cannot rid herself of the persistent thought that she is turning into a man. This is an **obsession.**

(ii) Another patient with a slight excess of facial hair is constantly bothered by this, spends a great amount of time and money on various treatments aimed at its removal and feels sure that everyone she meets must be as aware of its presence as she is herself. She does not regard her preoccupation as in any way abnormal and is surprised that anyone else could view the matter as less vital than she does. This is an **overvalued idea.**

PSYCHIATRIC SYMPTOMS AND SIGNS

(iii) A third patient believes firmly that she has excessive facial hair, but inspection shows this to be quite untrue. No amount of persuasion, however, will convince her for any length of time that her own belief is incorrect. This is a **delusion.**

HALLUCINATIONS. Normal perception is the end result of brain cell activity which has been brought about by some stimulus acting on special nerve-endings in the retina, the internal ear, the nose or tongue, the skin or internal organs. Stimulation of the retina, for example, by a pattern of light results in our perceiving an object of a certain shape and colour. Some patients, however, experience perceptions in the absence of any such stimulation of these sense organs and these abnormal perceptions are known as hallucinations.

They may affect any one of the five senses; the patient may hear non-existent voices, see visions, and so on. Popularly he is said to be " imagining things ", but imagination is the faculty which we all possess of conjuring up in our minds certain impressions, usually visual, which we can then at will dismiss, recognising all the time their unreality; hallucinations are not under the patient's control in any way and are usually extremely real to him, often terrifyingly so. Like delusons, therefore, they involve a break with normal external reality and a failure of adequate ego function, and are dependent also on the mechanism of projection.

Auditory Hallucinations. Typically the patient hears voices, sometimes unidentifiable and lacking in clarity, often the voices of persons known to him, uttering single words or complete phrases. The hallucinations may provide merely a constant comment on his everday activities or may make accusations. give commands, utter obscene words and suggestions, threaten punishment or provide reassurance. In some instances the patient describes, not a voice, but a peculiar noise. Auditory hallucinations are most commonly found in schizophrenic illnesses, but are also found in psychotic depressive reactions and in some forms of organic brain disease.

Visual Hallucinations. The patient sees visions, usually of clearly defined people or objects, but occasionally flashes of light or representations of geometrical patterns. The accompanying emotion may vary from joy to terror; the best known examples of frightening visual hallucinations occur in acute alcoholic psychosis (delirium tremens or " D.T.'s ") in which the patient typically sees unpleasant animals and spiders. The occurrence of visual hallucinations is strongly suggestive of the presence of an organic psychotic reaction, but they may also be occasionally seen in schizophrenic and depressive reactions.

Olfactory and Gustatory Hallucinations. These are hallucinations affecting the senses of smell and taste respectively; they are often found together in the one patient. The smell is rarely a pleasant one; much more commonly it is said to be horrible, being likened to gas, anaesthetic, bodily excretions, or described as smelling like disease and decay. Gustatory hallucinations are often not complained of as such; instead the patient states that his food has a peculiar taste, from which he frequently deduces that he is being poisoned. In one type of epilepsy due to disease of the temporal lobe of the brain olfactory hallucinations may occasionally be described (p. 274); otherwise the presence of these symptoms is almost diagnostic of a schizophrenic reaction.

Tactile Hallucinations. These false perceptions may be felt on any part of the body's surface and at times bizarre sensations may be described in internal organs. Very commonly they affect the sexual regions; the patient may complain, for example, that she has feelings in her genital tract which indicate that sexual approaches have been made to her during her sleep. Such hallucinations are most common in schizophrenic and in acute organic reactions.

As was previously mentioned, the presence of hallucinations indicates a break with reality and therefore a diagnosis of psychotic illness. Two exceptions, however, must be made to this—firstly, some patients who are prone to use the mechanism of dissociation may at times hear what they describe as

PSYCHIATRIC SYMPTOMS AND SIGNS

"voices", but which on questioning they realise to be their own thoughts which have become in some way split off from their ordinary consciousness and have obtained an auditory type of representation in their minds. Secondly, fleeting hallucinatory experiences may occur in normal people in a state of exhaustion, in the twilight state between waking and sleep, and under the influence of strong emotion; a vision seen in a state of religious ecstasy is an example of this type of hallucination. Finally it should be pointed out that the visual images which we all at times see in our dreams are very similar to hallucinatory experiences; all people thus possess the capacity to have their unconscious wishes and thoughts represented in visual or other sensory form, but only under exceptional circumstances or in the presence of frank mental illness does this occur when the individual is fully conscious.

ILLUSIONS. These are also false perceptions, but differ from hallucinations in that they arise in response to a definite external stimulus which is, however, wrongly interpreted. The anxious or confused patient who hears the rustle of leaves outside his window is actually receiving a stimulus to his auditory mechanism, but misconstrues this as being a noise made by people coming to attack him. Similarly, a coat hanging behind the bedroom door may be wrongly identified, particularly in darkness, as a man waiting for some sinister purpose. These experiences are common enough in anxious children and in otherwise normal adults under acute emotional stress; when they are seen in psychiatric patients they are much more persistent and terrifying and are a special feature of acute organic reactions.

PHOBIAS. A phobia is defined as an "irrational fear". The fear is irrational because the object or situation which is feared is not one which causes a similar degree of apprehension in normal people. As with obsessions, the phobic patient himself realises the absurdity of his fear, but is powerless to fight against it. This symptom comes about through the mechanism of **displacement** (p. 97); some basic conflict, which would cause the patient overwhelming distress if it were to become fully conscious, is defended against by avoiding situations which are in some way linked with the conflict or which might intensify it. In other instances the phobia results from a defensive camouflage of an unacceptable wish which is " turned into its opposite " by **reaction formation** (p. 95) and appears in consciousness in a totally reversed but socially acceptable form. It has already been mentioned that a conflict might arise from hostility felt unconsciously towards a person who is consciously believed to be loved; emergence of this hostility into open awareness would be unbearably threatening and is defended against by a grossly exaggerated, irrational fear that some harm might occur to this person.

Minor phobias are quite common in otherwise normal adults, and are seen also with great frequency for brief periods during the development of many children. When of clinical severity they are found most typically in that form of neurotic illness known as a phobic reaction, but they may also occur in virtually any other type of psychiatric disorder.

HYPOCHONDRIASIS. A substantial number of patients make numerous detailed complaints about some aspect of their bodily function; they are popularly known as " hypochondriacs " and show the symptom of hypochondriasis. Sometimes they have some definite organic bodily disease, though often of a very minor kind, about which they are excessively concerned; more frequently they are preoccupied with functional disturbances such as indigestion, palpitations or constipation. They may show a morbid interest in their heart rate, their blood pressure or the frequency, regularity and consistency of their bowel actions; others are " vitamin cranks " and develop odd food fads; others again grossly overemphasise the importance of physical fitness and spend large amounts of time and money on the cultivation of " the body beautiful ".

Most of these patients are showing one or other of the forms of neurotic reaction, in particular the hypochondriacal reaction itself (p. 194), but it has already been mentioned under the heading "delusions of bodily disease" that some patients' complaints about their bodies are so fantastic that they indicate the occurrence of a break with reality. Even if not overtly psychotic, many of these individuals are so eccentric and "odd" in their behaviour as to warrant the additional diagnostic label of schizoid personality (p. 229).

MOOD

The term mood is used to describe an emotional state which lasts for any substantial period of time. The word **affect** for all practical purposes has a similar meaning. Normal mood varies over a reasonable range from cheerfulness to occasional mild sadness and is responsive to happenings in the environment; bright company, a personal achievement or good news leads the normal person to react with happiness, whereas a personal failure or set-back or the loss of a loved person normally would induce sadness. Such fluctuation of feeling in keeping with the events around us is described as an **appropriate mood**. To feel miserable, therefore, is not in itself abnormal if the state of misery is not excessively intense or long-lasting and if it can be seen to be an understandable response to some external stress.

Depression. A state of sadness becomes a psychiatric symptom when it occurs as a mood of such persistence and severity that it interferes for a substantial period with the person's daily routine and adjustment to life. In these circumstances it is usually accompanied by feelings of anger and guilt (though these may not be immediately obvious), or in other instances by an overwhelming sense of complete hopelessness and helplessness. The possibility of **suicide** is very real in the presence of such feelings. At times depression can be clearly understood as an exaggerated and unduly prolonged response to an obvious stress situation; in other instances the precipitating factors are much more obscure, and sometimes not evident at all without a detailed knowledge of the patient. Individuals in the latter category are sometimes said to have an endogenous depression, on the assumption that the mood change is primarily due to some internal biochemical or physiological factor, quite unconnected with the patient's personality and life situation; proof for this notion has not as yet been forthcoming.

Many severely depressed patients show a pronounced retardation in both speech and general activity, though in other instances they may be extremely restless and agitated. In the psychotic varieties of depression delusions of guilt or of a nihilistic type are not infrequently present. Many patients with depression show their abnormal mood as part of a neurotic reaction, in which case other neurotic symptoms such as phobias or obsessions may be associated findings.

Elation. This term is used to describe an elevation of mood above the normal range; the patient is abnormally cheerful and optimistic in circumstances which in no way justify this. He frequently over-estimates his own capabilities and makes plans for his future quite out of keeping with any realistic view of his situation. Less marked states of elation are known as **euphoria**, where there is simply an increased sense of personal well-being, confidence and enthusiasm. In rare instances elevation of mood may proceed as far as a state of **ecstasy**, where the patient's feeling is one of complete rapture and bliss, often as part of a mystical or religious experience. All these mood elevations occur most frequently in manic reactions, but may also occur in organic psychotic reactions and in some schizophrenic patients.

Anxiety. A most important affect in psychiatric illness is that of anxiety, which may occur at some time in almost every type of disorder. Some of the sources of anxiety, and the ways in which the individual may defend against it, have already been considered in the previous chapter. The presence of an anxious affect in consciousness is a sure sign that the individual is faced with a situation which his usual defences are incapable of handling. These situations are of almost infinite variety and may stem from changed external life circumstances (for example, the threat posed by an impending surgical operation), pressure from the individual's instincts (for example, a sudden awareness of sexual feeling), or some combination of circumstances which represents both an external and an internal threat simultaneously (for example, awareness of the impending onset of old age, which may bring substantial practical difficulties as well as raising anxiety on account of failing mental and physical efficiency).

The state of anxiety has certain well-known bodily accompaniments such as tachycardia, sweating, dryness of the mouth and so on, and is often apparent by reason of the individual's muscular tension and general restlessness, even when no clear-cut complaint of anxiety is made. The nurse must be alert for such signs; the patient's cold, sweating palms may tell her more about his mood than any words he utters. When anxiety is accompanied by very definite restlessness it is usual to speak of **agitation**; in its most severe form it is known as **panic**, in which state the apprehension is so profound as to appear likely to disrupt completely the patient's equilibrium.

Hostility. Obviously it is not necessarily abnormal to feel or to express anger, which is a completely healthy response in certain situations. But if the feeling of anger persists as a sustained mood then this can fairly be regarded as a psychiatric symptom, though not one which is characteristic of any particular illness. Particularly is anger abnormal when it is experienced for reasons quite unknown to the patient; in other instances it arises in response to an apparently insignificant stimulus. Sometimes the patient deliberately tries to hide his rage, or may even keep it out of his own awareness, yet he demonstrates his feeling clearly through the look in his eyes, his tone of voice, his clenched fist or angry gestures. Such a patient may refuse to acknowledge the existence of hostility inside himself, yet sit sulkily in his room tearing a match-box or a handkerchief into small pieces in an obviously aggressive, destructive fashion.

Hostility may also be displayed in much more subtle ways by unco-operative behaviour, stubbornness or chronic mild irritability. Such patients are usually very trying nursing problems; even while being generally "difficult" and argumentative their external appearance may be pleasant, even charming, and the nurse may be puzzled as to why she finds the patient so hard to manage. When she detects her own irritation mounting without any obvious cause it is always useful to consider the possibility that she may be herself responding unwittingly to the aggressiveness which is unconsciously recognised by her in the patient's attitude. Such forms of veiled hostility are described as **passive aggression** and are extremely common ways in which psychiatric patients express anger and resentment.

Inappropriate (Incongruous) Affect. This term is used to describe the peculiarity of mood noted in many schizophrenic patients when they respond to particular events in a way strikingly different from the normal. They may recount horrifying delusions of persecution, or discuss threatening "voices", with a completely inappropriate cheerfulness; brought bad news they may react with fatuous and often mirthless laughter. Though they may accuse the nurses of detaining them in hospital without cause, they may accept continued hospitalisation with good humour.

This particular abnormality requires to be distinguished from a curious feature noted in some patients with conversion reactions who appear totally unconcerned about what the normal person would regard as serious physical disabilities. This incongruous cheerfulness, known as "la belle indifférence", is described more fully in Chapter 9 (p. 184).

Apathy. Though we may all at times feel apathetic and disinterested for brief periods the term apathy when applied to psychiatric patients refers to a flatness of mood which is much more severe and long-lasting. Such patients show no significant emotional response to any type of life experience, being equally indifferent to their own symptoms and to pleasant or unpleasant external situations. This absence of emotional response is often reflected in the patient's face, which appears dull and devoid of normal expression. It should not be thought that this flattening out of affect represents any true loss of the capacity for feeling—rather is it a defence against hurt, erected unconsciously by the patient as part of his illness, which is usually of schizophrenic type. Not infrequently apathy of perhaps many months' duration is interrupted by a temporary outburst of uncontrolled emotion which, even if inappropriate, indicates that the deeper affective capacities of the individual are not impaired.

Lability. This term is used to describe the extremely rapid, wide fluctuations of feeling which may be seen in some brain-damaged patients. The patient overreacts to some minor stress with a brief period of deep and genuine depression, often with copious tears and lamentations, but a few moments later is laughing uproariously and excessively at some very mildly amusing remark. This sign occurs as a result of a lessening of the normal control exercised by the cerebral cortex over basic and primitive emotional responses and is most frequently encountered in cases of senile brain disease (p. 263), where it represents only an exaggeration of the usual tendency to easy emotionality seen in very old people.

MEMORY

The ability to store knowledge and experience by means of the function we know as memory involves three steps—firstly, the **registration** of a particular impression, either derived through the sense organs or as the result of a thought process; secondly, the **retention** of such an impression over a period of time, which may be many years; thirdly, the **recall** of the stored information when the situation requires it. It has been already noted in our discussion of the unconscious levels of mental activity that many impressions may be registered and retained which are not able to be recalled at some later time because they are subject to repression and censorship (p. 82);

the entire emotional state of the individual thus affects his memory function, it being a general truth that "we only remember what we wish to remember" or, more accurately, "what we are able to remember without discomfort".

When we speak of "disturbance of memory" in psychiatric patients, however, the phrase is usually used to refer to relatively major alterations in the individual's capacity to register, retain and recall information.

Amnesia. This means "loss of memory" and is of several types. In the typical memory loss of old people there is a gradually progressing inability to recall past events and knowledge, a loss which is at first patchy, but which later spreads in severe cases to involve almost the entire range of the patient's previous information. In such cases it is extremely typical for recent memories to be lost much more extensively and much earlier than the memories of remote times; even relatively well-preserved old people may find considerable difficulty in recalling the happenings of the day just past, yet be able to converse with a wealth of fine detail about the events of their own childhood and adolescence. This type of memory loss is not confined to senile patients, but may be seen in any variety of organic psychotic reaction.

Amnesia may, however, also occur as a neurotic symptom with the clear, though unconscious, purpose of protecting the patient from painful memories. Amnesias of this type are described in more detail in Chapter 9 (p. 182). It is at times difficult to distinguish such an amnesia from an apparently similar loss of memory which may occur following a head injury or in some patients with epilepsy.

Hypermnesia. This term, the opposite of amnesia, describes an excessively retentive memory; events are recounted with an extraordinary wealth of detail. It is virtually only seen in manic reactions.

Confabulation. A patient suffering from marked memory loss due to organic brain disease may attempt to fill in the gaps in his story by inventing what appear to him to be suitable memories as replacements. Thus a patient who had been in hospital for several weeks, unable to remember how he had spent the previous evening, produced the absurd story that he left his bed and went to a night-club; encouraged to elaborate this, he plunged into wilder and wilder detail, describing the blonde who partnered him and giving a vivid description of the floor-show. This symptom may occur in several varieties of organic psychosis, but is most typically associated with the special form of mental deterioration due to alcohol known as Korsakow's psychosis (p. 264).

"**Déjà Vu.**" This French term can be translated literally as "already seen"; it describes the feeling, not infrequent in absolutely normal people, that a completely new scene or experience has been witnessed or lived through on a previous occasion. As a symptom of psychiatric illness, when it is likely to occur with much greater frequency and with an affect of unpleasantness, it is liable to indicate the presence either of a schizophrenic reaction or of that form of epilepsy associated with disease of the temporal lobe of the brain.

ATTENTION AND CONSCIOUSNESS

The normal individual is able to direct his attention to those elements in his present experience which are to him of greatest importance, while to a large extent ignoring those stimuli which are of little or no significance to him at the particular time. He is able, for instance, to read an interesting article in his evening paper during a bus ride while virtually completely disregarding conversations around him and the persistent noise of traffic. This ability is known as **concentration**; failure to be able to devote attention to some specific task, so that he is bombarded by a wide variety of stimuli, to all of which he feels the need to give some attention, is known as **distractibility**. With some patients it is almost impossible to gain their undivided attention for a continuous period, however brief.

When attention is interfered with by some damage to or disease of those brain mechanisms through which information is received and stored, then some degree of disturbance in the patient's consciousness and awareness is likely to occur.

Confusion. The truly confused patient usually reveals this quite clearly in his outward appearance; his face shows perplexity and bewilderment, often associated with considerable distress. There is a varying degree of disturbance in his intellectual functions, so that his judgement is faulty, his memory is to some extent disorganised, he is slow to grasp what is going on around him and finds it difficult or impossible to express himself logically. There is usually some degree of disorientation (see below). In some instances his difficulty in self-expression is so great that he is able to utter only disconnected words or incomplete fragments of sentences.

Confusion of this type, sometimes referred to as **objective confusion** because it is apparent to an outside observer, is found only in the presence of brain damage or some toxic agent interfering directly with brain function. Many anxious or depressed patients, however, will also complain of feeling " confused ", by which they mean that they feel themselves to be disorganised, forgetful and without clear aim or purpose. If they can be distracted from their mental preoccupations and engaged in concentrated conversation, it will be found that in fact they show none of the above features of objective confusion and that their intellectual functions, memory and general grasp of the situation are quite intact; they are thus suffering from a purely **subjective confusion.** Some schizophrenic patients also may give the impression of great bewilderment and intellectual disorganisation; the nurse, however, will be surprised to find that such patients, provided they can be brought into adequate contact with their surroundings (which may be extremely difficult), do not show disturbances of intellectual function of the type which would justify their being labelled as objectively confused.

Disorientation. The normal person knows who he is, where he is and to whom he is talking; he knows the approximate time of day and can give the correct date within one or two days. These capacities are known collectively as "orientation" and, if any one of them is absent, the patient is said to be disorientated for person, place or time as the case may be; he may be, and frequently is, disorientated in all three ways at the one time. Some patients who are exceedingly tense or depressed, or who are distracted by hallucinations, may find it so difficult to concentrate on their surroundings that they are unable to orient themselves fully. But by and large, if the patient is co-operative and concentrating on the questions asked him, the occurrence of disorientation is a definite pointer to the presence of some organic process affecting brain function.

Stupor. In some confused patients the condition may advance to a stage where their level of awareness is interfered with to such an extent that their contact with the outside world is progressively diminished. When the stage of stupor is reached the patient no longer makes any purposeful response to stimulation and is mute and motionless; a phase of noisy, violent restlessness may have preceded this. In some cases the condition may further progress to the stage of **coma**, in which the patient shows no response to stimulation of any kind, even pain. Such a progressive loss of consciousness may occur in many kinds of organic illness, such as acute generalised infections, meningitis, encephalitis, disorders of metabolism such as diabetes mellitus, and in various types of brain disease such as tumour or following head injury.

Stupor, however, may occur without a physical basis in some cases of schizophrenia, in very severe depression, and (very rarely) as a symptom of neurotic dissociation. In instances such as these the complete shutting out of the external world clearly represents the defensive function of withdrawal carried to the highest possible extent. These conditions were mentioned earlier in this present chapter (p. 108).

INTELLIGENCE

Though a precise assessment of intelligence can only be obtained through psychological testing, the nurse should form the habit of attempting to gauge the patient's intellectual level; this she will do partly through casual conversation, noting the words he uses and the way he uses them, partly through finding out his educational background, partly through noting his capacity to deal with ordinary situations requiring intelligent behaviour. Some rough estimate of his intelligence is of assistance to the nurse for two reasons—firstly, she will want to know whether, in his illness, he is showing a level of intelligent behaviour consistent with his past life or whether he shows some evidence of **intellectual deterioration**; secondly, knowledge of his intellectual level will assist in planning the day-to-day details of his nursing care and in finding occupations in keeping with this level which will be of use to him following his discharge from hospital.

For some psychiatric patients the major problem arises from their below average level of intelligence. This situation is considered at length in Chapter 14, where the measurement of intelligence is also discussed.

ATTITUDE TO ILLNESS

An appreciation of the mental state of the psychiatric patient is not complete until some estimate has been formed of his attitude towards his own illness. It is usual to state whether or not the patient shows **insight,** or understanding of himself, but this term has several levels of meaning.

1. The patient may show no insight at all into the fact that he is sick. Despite perhaps compulsory detention in a psychiatric hospital he insists on maintaining that he is perfectly well; other patients may state that their suffering does not indicate illness but is a form of punishment by God for their wrongdoing.

2. He may agree that he is sick (that is, he has insight up to a point) but may yet see his illness entirely in physical terms. Many neurotic patients, for example, have bodily symptoms for which, in the first instance at least, they refuse to believe that there is any explanation other than physical disease. Other patients may state glibly that their difficulties are due to " nerves " or a " nervous breakdown ", but as they talk they make it clear that this state means to them some sort of physical affliction quite unconnected with their personalities or their problems in life.

3. A deeper level of insight is shown by those patients who not only acknowledge the fact of their illness but who can also see, at least in part, that it is bound up with various factors in their past experience and their present relationships with other people. These patients are capable of co-operating in a treatment situation in a quite different way from those described in the preceding two paragraphs.

CONCLUSION—SYMPTOMS AND SIGNS AS DEFENCES

Both symptoms and signs must at all times be seen as the end products of various forces within the individual. That is to say, the nurse must not be content with mere description of what she sees and hears, but must be constantly alert for clues to the meaning of the abnormality which she is noting. For example, a depressed mood needs to be carefully observed and recorded for the patient's own protection and as a very beginning to the planning of his nursing care, but the nurse should not be content to leave it at that; she must also be on the alert for evidence of any underlying factors which may be accounting for his depression and should be attempting to understand the stresses and conflicts to which his mood is a response. In some instances symptoms will have developed as a direct result of some physical cause such as damage to or poisoning of brain substance; even here, however, the type of abnormal behaviour which is released by brain damage may reveal a great deal about the patient's previous personality and problems (p. 261). More frequently the feeling or behaviour is a result of the employment of the various defence mechanisms against anxiety which have been described in the previous chapter.

The abnormal talk, feeling and behaviour of psychiatric patients must, therefore, be looked at wherever possible in terms of its underlying meaning. Take, for example, the patient with a fixed delusion; it is essential for the nurse to be able to recognise and describe this, but after this step several other questions should arise in her mind. "What sort of life situation is he in that makes it impossible for him to cope without developing this symptom?" "Against what sort of underlying anxiety does this symptom protect him?—if he lost it, what might he have to face about himself?" "What can I learn about this patient from the form of his delusion?" "In what ways might we help him so that his delusion might become less necessary for him?" The answers to such questions are never easy, and may in some instances be impossible to find, perhaps due to lack of information about the patient, perhaps due to a complete inability to develop any sort of relationship with him. But only constant alertness for those clues which may lead her to a deeper understanding of the reason and purpose behind abnormal human behaviour will give the nurse a real feeling for her task and genuine interest and satisfaction in its performance.

7
FACTORS IN THE DEVELOPMENT OF PSYCHIATRIC ILLNESS

IN dealing with any sick person, an appreciation of the cause or causes of his illness greatly aids our understanding of him and his management. Nowhere is this more true than in psychiatry—and nowhere is it more difficult. In very many medical and surgical diseases, though by no means all, we now have definite knowledge of the major factors which operate to bring the illness about and treatment is planned accordingly; for example, antibiotic drugs such as penicillin are used to attack certain known bacteria. In psychiatry the so-called organic reactions are somewhat of this nature, in that they can be shown to be due to definite pathological changes in the brain—even here, however, as is discussed in Chapter 12, the patient's personality and the sort of life experience he has had will contribute to the form of the illness and may affect its treatment. The same is true for those individuals who are mentally retarded from birth or from an early age. But the great bulk of psychiatric illnesses do not fall into this category, being of the so-called "functional" type—that is, they represent a disorder of the function of the brain and not of its structure.

About the causes of this large group there is still a good deal of argument, often very heated. A substantial number of people hold the view that in at least some of these illnesses further research will show definite abnormalities in physiology or body chemistry which will explain their development. Some of these doctors do not necessarily discard the possibility that psychological and social factors could also have some importance, but there are others who seem to believe that abnormalities that can be expressed in physical terms are the only findings that could possibly be significant. This comes down to an understanding of the relationship between mind and body (p. 313); there is no need to assume that a measurable drop in the level of a certain brain hormone is necessarily more fundamental than, or more important than, a recognisable drop in the level of that person's self-esteem. There is mounting evidence that a wide range of abnormalities can be demonstrated in the blood and urine of patients with psychiatric illness; some of these findings are clearly secondary to the illness itself, others may reflect some inherited abnormality of the body's metabolism which may turn out to be a necessary but not sufficient " cause " of the illness.

Another group of research workers maintains with equal vigour that the causation of psychiatric illness (excluding the " organic " group) can be entirely understood in terms of the individual's psychological development, the interactions within his family particularly in early childhood, his experiences at home and within society, and the characteristics of the society or culture within which he lives. Some of the more extreme members of this group seem totally to reject the notion that hereditary or physical factors could play any part at all.

The point of view adopted in this book is the one for which there seems to us to be the most convincing evidence—namely, that the development of certain illnesses may require the presence of a particular hereditary constitution and associated biological abnormality, but that in virtually every case the patient's personal development, social network and life events will be found to have played an uniquely important role. The nurse should be wary of the occasional extremist she will encounter who will try to persuade her that the causation of all psychiatric illness can be understood by using some single, relatively simple formula; one-sided theories in psychiatry nearly always turn out to be misleading and dangerous.

Psychiatric Illnesses have many Causes

The idea that one single cause can be held responsible for his illness is often advanced by a psychiatric patient and almost

THE DEVELOPMENT OF PSYCHIATRIC ILLNESS

invariably by his relatives. Commonly the blame tends to be laid by them on some particular factor of a type which helps them maintain self-esteem and which removes the responsibility for illness from the patient himself or his family—such events as a "broken love affair", "overwork", "business worries", "war service" and so on. Other people, particularly those who have had no contact at all with psychiatric patients, show their ignorance (and their lack of tolerance and understanding) by labelling all psychiatric illness as due to "weakness of character", "no will-power", or to plain straightforward "bad living". But there is no isolated cause for any emotional disturbance—always a series of factors which combine to make the person behave in a way we label as "mentally ill". Even in many organic cases this is true—certain patients with brain damage have had this damage brought about by excessive alcohol consumption, so that alcohol is in one sense the "cause" of their illness. But what were the earlier situations which led up to the patient becoming an alcoholic? A small number of women develop a psychiatric illness following childbirth, but child-birth in this instance is not the one and only cause—what factors make child-bearing such an overwhelming stress for this particular group of people, in contrast to the vast majority of women on whom it has no such effect?

PREDISPOSING AND PRECIPITATING FACTORS

The answers to the type of question posed in the last paragraph come from an understanding of the fact that every psychiatric illness has two varieties of cause, a **predisposing cause** and a **precipitating cause**. What the layman usually talks about as *the* cause is only the precipitating cause, that incident or set of circumstances which has acted as a trigger to set off various patterns of abnormal behaviour. Similar circumstances (child-birth is still a good example) acting on a person not already predisposed to develop psychiatric illness will have no abnormal effect. This is not always true when the precipitating cause is of a gross, physical kind—for example, an extremely severe head injury or an extensive "stroke" may lead to a disturbance of mental function regardless of what has previously happened in the individual's life. (Even here, however, the nature of his previous personality will influence the form of the illness which results from the injury.) More minor head injuries, however, may or may not lead to emotional disturbance depending on the current state of the individual's anxieties, needs and conflicts, which are themselves in part the products of situations occurring during the course of his development.

COMMON PRECIPITATING CAUSES

These will be divided for convenience into **(1) physical causes** of a definite, concrete kind, and **(2) psychological causes,** in which the significant element is some conflict arising between the individual's needs and his environment. As will be seen, many incidents in a person's life have significance in both a physical and a psychological sense.

Precipitating Factors—Physical

Brain Injury. Damage to brain tissue brought about by physical injury commonly leads to some degree of mental impairment. Such damage most commonly arises from an industrial or traffic accident, but the same type of effect may occasionally be seen following extensive brain operations. (Injuries to the head may, however, frequently produce emotional disorder without there having been any interference with brain substance. The fact that such an injury may act as a serious psychological stress is hardly surprising when one considers the enormous importance we attach to our own head, knowing as we do that it contains the organ with which we think and feel and with which we earn our livelihood.)

Brain Disease. Any type of brain disease may lead to mental disturbance, though many may not do so until an advanced stage has been reached (for example, multiple sclerosis). The

THE DEVELOPMENT OF PSYCHIATRIC ILLNESS

list includes brain tumour, brain infections (for example, syphilis), degeneration of the brain due to old age or to inadequate blood supply, brain abscess and many others. Such disease processes are more likely to lead to frank psychiatric illness, or will do so more quickly, in the presence of an unfavourable life situation or when occurring in emotionally immature persons.

Toxic Factors. Any substance which acts as a poison to brain tissue may give rise to mental symptoms. One large group consists of drugs or poisons taken into the body; alcohol is the most common one, but the list includes barbiturates, bromides, amphetamines, certain industrial gases, digitalis, cortisone and many others. Bodily infections also set free toxic substances which in some instances may act on the brain to produce psychiatric illness, for example, pneumonia, septicaemia.

Bodily Illnesses. Some illnesses which affect the body generally, and which indirectly disturb the metabolism of the brain cells, may give rise to mental symptoms. Examples of these include thyrotoxicosis, vitamin deficiencies, congestive cardiac failure, kidney or liver failure and diseases affecting the level of blood sugar. But the significance of bodily disease in precipitating psychiatric disturbance lies more commonly in its psychological effects. Illness poses numerous threats to the person's overall adjustment, particularly if some or all of the following circumstances operate:

(a) *chronic illness,* which may seriously interfere with the patient's working capacity and bring, not only genuine financial hardship, but an associated loss of self-esteem and the anxiety or guilt which may be associated with having to depend on others (p. 380);

(b) *hospitalisation,* especially if prolonged, which may be a serious psychological stress, particularly in children, who have in most instances to tolerate not only separation from mother and family but also the anxieties aroused by a strange and often very frightening environment (p. 385);

(c) long-continued *pain*, the patient's defences being worn down by constant unpleasant stimuli with which he is powerless to deal;
(d) illnesses which result in *disfigurement or mutilation*, particularly if they involve the loss of a body part, which may provoke grave anxiety (not always conscious) because of the threat to the person's long held mental picture of himself (that is, his body image—p. 41);
(e) illnesses which involve a direct *interference with sexual capacity*, for example, paraplegia, which is a source of special stress, particularly to a young person. Even illnesses which do not in actual fact interfere with sexual function but which seem in the patient's imagination likely to do so may lead to serious anxiety. Emotional disturbance, for example, is more common after hysterectomy (removal of the uterus) than after cholecystectomy (removal of the gall-bladder).

Other aspects of this matter are discussed in the section on traumatic neurosis (p. 181) and also in Chapter 15 (p. 332).

Precipitating Factors—Psychological

Almost any type of life situation can act as a precipitating cause of psychiatric illness if it disturbs the particular person's adjustment and stimulates his underlying conflicts. In some individuals, heavily predisposed, the final breakdown of defences seems to come about due to nothing more than the ordinary stresses and strains of everyday living. More commonly, however, there is found in the history some definite event, or a series of events, from which the illness can be dated.

Critical Life Periods. Three particular phases in the individual's development pose special stresses:
(a) *adolescence*, with its upsurge of sexual feelings, coupled with the need for the gradual breaking of previous total dependency on the family and a more or less definite establishment of one's own identity (p. 57);
(b) *middle age*, with the decline of physical attractiveness and vigour, cessation of menstruation in the female and often the departure of children from home (p. 70);

THE DEVELOPMENT OF PSYCHIATRIC ILLNESS

(c) *old age,* with its many physical handicaps even in the absence of definite diseases, an awareness of declining importance in the world and often an increasing isolation and loneliness (p. 72).

During each of these three periods bodily changes are of course taking place, but it is considered to be the psychological impact of these, rather than the changes themselves, which is of importance. The menopause, for instance, has a different significance for a childless spinster than it has for a happily married woman with several children.

Psychiatric illness occurs particularly commonly at these three periods of life.

Marriage and Parenthood. It is not uncommon for psychiatric illness to become obvious shortly after marriage, during pregnancy or following confinement. In the first situation, full participation in sexual life seems to have reawakened buried anxiety and guilt concerning sexual matters, with or without further anxiety brought about by final separation from the parental home. The importance of the sexual factor is shown by the frequent occurrence of emotional disturbance which on close study is found to be related to the first conscious awareness of the sexual impulse.

When a woman's defences break down during the process of child-bearing it is often found that an important aspect is the stimulation of old unconscious conflicts concerning the mother-child relationship, anxiety having arisen initially from her own feelings about mother when the patient herself was a child. There is no evidence that physical factors play any part in this stress—in fact, the husbands of pregnant women, who certainly have no added physical burden during pregnancy, may themselves become emotionally disturbed at this time.

Unhappy marriages are often quoted as major causes of psychiatric illness and do indeed provide many individuals with a chronically difficult environment. One must remember, however, that the individual's own immaturity will almost certainly have contributed substantially to the marital unhappiness—in other words, unsuccessful marriages are more truly a result, rather than any basic cause, of emotional disturbance, though they will also add to the problems which the person has to face.

The incidence of psychiatric illness is substantially higher in the single and the divorced than in married people. This is almost certainly due to the fact that men and women with serious personality problems (of a kind which would predispose them to a later major disturbance) are less likely to form a permanent marriage relationship, and are therefore more liable to experience also the stresses of loneliness and isolation.

Occupational Stresses. " Overwork " is probably the most popular of all explanations for psychiatric illness—and is, of course, a very socially acceptable one. But there is no evidence to support its popularity; a history of recent overworking may be in itself a sign of emotional disturbance, or in other instances an overconscientious, self-driving pattern of activity may have been developed long before as part of the patient's defensive system against anxiety and inferiority. Other types of stress, however, can frequently arise on a man's job; competitive striving for advancement may bring its own problems, some predisposed individuals reacting badly when passed over for promotion, others (less commonly) being threatened at the prospect of passing over others and becoming " the boss ". Loss of a job can be serious, both in terms of the financial problems which may arise as a result but also (and often more importantly) because of the loss of self-esteem involved. Undoubtedly the nature of many occupations in an increasingly automated world creates major feelings of stress, frustration and tension, the monotonous and unvarying routine giving the individual little or no opportunity for any real self-expression or personal satisfaction in his work.

As with marriage, many stressful occupational situations are results, rather than causes, of emotional disturbance; many (perhaps most) individuals who have serious problems in their working lives contribute heavily to these through their own personality difficulties.

THE DEVELOPMENT OF PSYCHIATRIC ILLNESS

Combat Situations. The extreme stress of active service in the fighting forces in wartime led to many acute psychiatric illnesses, even in individuals who would not be regarded as strongly predisposed. Six *per cent.* of all admissions to British military hospitals during World War II were for psychiatric illness, and a third of all medical discharges from the Services were for this reason. The factors involved are many and various, the most obvious being the direct threat to personal safety which opposes the instinct of self-preservation; conflict develops between the desire to run away and the sense of patriotic duty and loyalty to comrades, as well as the necessity to maintain esteem in their eyes. Individuals with major underlying problems of aggression may be seriously threatened by being provided with weapons with which they can translate their unconscious destructiveness into action. In addition, the almost complete absence of feminine company may bring latent homosexual feelings to the surface, with resultant anxiety; factors of this kind were of importance in precipitating those numerous breakdowns which took place far from combat zones.

Bereavement. Many patients give a history of illness which clearly dates from the death of a close relative or friend—in particular a parent, spouse or child. Certainly it is normal for a person to experience profound grief following a major loss of this kind (indeed an absence of grief would be the abnormal state), and thereafter to undergo what may be a relatively prolonged period of painful readjustment to life without the dead person. But for some individuals the response is not normal grief and mourning but the development of a major psychiatric illness, commonly with profound depression as one of its outstanding features; there is also evidence to suggest that physical illness may sometimes be precipitated by bereavement.

Bereavement is a most severe stress for those persons who have always relied excessively upon the love and protection of others, who either were uncertain of being loved in childhood or who, through a parent's death or desertion, found supplies of love suddenly taken away from them (p. 86). Sometimes the relationship existing between the patient and the dead person was of a complicated kind, in which elements of unconscious rivalry and aggression contaminated the loving feelings. It has also been demonstrated that the outcome following bereavement is likely to be unfavourable when the death is closely associated in time with another major crisis—for example, the death of a woman's husband at a time when her mother is also gravely ill. But very importantly, and very practically, the outcome of bereavement has also been shown to be related to the quality of the emotional support which the bereaved person has available in the few months immediately following the loss. Successful adjustment is more likely to ensue when such support provides an opportunity for the free expression of feelings of grief, bitterness and sometimes guilt, and when there exists a relationship in which the bereaved person can talk openly about the death and the dead individual. Where this support is not available and where the individual is discouraged from feeling and talking about feelings, perhaps being given substantial doses of sedatives to suppress rather than express his emotions, then distinctly unfavourable consequences are certainly more likely to ensue.

PREDISPOSING FACTORS

Heredity. The exact part played by inherited factors in psychiatric illness is still in dispute. If an adolescent, for example, consults a psychiatrist and it is discovered that his mother spent some period of time in a psychiatric hospital during his childhood, one is certainly not justified in glibly assuming that the boy has simply inherited the mother's illness. Inheritance *may* play a part in such a case, but in addition the mother's basic personality is very likely to have been so abnormal that she was unable to provide him with normal mothering, quite apart from the effects on him of the period of time during his development when he was separated from her due to her hospitalisation. It is wise always to be cautious

THE DEVELOPMENT OF PSYCHIATRIC ILLNESS

in one's estimate of the importance of the hereditary factor in any particular case, for too great an emphasis on inherited defect is likely to lead to unnecessary pessimism and a defeatist attitude in treatment. " Mental illness runs in families " is an often-quoted and very true phrase, but this state of affairs is possibly less due to inherited factors than to the learning of unhealthy patterns of behaviour in the home environment.

Despite these cautions, there is no doubt that hereditary factors do play a definite part in some types of mental retardation (p. 302), in manic-depressive (p. 244) and in schizophrenic reactions (p. 226). There is little or no evidence that they are of any importance in neurotic illnesses, including the various personality disorders or character neuroses, though they may have some significance for the development of psychosomatic reactions (p. 316). In any event, the presence of inherited defect only lays down a *tendency* to develop a certain form of illness, a predisposition to react to stress in a certain way; it by no means indicates that the later development of illness is inevitable. Experiences on the road to maturity will determine in such a person whether or not a psychiatric illness develops.

Childhood Experiences

Chapter 3 has shown clearly the overwhelming importance attached to the quality of childhood experience for the later development of personality. In his early relationships with mother and other family members the growing child may or may not find satisfaction for his dependency; later he will learn that he must handle his aggressive feelings, and to deal with these and with his sexual drives he will develop certain defences of a healthy or unhealthy kind, as described in Chapter 5. Though later events may lead to substantial modifications in many of his surface characteristics, the main structure of his personality is laid down by the time he passes out of the Oedipal period at the age of six or seven.

The extent to which he is predisposed to later mental illness is determined by the adequacy of the ways in which the clash between his basic needs and the demands of his family and society has been resolved. The more that sublimation (p. 91) and direct discharge are employed to deal with his drives the more healthy is his personality, and the less likely is it to break down later in life. But if early experience has left him, for example, with an excessive amount of aggressive, destructive feelings which cannot be discharged directly and to deal with which sublimation is inadequate, mechanisms of an undesirable nature such as reaction formation (p. 95) or projection (p. 100) must be used by him. Such mechanisms, when stressful situations arise later in life, may give way or be replaced by even unhealthier ones, with psychiatric illness as the result. Some of these mechanisms may hide for years (in some instances for a lifetime), even from the person himself, the fact that his inner life is full of conflicting needs and wishes, incompatible with the rules of society or of his own morality.

Dependence. Excessive needs for dependence remaining in the adult personality arise either out of an excessive frustration of or, less commonly, an excessive gratification of the ordinary dependency wishes of the infant and young child. The first situation tends to be the result of an openly or subtly rejecting mother, to some extent aloof, mechanical and impersonal, or perhaps develops out of actual separation from the mother for some substantial period for any of a variety of causes (p. 40). Excessive gratification of childhood dependency is seen when the mother, by reason of her own immaturity, maintains the child's attachment to her beyond the usual period, discourages his independent personality growth and fosters, consciously or unconsciously, babyish habits and patterns of behaviour. Other parents again, fundamentally rejecting, may produce a different sort of basic conflict by prematurely thrusting a young child into responsible situations and forcing him to act in a more mature manner than is justified by his years.

A few of the possible unconscious problems in this area, and the ways in which they determine the significance of events later in life, may now be listed:

(i) The adult who still has an intense need for almost totally dependent relationships will be seriously threatened if he should develop such a relationship and it be subsequently broken; he will react with anxiety which may be overt or which may be dealt with by his customary defence mechanisms or by new and less healthy ones.

(ii) The individual, usually male, with intense unsatisfied dependency needs, who is thrust into a situation of chronic conflict when he is required to act as a permanent support to a wife and children.

(iii) Some adults need to deny any particle of dependence at all, due to the fact that childhood experiences of dependence have been felt to be intensely painful, humiliating and frustrating; if life should force them into a situation where dependence on others is inevitable (for example, due to serious physical illness), they may feel overwhelmed and helpless.

(iv) If childhood dependence were broken by the death or departure of the person depended upon, then such a child may in later life rigidly avoid, usually unwittingly, any situation in which a similar circumstance might arise; he says, in effect, " to be close to somebody means to depend on them to some extent—this could be dangerous because they might let me down, therefore I will be close to nobody ".

Aggression. Frustration of basic needs in early childhood produces a primitive, angry response; the most elementary observation of infants and very young children placed in frustrating situations shows this to be true. Because the child has to be taught social behaviour it is inevitable, however happy his family life, that curbs are placed on his desire to satisfy his basic needs and, therefore, equally inevitable that he will become angry; if exposed to unnecessary or excessive frustration he will become angrier still.

Some of this aggression arises from the checks placed on his natural inquisitiveness, checks which are meaningless to him; a good deal more develops out of the demands made by adults that he should partly abandon the pleasure principle, for he enjoys making a mess of his toys and of himself, and cannot appreciate why his parents wish him to be clean (see section on toilet-training, p. 42). The most basic frustration which may give rise to anger in the child is frustration of his need for love, which as we know is originally closely tied up with his need for food (p. 37). The baby who finds the supply of milk from mother's breast to be unsatisfactory will frequently be found to bite the nipple. Later he will resent separation from mother to a varying extent and will not at first be able to realise fully that she is not his alone, but has to be shared with other people. A special case of this resentment stems from the situation of sibling rivalry (p. 45).

Aggression arising in these and other ways is most healthily dealt with by sublimation, through which mechanism it becomes transformed into normal self-assertion and competitiveness. If it is handled by other mechanisms which do not transform it but simply bottle it up within the personality, later situations which reawaken this unconscious anger or which provide a temptation to discharge it may act as a trigger for psychiatric illness. Some examples follow:

(i) Military combat, as previously mentioned (p. 141).

(ii) In situations where an individual is threatened with physical violence by another person he may experience extreme anxiety, partly because of the threat to his own body, but often more particularly because of the unconscious fear that his own great destructiveness may be released by the other's assault.

(iii) Some adults have had the unfortunate experience in their past life of feeling or expressing strong anger against another person who very shortly afterwards has died or suffered serious injury or illness. In their imagination, life seems to have given them convincing proof of how destructive to another person their own anger can be; thereafter they unconsciously attempt to avoid any situation which might arouse angry feelings and may become extremely anxious if these attempts are unsuccessful.

THE DEVELOPMENT OF PSYCHIATRIC ILLNESS

(iv) Anger is seen as particularly threatening if it is felt towards another person on whom the individual is still strongly dependent. In these circumstances anger must be suppressed or repressed at all costs, for to show it may mean that the much needed support of the other person is lost; " if I am angry with him he will stop looking after me ". The seeds of this situation may have been sown in childhood by parents who threatened to withdraw their love from a child when he was angry and rebellious.

(v) Unconscious memories of childhood temper tantrums may lead to the state of anger being felt to be one of complete helplessness, disorganisation and chaos, in which one is wide open to the power of others; here again the individual finds it necessary to maintain elaborate defences against the possibility of feeling aggressive.

Sexuality. Psychiatric illness in adults is never found in association with a completely mature pattern of sexual life; though many patients may state (and believe) that their sexual adjustment is satisfactory and that their pleasure in sex is adequate, closer acquaintance will invariably show this belief to be based on deliberate or unwitting self-deception (or perhaps ignorance). It has been said, neatly and truly, that " happily married women never suffer from nervous troubles ", the term happiness here including an adequate sexual adjustment.

The work of **Sigmund Freud** was of major importance in our understanding of the enormous significance of early childhood development. His view essentially was that the development of mental stability depended upon the smooth progression through the various stages of what he called **infantile sexuality;** the word " sexual " was however used by him to include all varieties of pleasure derived from the body. In particular he focussed on the oral (p. 37), anal (p. 42) and phallic (p. 46) phases of development and introduced the term **fixation** to describe that process whereby too much mental energy may remain attached to these early forms of pleasure, with a resulting immaturity of sexual development, however carefully this is concealed. Above all, he emphasised the importance of the satisfactory overcoming of the Oedipus complex without which mature, guilt-free sexual feeling cannot develop; in all cases of psychiatric illness, he maintained, one would find evidence of unhealthy ways in which the triangular situation between the small child and his parents had persisted.

In those persons predisposed to later psychiatric illness substantial elements of immature attitudes towards sex persist in the adult personality, for example:

(i) There may be a pronounced exhibitionistic component in the individual's make-up, either expressed in sublimated form (especially in women) or in more direct sexual exhibitionism (virtually exclusively in men).

(ii) From childhood incidents, usually repressed, sexual behaviour may be felt to be an aggressive, destructive action, and may become linked in either sex with ideas of cruelty, punishment or damage.

(iii) Through faulty early training and experience, the adult may be unable to see sex and love as compatible; some immature men may only find sex desirable and interesting with promiscuous women or in any setting where a close emotional relationship is not involved, being disinterested or even sexually incapable with a loved person.

(iv) The child may, for any of a variety of reasons, have come to form a close association between the idea of " sex " and the feeling of " naughtiness " or " badness ". Sexual need in later life may then have to be totally repressed because of this connection, or can be gratified only in forbidden, " naughty " ways.

(v) Life experience, and particularly attitudes towards and feelings about parents, may in later life lead the adolescent or adult to doubt (unconsciously) just how masculine or feminine he or she really is. A major motivation in life may then become the need to prove that which is in doubt, commonly by means of numerous, insubstantial sexual affairs.

(vi) In both sexes, but much more commonly in girls, there

may be substantial envy of members of the opposite sex and a desire to be like them, perhaps partly because her life experience seems to the girl to have shown that to be a boy brings greater rewards and pleasures, but usually arising more directly out of the anxieties connected with the recognition of sexual differences (p. 47). Masculine envy of the female role is usually based less on a direct sexual envy and more commonly on the perception of a woman as being more able to give in to dependent needs.

These represent but a few of the ways in which problems in sexual life—using the term in its widest sense—may predispose to psychiatric illness. Based on one or other of the above types of conflict, or on other conflict situations too numerous to detail, the adolescent or adult may come to feel that his own sexual need is a frightening, dangerous thing; he may fear those impulses which he experiences inside him and may avoid situations which might arouse him sexually, becoming acutely anxious if these avoidance mechanisms fail and desire is experienced in consciousness. A particular form of unconscious anxiety seen chiefly in women is due to the fear that, should desire be aroused, it may become uncontrollable and lead to promiscuous behaviour.

While not necessarily disputing the importance of sexual development (for which the nurse will find ample evidence during her training), many later members of the psychoanalytic school have emphasised the even more fundamental importance of the nature of the child's initial relationship with his mother. Recent interest in the early years of growth has focussed very strongly on the process of **ego** formation (p. 83), the normal development of which, as we have seen, is clearly very much dependent on the child's deriving emotional warmth and a feeling of security in his experiences of mothering. Unsatisfactory ego development, leading to what is sometimes called a " fragile " ego because of its liability to break down in times of later stress, appears to be of primary importance for the later development of schizophrenic, paranoid and manic-depressive disorders. Grossly abnormal ego function is also found in patients with some forms of antisocial behaviour, for example in some sexual deviates who lack the capacity for impulse control which is shown by the normal person or by individuals with other types of neurosis.

After Freud, the most valuable contributor to the theory of psychiatric illness from the viewpoint of the nurse has been **Harry Stack Sullivan.** He focussed rather less on the individual person and much more on the nature of the human relationships which the person developed, seeing illness in terms of a breakdown of these relationships or the replacement of mature by immature ways of relating to others. He studied the ways in which one individual could communicate with another and pointed out that adequate communication between persons was essential for healthy mental life, but would be interfered with by anxiety. From this work developed the useful notion that many psychiatric symptoms represent unhealthy, immature and roundabout attempts at communication when no other method seems acceptable or possible to the patient; many times in this book it will be noted how a delusion, a phobia or a depressed mood can be seen to be a way of " getting across a message " which the patient for some reason or another is unable to express in any other fashion. (For example, that variety of suicidal attempt which represents, not a wholehearted desire to die, but a thinly concealed way of conveying the person's desperation and distress to others.) These viewpoints have led to the development of the so-called " science of interpersonal relationships " which is associated with Sullivan's name.

Two important practical points arise from this. The first is the clear implication from Sullivan's work that psychiatric illness, far from being some mysterious " thing " living within certain people and occasionally bursting out, is a description of such a person's " way of life ", his own abnormal mode of dealing with stress and of communicating with others. The causation of illness, in that great majority of cases where no

THE DEVELOPMENT OF PSYCHIATRIC ILLNESS

physical disease process is involved, boils down then to an understanding of why it should be necessary for him to abandon normal ways of doing the above things, or why in some instances he failed ever to achieve normal methods of relationship and communication. He becomes ill, in short, not because he chooses, but because all the factors in his development have left him with no other way of living in a stressful situation.

Secondly, if psychiatric illness involves a breakdown in interpersonal relationships, treatment to be successful must involve in some way and in some degree a reconstruction of the patient's capacity for relationships in a less anxious and therefore less defensive and distorted manner. This is by no means as easy as it sounds, as the nurse will quickly find out; though every psychiatric patient yearns at some level of his being to re-establish more normal, give-and-take human contacts with others, he has found these painful in the past (otherwise he would not have abandoned them) and defends himself in all sorts of ways against future hurt. But despite the difficulties, and notwithstanding the enormous value and importance of physical methods of therapy in modifying distressing symptoms and making patients more approachable, assistance in the development of newer and healthier ways of living and communicating is the prime task of psychiatric treatment, a task in which the nurse plays a major role.

There is currently a considerable vogue for the theories of **R. D. Laing,** a British psychoanalyst who has written extensively about the origins of schizophrenia, attributing this illness almost entirely to disorders of communication between parent and child, arising very early in life but continuing into the illness itself. He lays particular stress on what he calls the mystification which may be induced in a child by the receipt of messages which simultaneously have more than one level of meaning—for example, the mother's words may indicate that she approves of her child behaving in a certain way, yet the context in which she says this and some of her gestures and inflexions convey strong disapproval, leaving the child perplexed and bewildered. A very similar concept is conveyed by the use of the term **double bind**. Laing's theories are useful insofar as they provide a powerful counter-attack on those who are totally preoccupied with organic theories of mental illness, and who will not face up to the realities of communication problems arising within disordered families, but much of what he says is not really new and a great deal of it is stated in such extreme terms as to provide an almost ludicrously over-simplified picture of the nature of schizophrenia and its treatment. In more recent years he has gained importance from his status as a political rather than as a scientific figure.

CONCLUSION

Psychiatric illness cannot be understood as having " a cause " or even " a series of causes ". Various theories have been mentioned in this chapter, no single one of which provides a complete explanation for all the disorders which can be shown by the human mind; we are far, in fact, from having a totally satisfactory understanding of causation in some instances. But the overriding principle is clear—individuals develop psychiatric illness because a variety of factors, hereditary, physical or psychological in different proportions, interfere with their capacity to make a normal adjustment to the world they live in. Unhealthy methods of defence, originally developed early in life as a means of coping with childhood anxieties and frustrations, prove incapable at a later date of dealing with new stresses, whether these be physical or psychological. If the predisposition from childhood is strong, comparatively minor stresses in adolescence or adult life may set off abnormal modes of thought, behaviour and feeling. These will represent the patient's way of " reacting "—the only way he knows—to the problems of living in the world. This idea of psychiatric illness as a " reaction " is developed more fully in the next chapter.

8
CLASSIFICATION OF PSYCHIATRIC ILLNESS

IN Chapter 6 it was said that the symptoms and signs of psychiatric illness tend to occur in particular combinations or patterns. It is to these patterns of disturbed thinking, feeling and behaviour that we attach diagnostic labels, just as is done in the various forms of physical disease.

But immediately there must be stressed several important differences in the manner of diagnosis of physical and psychiatric disorders. Take the following example of diagnosis in physical illness: a middle-aged man, without any previous history of intestinal disorder, complains of increasing constipation and rectal bleeding, together with episodes of abdominal pain. Physical examination by the doctor, together with X-ray investigations, suggests the presence of a carcinoma of the colon and at operation this diagnosis is confirmed. A definite, visible disease process has been found to be responsible for the symptoms; treatment can therefore be immediately directed at the diseased area and, if removal of the carcinoma is successful, symptoms will disappear.

In diagnosing psychiatric illness rather different considerations operate and the following principles need to be firmly grasped.

Psychiatric Illnesses are not "Diseases"

Three important differences can be noted between the concept of carcinoma of the colon as a disease and the concept of psychiatric illness. Firstly, the symptoms of the carcinoma can be shown to be due entirely to a clear-cut bodily change, recognisable to the naked eye and under the microscope; such is far from the case with most psychiatric illnesses. Secondly, the great majority of the disturbances seen in psychiatry represent the end results of a combination of many circumstances which involve the patient's entire life experience; though there is often a definite starting point for the actual illness very many things which have gone before have contributed to the development of the disorder. Thirdly and most importantly, the preceding chapter has pointed out that psychiatric symptoms can only be understood if they are seen as arising from conflicts within the individual and from his unhealthy ways of trying to adapt to them. We cannot therefore hope to " remove " or " repair " the hallucinations of a schizophrenic patient or the phobias of a neurotic in the same sense that we can attempt to unite a fracture or cut out a cancerous growth; the psychiatric symptoms are the visible evidence of the patient's defences, representing the way (however abnormal) in which for the time being he is " getting by " in the world.

If one objects that in the organically caused psychiatric illnesses the above differences do not apply, at least to the same extent, it must be pointed out that even here there is not the same type of cause and effect relationship between brain disease and abnormal behaviour as exists in physical illness. This point is considered more fully in Chapter 12 (p. 261).

Psychiatric Illness arises out of Personality

One descending colon is very much like another descending colon and most carcinomas in this site have very similar symptoms and tend to behave in a rather similar way. Other things being equal, the response to surgical treatment is much the same whether the patient is a Prime Minister or a peasant, a Tasmanian or a Turk, a priest or a prostitute. But no two personalities are identical—great and obvious differences can be detected between all the members of any group of people, for example, between the nurses in a training school. As psychiatric illness arises out of and is very much coloured by the whole personality of the patient, then every individual case will have some distinctive features depending on the past habits, feelings and life experience of the patient concerned. Moreover, the plan of treatment may be very much influenced by the patient's intellectual level, social background and personality traits. This is true even in those illnesses which are related to definite brain injury or damage—here too the personality of the patient is of great importance in determining the form and severity of the resulting symptoms.

Another complication is introduced by the fact that the personality of the nurse, or of anyone observing the patient, may make a significant difference to her conclusions about him. If one has a physical illness oneself, such as arthritis, this does not interfere with the capacity to recognise arthritis in another person—yet an individual with strong but unrecognised hostile feelings towards people in authority may completely fail to detect similar feelings in a patient, or may perhaps detect them yet overlook their significance for his personality and illness.

Psychiatric Illness has Connections with Normal Mental Life

There is, for all practical purposes, no intermediate stage between having a colon which is normal and a colon which is the site of carcinoma; the definite features indicating carcinoma of the colon are never under any circumstances seen in a normal person. In terms of psychiatric illness both these propositions are untrue—firstly, there are all grades of disturbance between complete normality on the one hand and the severely ill hospitalised patient on the other. Secondly, many of the mental processes which appear on the surface in, for example, a person with a schizophrenic disorder may be detected in normal people at other times and in other circumstances—notably in dreams (p. 119). There are then no clear-cut dividing lines in psychiatry between the normal, the moderately ill and the severely ill; many otherwise normal people can show pieces of obviously abnormal behaviour when under severe stress. Various drugs, notably mescaline and lysergic acid diethylamide, can induce states remarkably like schizophrenia when given to normal volunteers.

Schizophrenia, for all these reasons, is not a disease in the usual medical sense of the term, but a description of certain ways in which some sick people think, feel and behave. It is one of the various abnormal ways in which an individual may *react* to any unbearable stress, whether this stress comes from inside himself or from outside. Such a person is therefore best diagnosed as having a *schizophrenic reaction*. Another individual, reacting to stress with symptoms mainly of anxiety, is given a diagnosis of *anxiety reaction*. *The diagnosis of a psychiatric illness is a description of the unhealthy reaction of a person to a situation of stress,* indicating the specific abnormal ways in which he is currently dealing with it.

Bearing these ideas in mind, the nurse will not be surprised to find that many of her patients do not fit precisely into any of the usual " pigeon-holes " of diagnosis, their illnesses not uncommonly showing features of two or more types of reaction at the one time. She will understand more clearly why it is that each illness she sees has some unique features, each individual's " reaction " being a little bit different from every other one because he has some unique features in his personality. Above all, it is hoped that she will see the uselessness, indeed the positive harmfulness, of drawing any far-reaching conclusions from the diagnostic label which she hears applied to a particular patient. One of the worst errors into which she can fall in her ward work is to develop a permanent mental picture of her patient Miss Jones as " the schizophrenic " or, worse still, " the new case of schizophrenia " or, worst of all, " the schiz ". Using labels in this way results in her own thinking about Miss Jones and her attitude towards her becoming set in mental concrete. What she should be thinking, and what should be determining her approach, is something like the following: " Miss Jones is a young woman, with a certain family background and life experience and particular

CLASSIFICATION OF PSYCHIATRIC ILLNESS

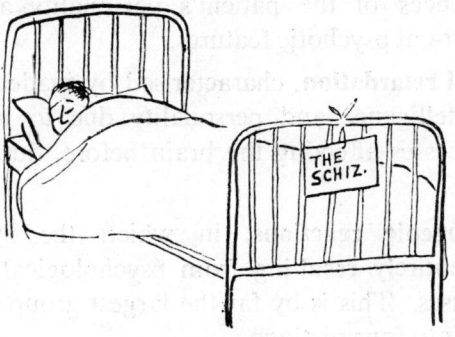

Fig. 10
One of the worst errors into which the nurse can fall.

current problems, who is at present reacting to her environment in a schizophrenic manner." Such an approach, to Miss Jones and to all her other patients, will obviously not be brought very often into the nurse's own conscious awareness, but it should at all times be part and parcel of her underlying attitude towards people with a psychiatric illness.

THE FORMS OF MENTAL ILLNESS

Despite all that has just been said, it is clearly necessary to have some system in which one can classify the most common forms of reaction. Identifying one's patient, however loosely, in one of the common categories of psychiatric illness leads to certain useful ideas about the severity of the disorder, the treatments likely to be effective and the possible outcomes, both in the near and the distant future.

Details of schemes of classification vary from country to country, sometimes from one hospital to another. All, however, recognise three broad groupings:

1. Organic reactions, those forms of psychiatric illness dependent upon some definite change in the structure or function of the brain tissue. These commonly show the symptoms characteristic of a psychotic reaction (see below), but in many other instances the disease process is manifested by disturbances of the patient's personality and behaviour without clear-cut psychotic features.

2. **Mental retardation**, characterised by inadequate development of intelligence and personality due to heredity or to disease processes affecting the brain before, during or shortly after birth.

3. **Psychogenic reactions,** in which the symptoms are largely or entirely resulting from psychological and environmental stresses. This is by far the largest group and is further subdivided into four sections.

(a) FUNCTIONAL PSYCHOTIC REACTIONS. The word psychotic describes a form of mental disorder severe enough to involve a grave disorganisation of the personality and which results in some degree of disturbance in the appreciation of ordinary reality. Symptoms such as delusions, which always involve an idea of reality different from that of the normal person, are thus only found in psychotic reactions. In many instances the behaviour of a psychotic person is very obviously abnormal. These are the patients thought of by the popular mind as "mad", "crazy" or "insane" (none of which terms, of course, are suitable for the nurse to use).

(b) NEUROTIC REACTIONS. The word "neurotic" is extremely hard to define. It describes all the various types of reaction to conflict which are not, on the one hand, normal, yet which are not of a kind to be labelled psychotic as just defined. Neurosis represents the result of immature attempts to adjust to the stresses and strains of life and always leads to the partial or complete blocking of some of the individual's talents and instincts. Nevertheless, except in rare instances, the observed behaviour of the neurotic patient does not differ greatly from that of the normal person.

The two major divisions of neurotic reactions, **symptom neurosis** and **character neurosis,** are described in detail in Chapter 9; from the numerous examples given in that chapter the concept of neurotic disorder will be more clearly grasped.

CLASSIFICATION OF PSYCHIATRIC ILLNESS

(c) PSYCHOSOMATIC REACTIONS, in which the principal symptoms are of a bodily kind (for example, asthma, duodenal ulcer), these having been produced, at least in part, by psychological stress.

(d) ADJUSTMENT REACTIONS, forms of abnormal behaviour arising clearly out of severe current stress, usually somewhat less serious in their significance than the well-developed neurotic reactions, and likely to subside as soon as the stress is removed.

A fuller classification follows, in which will be mentioned all the forms of psychiatric illness referred to in this book. No attempt should be made to memorise this table, but in reading later chapters the nurse should repeatedly return to it to ensure that she understands the position in it of each form of reaction described. Terms which are alternative to those used in this book are given in brackets.

I. Organic Reactions

A. **Acute organic reactions** (confusional psychosis, toxic psychosis, delirium, acute brain syndrome):
— associated with generalised infection;
— associated with infection of brain or meninges;
— associated with alcohol intoxication (delirium tremens);
— associated with intoxication by other drugs;
— associated with head injury;
— associated with cardiovascular disturbance;
— associated with epilepsy.

B. **Chronic organic reactions** (dementia, chronic brain syndrome):
— associated with syphilitic infection of the brain (general paralysis of the insane, G.P.I.);
— associated with other infections of the brain;
— associated with chronic intoxication by alcohol (Korsakow's psychosis);
— associated with chronic intoxication by other drugs;
— associated with head injury;

B. **Chronic organic reactions** (dementia, chronic brain syndrome) *contd*.
— associated with cerebral arteriosclerosis;
— associated with other cardiovascular disorders;
— associated with epilepsy;
— associated with the brain changes of senility (senile dementia);
— associated with presenile brain changes (Pick's disease, Alzheimer's disease);
— associated with general metabolic or nutritional disturbance (for example, pellagra);
— associated with brain tumour;
— associated with other forms of brain disease (for example, multiple sclerosis, Huntington's chorea, Parkinson's disease).

II. Mental Retardation

(Mental subnormality, mental deficiency, mental handicap, amentia):
— due to hereditary factors;
— due to specific abnormality of the brain.

Note: The *degree* of mental retardation is usually included in the diagnosis, using the categories of **mild, moderate, severe** or **profound.**

III. Psychogenic Reactions

A. **Functional psychotic reactions:**
 1. REACTIONS PRIMARILY INVOLVING AFFECT:
  — manic-depressive reaction, manic type;
  — manic-depressive reaction, depressive type;
  — psychotic depressive reaction (i.e., a depressive reaction clearly of psychotic type but without the clearly defined features of the manic-depressive reaction);
  — involutional melancholia (involutional psychotic reaction).

CLASSIFICATION OF PSYCHIATRIC ILLNESS

2. SCHIZOPHRENIC REACTIONS:
— schizophrenic reaction, simple type;
— schizophrenic reaction, hebephrenic type;
— schizophrenic reaction, catatonic type;
— schizophrenic reaction, paranoid type;
— schizophrenic reaction, acute undifferentiated type;
— schizophrenic reaction, chronic undifferentiated type;
— schizophrenic reaction, schizo-affective type;
— schizophrenic reaction, childhood type;
— schizophrenic reaction, residual type.

3. PARANOID REACTIONS:
— paranoia;
— paranoid reaction (paranoid state, paraphrenia).

B. **Neurotic reactions:**

1. SYMPTOM NEUROSIS:
— anxiety reaction;
— dissociative reaction[1];
— conversion reaction[1];
— phobic reaction;
— obsessive-compulsive reaction;
— neurotic depressive reaction;
— hypochondriacal reaction.

2. CHARACTER NEUROSIS (personality disorder). This term covers an extremely wide range of abnormalities of feeling and behaviour. Some of the most commonly found forms are:
— schizoid personality;
— cyclothymic personality;
— paranoid personality;
— hysterical personality;
— compulsive personality;
— passive-aggressive personality;

---

[1] The term "hysterical reaction" ("hysterical neurosis") is sometimes used to describe both dissociative reactions and conversion reactions.

2. Character neurosis (personality disorder)—*contd*.
 — emotionally unstable (explosive) personality);
 — antisocial reaction (psychopathic personality);
 — sexual deviation;
 — drug or alcohol dependence (drug addiction).

C. **Psychosomatic reactions,** the most usual forms involving one of the following body systems: skin, muscles and joints, respiratory, cardiovascular, gastrointestinal, urinary or reproductive systems.

D. **Adjustment reactions:**
 — in childhood;
  — habit disturbance;
  — conduct disturbance;
  — neurotic traits;
 — in adolescence;
 — in adult life;
 — in late life.

POSTSCRIPT: THE NORMAL MIND

It was said earlier in this chapter that there is no watertight division between normal and abnormal mental life. All sorts of factors have to be taken into account—a certain piece of behaviour may be labelled as " sick " by a civilised society today, yet might be accepted as normal in an uncivilised native tribe, or might have been regarded as such 500 years ago. Even in the one big city the same type of behaviour may be viewed quite differently by two contrasting social groups; the famous studies by Kinsey on sexual behaviour showed, for example, that certain sexual practices regarded as grossly abnormal by one section of society were accepted as perfectly normal by other persons in the same society with a different education and social background.

Put in another way, we have few fixed standards of measurement in mental life against which we can compare a person's behaviour and say precisely whether or not it falls within the

CLASSIFICATION OF PSYCHIATRIC ILLNESS

normal range. With height, for example, we know the average height of adults in a particular country, we can measure any particular person and find whether his height is within, above or below the average range. The same is true for more complicated matters of physiology such as kidney function, blood volume, the number of white cells and so on. A few aspects of psychological function, such as intelligence, are capable of the same sort of measurement (p. 306), but it is a different thing altogether to talk about a " normal " amount of anger or to define what one means by the term " a normal mother ".

The word " normal ", then, presents so many difficulties that it is more useful to talk in terms of the rather broader concept of **mental health**. We can then ask—" what sort of behaviour is typical of a mentally healthy person? What sort of things does a mentally healthy person do and feel which distinguish him from a mentally *un*healthy person?" The answers include the following:

(i) The mentally healthy person is able to love, that is, to form a relationship in which another person's satisfaction and happiness are of as much importance to him as his own, and where the feelings between the two individuals are truly mutual. This mature, healthy love requires to be distinguished from a relationship which is based primarily on a need to obtain love from the other person, and from those situations where the major (even if unconscious) motive of the lover is to dominate and control.

(ii) He is able to adapt himself to a reasonable environment, or to change his environment if such a change is desirable and possible—that is to say, he does not submit passively to unfavourable external circumstances if these are capable of alteration.

(iii) He is able to form harmonious relationships with a number of people of both sexes; he is therefore able to function adequately in social and work situations.

(iv) He is able to achieve satisfaction, direct or indirect, for the basic instincts with which he was born and he is able to employ adequately the various talents and skills which are within him to be developed.

(v) He must be able to do all these things within the limits set by his own conscience, which must be reasonable enough to permit him to gratify his basic drives in socially approved ways.

All this can be summed up in terms of our previous discussions of id, ego and superego (p. 82). Every individual at every moment of his life has to strike a balance between three types of pressure—pressure from his id of instincts requiring satisfaction, pressure from his superego which sets limits to his

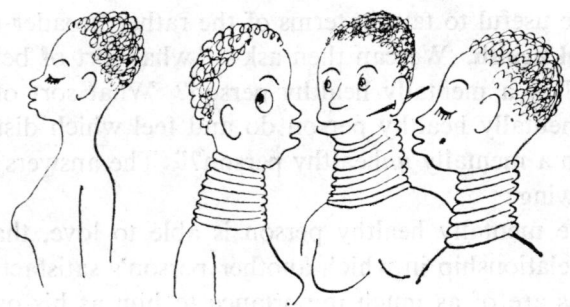

Fig. 11
Pressure to conform to the standards of society.

own behaviour and which causes him guilt if he oversteps them, pressure from the world about him which insists that he conform to the demands of ordinary reality and to the standards and laws of the society in which he lives. In diagrammatic form the situation can be represented in this way:

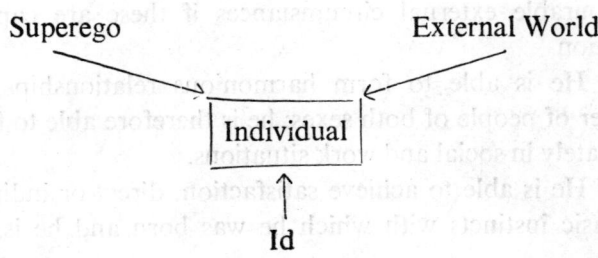

CLASSIFICATION OF PSYCHIATRIC ILLNESS

The mentally healthy person has developed ego functions which enable him to reconcile these conflicting pressures and to make a balance between them. It is useful, on the other hand, to consider a great deal of psychiatric illness as the result of unsatisfactory attempts to live with these three forces. To take only one example, the so-called delinquent youth achieves satisfaction for his aggressive or sexual instincts within limits that his conscience approves (at least temporarily), but at the price of offending against the rules of his society. Many more examples will be found in later pages of this book.

9

NEUROTIC REACTIONS

IT is extremely difficult to provide a precise definition of the word "neurotic". Unfortunately the term has crept quietly into ordinary English usage, where it has come to mean a variety of things, most of them wrong. It is sometimes employed, quite incorrectly, to describe a person who is consciously and deliberately behaving in certain "sick" ways to attract sympathy and to gain certain ends. Even more commonly the word is used in a moralistic fashion to describe a patient who constantly complains of a variety of bodily ailments, often with a good deal of self-pity; such a person may or may not have a neurotic illness (he may be psychotic), but in any event the speaker's tone usually makes it clear that he is not using the word to provide a concise clinical description, but in order to express his own criticism and disapproval of such behaviour, which he happens to find offensive. In fact, even in the hands of some doctors, the word "neurotic" may be a term of abuse more than anything else, used to label any behaviour of which the speaker personally disapproves.

Part of the problem of definition stems from the fact that it is difficult to rid oneself of the notion that neurosis is a fixed, static "disease process", similar to bronchiectasis or an ovarian cyst (see p. 153). Nothing could be further from the truth, and nothing could be more damaging to the nurse's understanding of neurotic behaviour. On the contrary, a person's behaviour may show neurotic features in some situations and not in others, so that some people (for example, his wife and children) realise that he does not think and react in a normal, average fashion, while others (for example, his workmates) see no evidence of any abnormality. Moreover, when under particular stress, a man may behave for a short period in ways that show markedly neurotic characteristics, though there has been little or no evidence of such characteristics in his previous life, and his normal ways of coping reappear when the current stress subsides.

This last notion returns us to the ideas brought forward at the end of the previous chapter—namely, that each individual, throughout his life, has to find ways of dealing with the conflicting demands of his own conscience, the external world, and his inescapable instinctual needs. In the normal person this task is handled, for the greater part smoothly and automatically, by ego functions which at times permit direct instinctual discharge and which favour the use of sublimation as a preferred mechanism to avoid an excessive build up of conflict and tension (p. 144). In other less fortunate individuals, for a variety of possible reasons, the adaptation of inescapable needs to equally inescapable environmental factors does not function as smoothly, and a variety of immature defences are brought into play, the operation of these defences being revealed as neurotic symptoms or behaviour.

Without then trying to provide a precise, easily memorised definition, it will be more useful to specify some of the **general characteristics of neurotic behaviour,** trying to distinguish it on the one hand from normal behaviour, on the other hand from the behaviour characteristic of a psychotic degree of disturbance in the individual's adaptation.

1. Neurotic behaviour results from an unsatisfactory attempt to resolve a conflict between the individual's needs, his superego and his environment. The conflict is moreover an unconscious one, of which the patient is therefore unaware.

2. The existence of the neurotic symptoms serves to enable the patient to avoid recognising the unconscious conflict, the presence and nature of which would be unacceptable to him and which would be likely to arouse extreme anxiety or unbearable feelings of guilt should he become aware of it. His intense fear of death, for example, may " protect " him from the recognition within himself of powerful aggressive, destructive impulses which would be unacceptable to his superego.

3. The neurotic symptom or behaviour, however non-rational it may appear on the surface, does however have a **meaning**, for it is determined in part by the nature of the conflict which the patient is attempting to solve, though its precise form will depend on the particular defence mechanism which the patient unwittingly brings into action. Repeated, compulsive hand-washing, for example (p. 190), may indicate in a highly symbolic way that the patient has deep-seated, largely unrecognised feelings of guilt based on a picture of himself as " dirty ", these feelings commonly being linked with complexes related to masturbation in childhood.

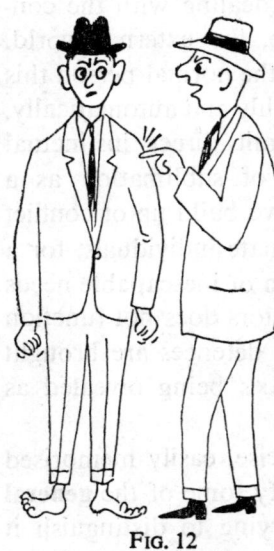

FIG. 12
" Just pull up your socks now ".

4. Because the behaviour has a defensive role in the patient's overall adjustment he will be reluctant to abandon it, even though it may be causing him considerable distress and although he believes at a conscious level that there is nothing he wants more than to lose his symptoms. It follows that he is quite unable to respond to the commands and advice usually given by his friends and relations—" just pull up your socks now . . . pull yourself together, man . . . your only trouble is that you need more self-control, more will-power ", and so on. These are commands that he has already given to himself, without effect.

5. The symptoms produced by the operation of the neurotic defences may *appear* to provide some solution to the underlying conflict—for example, loss of speech brought about by the defence mechanism of conversion may protect the patient from expressing in words his deep-seated angry feelings towards someone he cannot afford to offend. But because the underlying

conflict is not in any sense satisfactorily resolved by the formation of this symptom, nothing has really changed; in fact, sooner or later, neurotic symptoms lead to added complications in the patient's existence.

6. Similarly, because the conflict persists in a way which it would not do if sublimation were employed, the neurotic behaviour tends to be repeated, or one neurotic symptom may be replaced by another, with the real possibility that the patient becomes increasingly disabled and unhappy. Neurotic behaviour thus tends to be **repetitive;** the middle-aged housewife who has become dependent on barbiturate drugs returns time and again to her drug-taking habits, even though it is clear to other people (and at times clear to her) that this course of action can only end in frustration and disaster.

7. As has already been suggested, the neurotic patient has far less control over his symptoms and behaviour than is popularly believed. In fact, one very conspicuous and important feature of neurosis is that the patient's ability to select particular behaviour patterns, according to his own conscious wishes, is substantially impeded. Many neurotic acts are clearly recognised by the patient himself as logically unnecessary, non-rational, foolish or downright dangerous; this aspect is particularly clearly seen in some sexual deviants—they may carry out perverse acts which they know full well are against the law, for which they know their superego will make them suffer, for which they could be arrested and imprisoned, with grave effects on family life and career. Yet all these considerations may not be powerful enough to enable them to exert a normal measure of choice and control over what they do. Neurotic feelings, thoughts and behaviour therefore, unlike normal feelings, thoughts and behaviour, have an **obligatory** quality.

8. The neurotic patient does not falsify external reality in the way, or to the extent, which is characteristic of the psychotic individual. As in the example given in the previous paragraph, he may at times brush reality aside and act *as if* it did not exist for him, but in fact he has the same picture of the external

world as the normal person. Put in another way, he makes only strictly limited use of the ego defence mechanisms of projection (p. 100 and denial (p. 93).

9. Psychiatrists are not always able to explain the precise, detailed reasons behind the choice of one particular symptom rather than any other symptom, even though the nature of the underlying conflict may be clear enough. This is because various factors in the individual patient's experience and environment enter into the process of symptom formation; the external form in which a neurosis appears is likely to be different in a wealthy business executive from the way in which a basically similar conflict is resolved by a relatively uneducated, unsophisticated farm worker. Similarly, the clinical pictures of neurotic illness tend to vary from one country to another, and certainly have changed quite markedly during the past 50 to 100 years. These changes provide proof, if further proof were needed, of the dynamic nature of the neurotic symptom, an unsatisfactory and unsatisfying attempt to secure some compromise between the particular conflicts of an individual and the particular environment in which he is located.

10. Because the neurotic patient cannot develop a workable adjustment to the realities of existence without disowning various unacceptable parts of himself, it is likely in every case that there will be some degree of constriction of his personality growth and development, so that he fails to attain his full potentialities, either in human relationships, in the expression of his own particular talents and abilities, or in both areas.

THE FORMS OF NEUROTIC ILLNESS

The exact frequency of neurotic illness is extremely hard to estimate, though it is certainly safe to say that this particular group of disorders represents by far the largest proportion of all those patients suffering from psychiatric disturbance. The matter is very much complicated by the fact that some people whose behaviour displays evidence of many, perhaps most, of the characteristics set out in the previous section do not present themselves for treatment and may not be regarded as "sick" either by themselves or by their family and friends. Certainly many people who arouse no adverse comment from society (for example, the otherwise successful bachelor who throughout his life actively avoids all contact with women) must be regarded as showing definite neurotic features in their patterns of adjustment, and therefore classified as neurotic in the strict sense of the term. Even some persons whose behaviour tends to bring society's approval (for example, the young woman who renounces all other opportunities in life so that she can stay with a demanding and ungrateful mother) may well be labelled as neurotic by a psychiatrist in full possession of the appropriate facts. Perhaps, then, we all have some elements of neurosis in our make-up—it may be an isolated, irrational fear, or some small ritual which we need to keep us happy—insufficient, however, to interfere with our overall adjustment to life and therefore requiring no treatment.

In clinical practice, however, no such theoretical difficulties arise in the ordinary course of events. Patients who present for treatment are clearly suffering and unhappy, commonly causing considerable distress to others, and showing obvious handicaps in their personal relationships. But it will quickly be apparent that the concept of "neurotic illness" covers a very wide range of human behaviour indeed. Relatively few patients with neurotic reactions are admitted to the usual psychiatric hospital, unless they are quite profoundly disturbed and display an almost complete inability to adjust to the demands of ordinary living without disabling symptoms. Many more will be seen in outpatients' departments and day hospitals, in the psychiatric units of general hospitals and in private psychiatric clinics. Probably the majority of those who recognise that they need help do not approach a hospital at all, receiving treatment from a general practitioner or a specialist psychiatrist; many are treated by general physicians, or in the medical and surgical wards of general hospitals, for illnesses which are undoubtedly neurotic though not recognised as such, at least in the first instance. Over and above this, it is impossible to estimate the number of people who go through life with various forms of disturbed behaviour, sometimes spectacular, sometimes very humdrum, which are never regarded, either by the individual himself or by his friends, as being basically due to a neurotic maladjustment.

Some examples of the various facets of neurosis, all seen in a brief space of time by the one psychiatrist, may illustrate more clearly the range of the problem we are considering. In each instance, examination showed that the symptoms possessed all the characteristics of neurotic behaviour as previously defined.

1. A highly intelligent young woman, not yet 20 but already married and divorced, earning her living by prostitution and painfully aware of an almost complete block in her ability to express love for her child.

2. A housewife of 45 years complaining of long-standing feelings of depression, disinterest and irritability, who had more recently begun to disrupt her family life by excessive alcohol consumption.

3. A boy of 17, with an extremely disturbed family background and a history of many years in an orphanage, who without obvious cause or need began to indulge in petty thefts which brought him into sharp conflict with the law.

4. A married woman of 38 with fears of death of such intensity that she was almost completely unable to leave her home and who experienced repeated panics if she were left alone, even within her own four walls.

5. A young professional man with a speech impediment severe enough to interfere very greatly with his working life.

6. A 26-year-old single girl with obsessions and compulsions of almost disabling severity; she had regularly recurring and very frightening thoughts that she may in some way have harmed others and had developed very complicated and time-consuming rituals which she felt obliged to carry out in connection with the disposal of her bodily excretions.

NEUROTIC REACTIONS

Such a list could be continued virtually indefinitely; it has not included, for example, the chronically anxious, the drug addict, the cold and grossly reserved personalities, the sexually deviated and very many others. It must be stressed, then, that the field of neurosis extends far outside the walls of the psychiatric hospital and touches in some way nearly all of the problems of life.

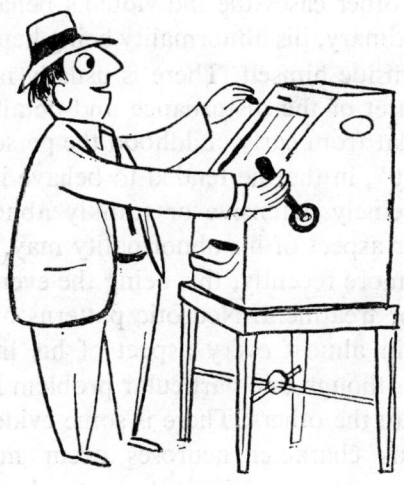

Fig. 13
The field of neurosis touches nearly all the problems of life.

Understanding will be easier if we define two broad groups of neurotic reactions:

1. **Symptom Neurosis.** The outstanding feature is the presence of one or more definite, specific psychiatric symptoms, usually beginning at a certain recognisable point in the individual's life history, and sometimes following a rather episodic course. Because most of the individual's conflicts are finding some sort of solution, however unsatisfactory, through this symptom or group of symptoms, he may function reasonably adequately in other areas of his life which are not directly involved in his neurosis. The illnesses described later in this present chapter come into this category.

173

2. **Character Neurosis.** Here we deal with individuals who, in typical cases, lack specific symptoms of the above type, but whose abnormality is shown in their entire character structure, or in large segments of it. They are sometimes said to be suffering from " personality disorders." Their illness may be apparent to the outside world by reason of an obviously disturbed pattern of life (for example, the delinquent or the drug addict), but in other cases the individual's behaviour may not be out of the ordinary, his abnormality being kept by him, often unrecognised, inside himself. There is usually no clear history of a definite onset of the disturbance and detailed study commonly shows that from early childhood the person was realised to be " different ", in that he tended to behave in an obviously immature, extremely defensive or frankly abnormal manner. Some particular aspect of his abnormality may, however, have only appeared more recently, this being the event which finally brought him for treatment. Neurotic patterns of reaction may be observable in almost every aspect of his life, if a proper history is taken, though one particular problem is usually more conspicuous than the others. There is some evidence to suggest that the various character neuroses occur more frequently nowadays than was the case in past years, whereas the prevalence of at least some of the symptom neuroses has probably declined. The most important and common patterns of character neurosis are described in the next chapter.

It should not be imagined that the separation of the neurotic illnesses into these two broad groups represents any watertight division. Many patients will be encountered who show the features of both types of reaction, and it is probably true to say that behind every symptom neurosis there is at least some degree of character abnormality, if it is sought, though the patient will possibly deny this in the early meetings with his doctor. Nevertheless the separation, despite this degree of overlap, is important in aiding our understanding and management. By and large, patients with a symptom neurosis experience more personal distress and discomfort; they are therefore more inclined to seek treatment and, partly because of their own dissatisfaction with themselves (but for other reasons as well) they are more inclined to respond favourably to psychiatric help. Patients with a character neurosis on the other hand —or patients with a very large component of neurotic character structure—tend more towards seeing their own behaviour as inevitable and fixed, sometimes even claiming that it is the desirable norm towards which others should aspire; they may in many instances derive a good deal of immature satisfaction from their own abnormality (for example, the alcoholic or the exhibitionist) and may in some cases actively oppose psychiatric referral and treatment.

These considerations lead to a situation unique in medical practice, in that the neurotic patient who actively seeks treatment must clearly be distressed by his own maladjustment in order to take the necessary steps to obtain help, yet he may not be as " sick ", in terms of degree of personality abnormality, as many others who are either unaware of or ignore their own need for assistance. The married woman with severe anxiety and phobias who presents for treatment is usually not the only disturbed member of her family group; one may not be able to persuade her husband to seek help for himself, but a fairly superficial acquaintance with him may reveal (for instance) that he is a cold, cruel person, incapable of showing his wife any warmth of feeling, having poor relationships with his workmates and carrying on numerous extramarital sexual affairs. In this example the personality disturbance (the " character neurosis ") of the husband is at least as great, perhaps greater, than that of the " patient ", though it is not of such a kind as to raise his own anxiety about himself. One of the factors which determines the possibility and form of treatment in neurotic illness is the individual's own ability to look at and face up, at least in part, to some of the problems in his own life. Lack of this ability is one of the chief reasons, for example, why criminals and delinquents, severely neurotically disturbed though many of them undoubtedly are, prove so difficult to reach through psychiatric treatment. In general it is only the neurotic patient who is intensely discomforted by his symptoms or seriously dissatisfied with the pattern of his own life who will be seen professionally by the psychiatric nurse, except in those programmes where other family members are required to become involved in the patient's treatment.

THE CAUSES OF NEUROTIC REACTIONS

There is little evidence that hereditary and constitutional factors play any significant part in the development of neurosis. It has already been noted (p. 142) that the occurrence of neurotic parents and neurotic children in the one family can be satisfactorily explained without resorting to any theory involving heredity. Some believe, because similar sorts of life experience seem to lead to neurosis in one person and not in another, that the affected person must have begun life with some basic predisposition towards the development of neurotic illness; it is impossible however for any two persons' life experiences to be really identical. In a family of two children, for example, one child grows up (say) in an environment containing a sister three years younger, the other has a brother three years older—a strikingly different situation, even if each parent has the same sort of feelings towards both children, which is probably unlikely, particularly when the children are of different sexes.

It is not believed that disturbances of body structure, function or chemistry play any part in the development of neurosis; many physiological alterations may however be seen as the result of neurotic illness, particularly in severely anxious patients.

As in all psychiatric illness, it is important to look for both **predisposing** and **precipitating causes** (p. 135). The latter are usually the more obvious, they are often at least partly known to the patient and are very frequently used unconsciously by him to obscure any understanding of more deep-seated personality difficulties and complexes. Let us be clear that precipitating causes do exist in every case and that they always have some importance; every neurotic patient is in a current stress situation, although some individuals with a certain amount of psychological knowledge may attempt to disguise this fact by concentrating their story exclusively on details of unpleasant childhood experiences. But, as we have seen in Chapter 7, the current stress very often only has real meaning in terms of the disordered personality background which preceded and perhaps created it. It can be again emphasised here in particular relation to neurotic reactions that the precipitating factor, whether it be in the marital, physical, occupational, or any other sphere, is only of significance in the vast majority of cases insofar as it reawakens and uncovers older conflicts or stimulates unresolved needs, guilts or anxieties which the patient's life situation had permitted to remain hidden up to that point in time. It should further be remembered that a fully conscious conflict is never in itself the whole cause of neurotic symptoms; either the surface anxiety exists in conjunction with other, unrecognised anxieties or the current stress is significant because of its link with deeper, unconscious complexes.

The predisposing causes of neurosis lie, as we have seen, in conflicts arising within the personality from the experiences and relationships of childhood, particularly in the areas of **dependence, aggression** and **sexuality.** Unfortunately, even without any added difficulties created by disturbed family relationships, our Western civilisation produces a most complex situation for the developing individual in each of these areas— independence tends to be overvalued and needed dependency despised; aggressiveness in ordinary social living is strongly condemned, yet in time of war is rewarded with an appropriate military decoration and in any event is needed in some measure for survival in our competitive society; many aspects of sexual behaviour continue to meet with disapproval from society's institutions, despite the existence of a generally more permissive attitude, while at the same time sexual drives are being constantly stimulated and indeed exploited in advertising, literature and films. (The fact that overt neurosis in men is strikingly less common than in women is due presumably, at least in part, to the fact that our society provides more opportunities for males to find direct or indirect outlets for sexual aggressive tensions without, or with much less, social disapproval.) Small wonder then that even the fairly well-adjusted parent finds considerable difficulty in helping her child deal with these basic impulses; it can be easily understood that the parent's task is much more anxiety-provoking and more liable to lead to confusion in the child when the latter's behaviour stirs up the parent's own unconscious anxieties in the area concerned.

In the early developmental history of many adult neurotic patients there will very frequently be found evidence of childhood emotional disturbances. The patient or his relatives may report that childhood was marked by bed-wetting, temper tantrums, gross nail-biting, excessive fears, poor school record, extreme shyness, cruelty and destructiveness, and so on. These symptoms will be further considered in Chapter 13; it must be stressed here that they are not causes, but rather the early warning signs of neurotic illness in later life.

CLINICAL PICTURES

It will by now be clear to the nurse that neurotic reactions are not " diseases " in the ordinary medical sense of the term, but ways in which certain predisposed persons react to stress and conflict. If this idea has been firmly grasped, then she will not be surprised to find that virtually each neurotic patient is different in some way from previous patients she has seen, so much does the illness depend on his type of personality and his experiences in life. It is far more important for her to attempt to understand why a neurotic patient has certain symptoms or behaves in such and such a way than to try to force his " case " into the nice tidy pigeon-hole of an exact diagnosis. Nevertheless certain patterns of symptoms and behaviour occur in combination with such frequency that they can be described as representing a certain type of neurotic reaction, and the most

common types will now be described. The nurse however will find numerous patients who do not conform to any one of the following descriptions, but who show some of the features of two, three or more of them.

PATTERNS OF SYMPTOM NEUROSIS
Anxiety Reaction

These are the patients in whom the basic underlying anxiety bursts out into the open in an obvious form, relatively undisguised by any of the various defence mechanisms which other neurotic patients use or which they themselves have previously employed. Often starting very acutely, frequently in relation to some definite precipitating event, they develop a general anxiety and fearfulness which may colour every aspect of their lives, interfering with concentration, appetite and sleep and associated with almost explosive feelings of inner tension and restlessness. Because their anxiety is diffuse and not related to one particular type of situation it is described as **free-floating anxiety.** Various special fears may be mentioned, particularly a fear of insanity, but these are not prominent features; patients who only experience anxiety and fear in relation to certain definite situations are said to manifest a phobic reaction, which will be described later in this chapter.

Bodily complaints are usually numerous and important. Energy tends to be markedly diminished, sexual interest dwindles or disappears entirely and various fleeting aches and pains of a vague nature are experienced. Sometimes one particular bodily system is affected; anxiety can give rise to palpitations and chest pain, these symptoms creating a fear that the heart may be diseased—as such a thought obviously increases the patient's anxiety, a vicious circle is set up. Other patients may suffer peculiar gastric symptoms; others again experience a disturbance in their pattern of respiration—they feel suffocated and begin to breathe more heavily and deeply and this breathing, by bringing about a disturbance in blood chemistry, produces further bodily symptoms including tingling sensations in the hands and feet, muscle cramps, dizziness and a feeling of impending faintness. Patients frequently complain of " headache " but questioning will very often show that they are not experiencing actual pain in the head but rather various " queer sensations ", sometimes described as " like a tight band around my head " or " like something pressing down on my skull "; such feelings may lead them to wonder about the possibility of a brain tumour (Fig. 14).

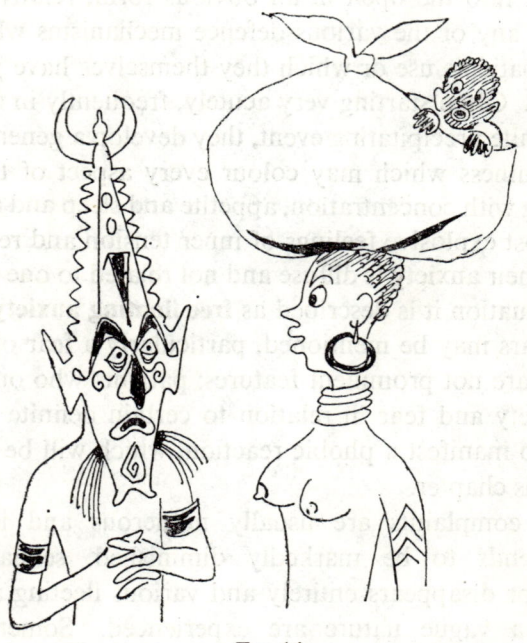

Fig. 14
" Like something pressing down on my skull ".

In the most acute form of anxiety reaction patients suffer from periodic attacks of sheer panic, in which they experience a host of unpleasant bodily symptoms all at once and at this time have the strong feeling that they are about to die.

Because of anorexia a substantial amount of weight is usually lost. Insomnia is almost invariably a serious problem and the patient may complain of frequent terrifying dreams.

Traumatic Neurosis. A special form of anxiety reaction may arise immediately following, or shortly after, some serious external threat to the patient's life which temporarily overwhelms him. Such a reaction, commonly known as a traumatic neurosis, may arise following severe battle stress in military personnel; in civilian life it occurs most frequently after serious traffic or industrial accidents, particularly those in which the patient could see disaster about to overtake him but was powerless to avoid it, or in circumstances where he was physically trapped in a painful, helpless situation for minutes or hours. Such patients, in addition to the full picture of the anxiety reaction just described, tend to have particularly horrifying nightmares in which the original precipitating situation is experienced again in all its agonising detail. The factor of financial compensation often complicates this situation and such patients tend to develop superadded conversion symptoms. (See section on compensation neurosis, p. 186).

Not all patients who show acute, readily observed anxiety belong in this category of anxiety reaction. In addition to the various other patterns of neurotic illness in which acute apprehensiveness is a striking symptom (notably in phobic and obsessive-compulsive reactions), many patients with early schizophrenic illnesses display periodic outbursts of acute anxiety. Anxiety may be a feature of some severe depressions, particularly in middle age, and may also be one of the early signs of organic psychotic reactions.

Dissociative Reaction

When the defence mechanism of dissociation (p. 98) is used against painful emotions, the result is a " splitting off " of some portion of the individual's personality which in some instances is able to function side by side with, but independent of, the remainder of his consciousness. Probably we can all in very minor degree do just this in our ordinary lives; some people in particular have a highly developed ability, for example, to read a book at the same time as the radio is playing, totally dissociating the sound of the music from the rest of the mind's activity and subsequently being genuinely unable to state what was being played.

Dissociative reactions may appear in any of the following forms:

Amnesia. Many neurotic patients complain of brief periods of loss of memory (p. 126); they suddenly realise that there has been a gap in their awareness and that they are performing actions which have no apparent connection with the last action they can remember carrying out. During this time they have most commonly functioned in an apparently normal manner in the opinion of outside observers, who probably have not noticed anything wrong. Usually of a few minutes' or a few hours' duration, rarely the amnesia lasts for days, weeks or months; even more uncommonly a large part or even the whole of the individual's previous life, even his name, is blotted out from his recollection.

Fugue. In a fugue the patient not only has amnesia for some segment of time but during this period he makes a journey, which may involve only a few suburban blocks but which may in other instances take him many miles from his original starting point into quite unfamiliar territory. During his wanderings his behaviour is well-organised and he usually shows no apparent abnormality to the casual eye. When finally he " wakes up "—hours, days or even weeks later—he has no recollection of his travels and can give no account of how or why he left home and reached the spot where he was found. Occasionally an amnesia for part or all of his life prior to the onset of the fugue persists for some time afterwards.

Double (or Multiple) Personality. This is a very rare form of dissociation in which, within the one individual, two or even more separate " personalities " may be developed, each with different characteristics, each being dominant at different times and being completely unaware of the existence of the other personality. The case dramatised in both book and film versions as " The Three Faces of Eve " has been the most startling example in recent years.

Depersonalisation. This is a distressing symptom which is not uncommonly a feature of neurotic reactions. The patient feels dissociated from his own body or his own emotions and has a painful sense of separateness from the outside world; his own self or the world about him, or both, seem to him to be unreal and somehow changed. He may describe himself as being in a constant " waking dream " and may feel that he is acting in a completely mechanical fashion. In contrast to some other states of separateness from the world, for example, schizophrenic withdrawal into fantasy, the patient with typical depersonalisation always stresses the severe unpleasantness of his condition.

The symptom of depersonalisation is not confined to patients with neurotic reactions; it may also be seen in some patients with early schizophrenic disorders and in some depressive illnesses.

Dissociation as a defence mechanism is used as an unconscious escape from situations which, if faced squarely, might lead to unbearable anxiety, guilt or depression; very frequently the patient has been clinically depressed just prior to the onset of amnesia or a fugue. Frequently there is a current painful situation of stress involving sexual or financial matters; an actual criminal act may be an occasional precipitant. A state of moderate drunkenness seems to aid the use of dissociation as a defence. Many of these patients give a history of having once had a head injury, perhaps some years before, and the loss of consciousness and amnesia of an organic kind brought about at that time by the accident seem to have laid down a pattern for the later employment of amnesia as a neurotic symptom.

The tendency to recurrence of states of dissociation is very high; it is a mechanism which, once used, tends to be resorted to with increasing ease in later stressful situations.

Conversion Reaction

In this form of neurotic illness the unconscious anxiety and conflict have been transformed, by a process which we are still very far from understanding, into a bodily symptom (p. 97). Because this mechanism of conversion seems to deal with anxiety more completely than any other, the patient's mood is often one of surprising cheerfulness and optimism, a mood which is traditionally referred to by the French term *la belle indifférence* (p. 124). Indeed, the presence of rosy confidence and the absence of anxiety or depression in a patient with a seemingly severe physical disability may often be a significant pointer to the realisation that the physical complaint has been brought about by the conversion mechanism.

The actual physical symptom which appears represents a disturbance or distortion of some function normally carried out by the central nervous system. Some of the most common symptoms are:

— disturbances of sensation: pain, numb feelings or sensory loss;
— loss, partial or complete, of sight or hearing;
— weakness or total paralysis of one, two or rarely all four limbs;
— muscle spasms, twitches or contractures;
— loss of speech, or inability to speak above a whisper;
— seizures of various kinds, in some forms of which the patient's consciousness is disturbed (due to the simultaneous use of the dissociation mechanism) and in which the resemblance to epileptic convulsions may be very close indeed (p. 278);
— disturbances in swallowing, often associated with a feeling of severe constriction around the throat—a symptom known as *globus hystericus*.

Why a particular patient develops one particular symptom is often very hard to determine. Sometimes the region affected is one which has previously been the site of organic disease—for example, a patient who in childhood had temporary weakness of one limb due to poliomyelitis developed in adolescence a similar symptom, this time without physical cause, as part of a conversion reaction. In other instances the symptom seems to have been unconsciously " copied " from another person, usually one close to the patient at some period of his life, who had the same disability either on an organic or a neurotic basis. Yet another possibility is that in childhood the patient passed through a period of emotional conflict while simultaneously suffering a physical disease, some unconscious link being forged between the two situations so that, in later life, further mental conflict tends to reawaken the old physical symptom, this time on a neurotic basis. Finally the symptom may have a simple or complicated symbolic meaning—for example, blindness may be a symbolic representation of a literal desire to avoid " seeing " some particular painful situation. (Further examples are given on p. 98). Here one can see clearly the defensive nature of the neurotic symptom and the way in which it attempts to provide some solution to mental conflict.

Secondary Gain. It may at times be exceedingly obvious to the nurse that a patient with a conversion reaction is achieving a more favourable life situation as a direct result of his illness. A common problem is posed by the unhappily married woman who develops some bodily complaint on the basis of conversion, the result of which is to attract, at least temporarily, the sympathy and added protection of a previously cold and distant husband. This may also apply in those situations where the basic complaint is of a purely physical kind (p. 324). Such a situation, of course, makes it in the long run doubly difficult for her to throw off her neurotic pattern and return to more mature living; not only must she then face the primary conflicts within herself which her neurosis had enabled her to avoid, but she must also abandon a powerful tool with which she has been unwittingly manipulating her environment. It must be stressed that these secondary gains are *not* conscious and deliberate; in those rare instances where the patient is believed to be fully aware of the beneficial effects of remaining ill she is described as a malingerer and she is not suffering from a true neurotic reaction at all.

Compensation Neurosis. A special example of the secondary gain problem may occur in the patient who is receiving, or who may receive, monetary compensation as a result of a traffic or industrial accident. Usually there has initially been a genuine physical injury, often coupled with a traumatic neurosis; if conversion symptoms develop, then the original physical disability is prolonged or exaggerated on a neurotic basis. In other instances no physical damage has occurred at any stage and the reaction is of wholly neurotic type from the very beginning. In either case the patient derives a special secondary gain from remaining sick; with present day standards of compensation he may be financially relatively secure, and can protect himself in this way from the anxiety associated with returning to work, where he might find that he is not in fact fully fit and has to accept reduced status or perhaps go off work again, this time without economic security. Obviously this problem will be especially pronounced in patients who have massive unsatisfied dependency needs, or who are hostile to authority figures in the person of employers or insurance companies—they tend to be, in short, the people who have always been inclined to believe " the world owes me a living ". Overenthusiastic medical and surgical treatment and investigation may worsen the situation, as may vague statements about his condition made to the patient or in his hearing. The whole problem is gravely aggravated by the enormous delay which usually ensues between the time of the accident and the final legal settlement of the insurance claim. By this time the neurotic patterns of behaviour may have become so firmly fixed that even the payment of a substantial lump sum of money does not reverse the reaction, although the converse is more commonly the case. It may be particularly difficult in some of these patients to decide whether an element of conscious motivation (*i.e.* malingering) is complicating the problem.

Similar difficulties arise in those patients who have been granted a pension, either for a purely neurotic reaction or for a physical disability with many additional neurotic features; the material and psychological rewards in remaining sick are so real that such persons are seldom able to be helped by psychiatric treatment.

Secondary gain problems, though they have been described under the heading of conversion reaction and are certainly most frequent and severe in patients with such symptoms, are by no means confined to this group and may be an additional factor in virtually every type of neurosis.

The Hysterical Personality. Over 50 *per cent*. of patients with conversion reactions have shown a particular type of neurotic character structure for many years prior to the development of their specific symptoms. Some or all of the following features may be noted: shallowness of true feelings associated with profuse display of spurious emotion, " showing off " and a generally dramatic quality in their behaviour and in their account of themselves, marked self-centredness and egotism, superficial protestations of religious feeling, flirtatious and " sexy " behaviour without any real capacity for sexual pleasure or gratification. They tend to be very demanding individuals, trying the nurse's patience by repeated requests for special consideration in all sorts of ways, and in so doing also showing the extreme dependence which is a feature of their personalities. Patients with well-developed forms of such behaviour will be among the most difficult, if not *the* most difficult, individuals which the nurse has in her ward; they tend much more commonly to be women. (Note that some people may show such a personality type without ever manifesting conversion symptoms—that is, they have one of the forms of character neurosis, on top of which there may or may not develop superadded neurotic symptoms.)

Phobic Reaction

The defence mechanism employed here is that of displacement (p. 97); anxiety arising out of unconscious conflict, instead of being free-floating as in the typical anxiety reaction, becomes connected to a particular object or situation, and it is only in the presence of this object or situation that the patient experiences anxiety or panic sensations. He is therefore reasonably comfortable as long as he avoids those conditions liable to provoke his fear but if, as is common, his fears gradually increase in number, then he may find his life becoming progressively restricted. At first, for example, becoming panicky only when in a train which enters a tunnel, later all riding in trains may become impossible because of anxiety attacks and later still any situation which brings him in contact with a crowd of people may set off a similar reaction.

Phobias are probably the most common of all psychiatric symptoms, though often they are of such trifling severity as to make little or no difference to the individual's life. They frequently arise for brief periods in childhood—for example, fear of the dark, fear of storms, or fear of animals (or of some particular animal). In adult life mild phobias are also common —for example, fear of storms, fear of heights, fear of closed spaces, though each of these may in some instances reach the status of a major symptom. (How many nurses of your acquaintance have an irrational fear of mice?) In patients seen on a psychiatric service phobias if present are usually major ones, and the following are some of the most common and important:

(i) fear of crowds, especially when the patient is unaccompanied, but sometimes felt even when with her husband or a close friend;

(ii) fear of being alone—in a mild form this may occur in many otherwise normal women, but in some instances may become a serious problem;

(iii) fear of dirt, usually with an associated fear of contamination by bacteria—there are all grades of neurotic disturbance between this type of phobia and a full-blown obsessive-compulsive reaction with handwashing rituals (p. 190),

(iv) fear of some particular disease—cancer and syphilis are the most common;
(v) fear of insanity, which may start from some small seed of doubt in the patient's mind and quickly reach terrifying proportions;
(vi) fear of harming others—this is again particularly common in women, usually taking the form of a fear of injuring their children, and may lead them to take elaborate precautions to hide from themselves any instrument with which aggressive actions might be carried out.

There is no easy way of determining the meaning and underlying significance of any phobia in a particular patient. Conflicts surrounding sex and/or aggression are usually of great importance, but these emotions have commonly been deeply buried in the unconscious segment of mental activity for many years. For example, the adult woman tormented by the fear of harming others is typically, though not invariably, a woman whose basic anger has always been dealt with by the mechanism of reaction formation (p. 95), and she has therefore appeared to herself and to others to be an exceptionally timid, submissive person incapable even of strong indignation, let alone aggression. Many phobias represent an unconscious defence by displacement against the patient's feared sexuality; here again the defence of reaction formation has often made the patient appear prudish, narrow-minded and almost totally lacking in sexual interest.

Obsessive-Compulsive Reaction

The simultaneous occurrence of obsessional thoughts and compulsive behaviour in the one patient is so common that such forms of neurotic reaction are labelled as obsessive-compulsive. The nurse would do well at this point to make certain that she fully understands the correct psychiatric meaning of the words obsession (p. 115) and compulsion (p. 109), for they are terms which are frequently loosely and wrongly employed.

Patients with persistently recurring obsessional thoughts tend to be among the most distressed and tense persons the nurse will see. One reason for this is that the thoughts are often felt by the patient to be totally opposed in their content to what he considers to be his true personality; for example, the deeply religious individual who finds his head constantly filled with blasphemous notions, or the prim single woman who cannot rid her mind of grossly obscene words or ideas. The harder the patient tries to rid himself of his mental preoccupation, the more strenuously the ideas seem to persist. Sometimes the thoughts are less anxiety-provoking in themselves and it is their very repetition which is so disturbing—for example, ceaseless uncontrollable rumination about the nature of God. One such patient, passing any common object such as a bus or a tree, would be unable to check obsessional preoccupation about the true nature of what he had just seen; he would have to ask himself, " Is that *really* a bus?—why do you come to that conclusion?" and could have no mental peace until he had precisely defined to himself the reasons for his decision.

Such obsessional thoughts are, like all neurotic symptoms, defences against underlying anxieties. Like all neurotic defences, they may prove inadequate after a period of time and are frequently joined by compulsive rituals which further attempt to control and keep out of awareness the unconscious conflict. A common example is provided by the patient whose illness begins with excessive concern about the possibility that unknown bacteria may in some way contaminate her; typically this leads quite quickly to the development of elaborate washing rituals following any contact with an object not scrupulously clean, and this may go on to involve full bathing and a complete change of clothes several times a day, perhaps with repeated scrubbing of hands and arms to such an extent as to interfere radically with her working capacity and to produce rawness and redness in the areas so excessively washed. Compulsions, however, may take almost any form and, like obsessions, tend to be associated with extreme

NEUROTIC REACTIONS

anxiety; carrying out the magic ritual may relieve the tension for a brief period, but it is in the nature of compulsive actions to require repetition almost as soon as the ritual has been completed.

A common form of obsessive-compulsive reaction is the *folie du doute* (the " doubting madness ") (Fig. 15). These patients are in a state of almost constant anxiety lest they should have forgotten to perform some necessary action; gas-taps and door-locks have to be repeatedly checked, a long and tedious trip has to be made back to the office to make completely certain that the safe has been securely closed, only to find on returning home once again that doubt still persists. An interesting example was seen in a pharmacist's apprentice; immediately after making up a bottle of medicine containing a dangerous drug, she was in an agony of apprehension lest she may by accident have put in double the dose of the poisonous component, and the mixture would have to be tipped down the sink and a fresh start made. But even after the fourth or fifth repetition of such a performance she could not achieve a feeling of complete certainty that she had carried out the correct instructions; the doubt and anxiety were never conquered.

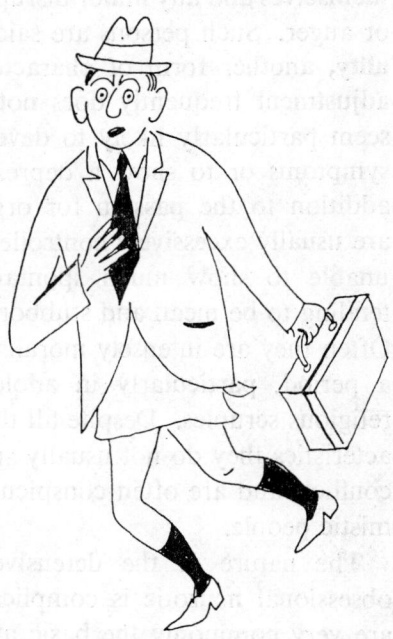

FIG. 15
Folie du doute—" did I remember to put on my tie?"

Obsessions and compulsions, like phobias, are common in childhood, usually in minor degree but occasionally of great severity. Many normal children's games have a compulsive, ritualistic quality—for example, the common pastime of walking along pavements scrupulously avoiding stepping on cracks, or perhaps counting every thirteenth paling in the fence. Many adults also show compulsive features in their behaviour; there are all grades of orderliness and neatness ranging from, on the one hand, the tidiness and organisation necessary for reasonable cleanliness and efficiency to, at the other extreme, the state of mind where order and system become ends in themselves and any minor disruption of the ritual brings anxiety or anger. Such persons are said to have a **compulsive personality,** another form of character neurosis; though their maladjustment frequently does not proceed past this point, they seem particularly likely to develop later obsessive-compulsive symptoms or to show a depressive illness in middle life. In addition to the passion for organisation just described, they are usually excessively controlled persons in all their activities, unable to show much spontaneous emotional warmth and tending to be mean and stubborn in their human relationships. Often they are intensely moralistic and intolerant and may for a period, particularly in adolescence, have difficulties over religious scruples. Despite all these defensive personality characteristics they do not usually succeed in dealing with all their conflicts and are often conspicuously anxious, tense and pessimistic people.

The nature of the defensive measures employed by the obsessional neurotic is complicated. Intense feelings of guilt are very commonly the basic affects, and many of the persistently repeating thoughts and actions can be understood as magical, symbolic rituals unconsciously designed to attempt to abolish these hidden painful feelings. When Lady Macbeth compulsively washed her hands she was endeavouring to remove, not only the blood of the man she had killed, but much more importantly, even though unconsciously, the guilt she felt arising out of her murderous action. The defence mechanism of **undoing** is significant here—one good thought or action is used in an attempt to atone for or wipe out another bad thought or action. But as the guilt-laden wish based on an instinct keeps repeating itself, so the counterbalancing obsessional thought or compulsive action has also to be repeated, and thus the process goes on incessantly. Such patterns of thought are typical of the obsessional neurotic and show clearly a primitive, magical quality which has certain similarities both to the thinking of uncivilised native peoples and to the basic assumptions of some religious rituals. Many obsessive-compulsive patients show such characteristics in their intensely superstitious way of life, believing implicitly in the danger of " Friday the thirteenth " and the awful consequences of a broken mirror or an umbrella raised inside the house.

It has already been inferred that the obsessional patient, like the phobic, has a personality structure in which many features are determined by reaction formations against feared basic instinctual drives.

Neurotic Depressive Reaction

Some neurotic illnesses show depression as their chief symptom, usually in association with other complaints such as phobias. Such depressions are sometimes termed " reactive ", indicating that they arise as a " reaction " to some external, depressing situation; this seems a bad term, as it can be a perfectly healthy response to " react " with depression to some external stress, such as a bereavement, whereas on the other hand some depressive reactions to external catastrophe take a clearly psychotic form.

The patient with a neurotic depressive reaction may in some instances be very gloomy indeed, though his mood is commonly able to be temporarily lightened by a cheerful environment. He may cry a good deal, lose interest in his surroundings, feel generally fatigued, and he usually eats and sleeps poorly. The possibility of suicide is a real one in severe cases; suicidal attempts not uncommonly have a somewhat attention-seeking quality, but in many instances they are genuinely self-destructive and are occasionally successful. (The nurse should disregard the commonly given but totally incorrect advice that patients with a diagnosis of neurotic reaction are never genuine suicidal risks). There is no retardation in the true sense of the term, only inertia and disinterest, and delusions of course are never present. (For a summary of the clinical picture of the neurotic depressive reaction and its points of difference from psychotic forms of depression the Table on p. 247 should be consulted.)

Depressions of this type commonly arise as a sequel to some quite definite external event which can usually be discovered without too much difficulty. More often than not the significance of this event lies in its interpretation by the patient as an indication that he is not loved, or that love he has previously received will no longer be available; such incidents as the loss of a job, a broken engagement, a real or imagined rejection by a relation, may all be experienced by him in this way, although this significance is probably not appreciated at the conscious level. What has been called in Chapter 5 anxiety over loss of love is often, therefore, the basis of this reaction. The anger and destructiveness which have been stirred up by this rejection are not expressed and are turned in on the self, leading to the depressed mood, the mechanism of introjection (p. 101) being commonly employed. Patients with this type of depression have been aptly described as being in "a state of frozen rage".

Hypochondriacal Reaction

Many psychiatric patients make frequent reference to their belief that all is not well with their bodily functions. Some of these symptoms may best be understood as manifestations of a conversion reaction (p. 184) whereas others are clearly produced by psychosomatic mechanisms (p. 313) and are best classified as such. Complaints of bodily distress may also represent the outward signs of some delusional belief concerning an alteration in the shape, size or function of some particular organ or system (p. 114), such patients being by definition psychotic, usually having a schizophrenic illness. When all these possibilities have been excluded, however, there remains a small but definite group of patients in whom the outstanding feature of the illness is an anxious preoccupation with some aspect or aspects of their physical health, and who can not be reassured that they are not seriously ill despite the evidence of numerous negative investigations and the confident pronouncements of an army of specialists. In some instances a minor organic abnormality does in fact exist, or has existed in the past, but on to this the patient attaches a quite abnormal amount of interest and concern. An excessively cautious statement by a previous physician may well have exaggerated this tendency, though it would not have been a primary cause. The condition tends to be a chronic one, and the unfortunate patient frequently succeeds in antagonising his doctors and nurses, who sometimes find it hard to believe that his distress is genuine and are unwittingly irritated by the way he seems so stubbornly to cling to his symptoms despite the abundant reassurance he is given. The nurse will quickly discover, in fact, that ordinary reassurance may well make him *worse,* as he interprets this to mean that people believe he is " imagining " his complaints and is not really suffering at all, so that he has to redouble his efforts to convince people whom he now takes to be unsympathetic and lacking in understanding. Such patients are amongst the most difficult that any doctor or nurse is called upon to treat.

10

NEUROTIC REACTIONS
(continued)

PATTERNS OF CHARACTER NEUROSIS

THE types of neurotic character structure with their resulting abnormalities in feeling and behaviour are almost limitless in their variation; only the most common and serious patterns will be outlined here.

DRUG DEPENDENCE

When we say that a person is dependent upon a drug we are describing a state in which he experiences a strong and sometimes overpowering desire to take the particular substance, regardless of any ill effect which it might be having on him, because he craves the special mental and/or physical sensations which he knows it will produce. Until recently it has been customary to talk of some of these patients as **addicted** to drugs, which usually implies that there is a definite bodily craving for the substance, in the absence of which he will experience distressing and even serious physical symptoms. In such patients the dosage is usually steadily increased, as the body requires a progressively larger amount to produce the desired effect, or to ward off the unpleasant symptoms of abstinence; this phenomenon, known as **tolerance,** means that the truly addicted person may ingest daily doses of a drug such as morphine (*e.g.*, 1 gm. or more) which would be lethal for a non-addicted person. In other patients, using slightly less potent drugs, there is a pronounced psychological craving but little or no physical dependence, these patients commonly being described as **habituated** to drugs rather than truly addicted. In practice the distinction is not always an easy one

NEUROTIC REACTIONS (CONTINUED)

to make, so that the present tendency is to use the more general term **drug dependence** to include both types of abnormality. The terms " addiction " and " habituation " are still, however, in fairly frequent use, and in many instances there is absolutely no doubt as to which is the appropriate word; *e.g.*, patients certainly do not become merely " habituated " to morphine, nor do they become " addicted " to lysergic acid.

Obviously only a tiny handful of those many people who take drugs at one time or another become dependent on them. Predisposed persons appear invariably to have a markedly neurotic character structure. They are people whose early experiences have left them incapable of tolerating frustration and in whom the presence of any sort of painful tension leads to immediate demands for its relief; taking the drug leads to an experience of pleasure through relief of this tension, any sense of aloneness is abolished and a temporary state of peace with the world is achieved. Despite a mild or severe " hangover " phase, the initial pleasure is so great that its repetition is often a matter of urgency. In many severe addicts unconscious self-destructive motives are also very noticeable. The early experiences thought to be of major importance are those of the mother-child relationship; either through excessive frustration or excessive gratification of the infant's very early needs for love, the developing personality is one in which any experience of tension is unbearably painful and the need for pleasurable indulgence very great. Such patients tend to have very poor relationships at any real level with other people (though they may appear superficially bright and popular) and see the world very largely in terms of how much love it can give them. Often their personality disorder has been well-camouflaged before the addictive process sets in. Social factors, particularly those found in delinquent subcultures, may certainly be important in inducing some young people to make an initial experimentation with drug-taking, particularly involving the use of marihuana and the amphetamines, but clinical experience suggests that those relatively few members of this group who become dependent on these drugs, or who progress to using more dangerous narcotics, will be found to have basic personality characteristics of the type just described.

Chronic Alcoholism

The drinking of alcohol is an extremely widespread custom and its users range all the way from the person who drinks only moderately on certain social occasions to the full-blown chronic alcoholic, who is drug dependent in every sense of the term. It is often hard to say precisely when true alcoholism has begun —the patient is often the last person to realise that he has gone past the stage of being a " social drinker ". Perhaps the most useful criterion is that true dependence can be recognised when the individual is unable to do without the support of alcohol if he is to cope with his normal round of work and pleasure. Giving in to the need to drink when alone is usually a serious warning sign. Many years of moderate but steadily increasing drinking may have preceded the development of alcoholism proper; less commonly the problem starts more suddenly in adult life or middle age following some serious personal crisis.

In most Western communities some two, three or four adults in every 100 can be classified as alcoholics; the rate varies from one country to another, being substantially higher, for example, in France, Scandinavia and the United States than in Great Britain. Men are affected at least four times as frequently as women (though for various reasons the outlook for the latter is usually worse). Cultural attitudes towards the drinking of alcohol greatly affect the number of cases in a community; alcoholism is, for instance, relatively rare in Jewish people and among the Japanese.

There is absolutely no evidence at the present time for the popular belief that alcoholism has some physical or organic cause, nor for the idea that the alcoholic is in some way 'allergic " to alcohol.

Clinical Picture. Alcoholic excess may arise as a secondary complication of other psychiatric illnesses; the distress of an

NEUROTIC REACTIONS (CONTINUED)

acute anxiety reaction, the misery of an intense depression, the chaos and panic of early schizophrenia—from all these the patient may attempt to escape into the false comfort of excessive drinking. Most cases seen in a psychiatric hospital, however, arise out of the previously mentioned type of personality disorder and no other clearly defined psychiatric illness is present.

With increasing use of alcohol, gradual but definite changes begin to appear in the personality. Moral standards slacken and previously repressed antisocial tendencies may appear such as lying, stealing or frank criminal behaviour; ordinary responsibilities, both in business and in domestic life, tend to be progressively neglected. Deterioration occurs, first in matters of dress, then later in ordinary personal hygiene. Food becomes less and less important and the standard of nutrition falls off, even though weight may be retained for a considerable period. Rationalisation (p. 99) of his own behaviour becomes the order of the day; the alcoholic usually is blind to his own shortcomings, finds absurd excuses for his errors and blames others for his misfortunes. Judgement may become seriously impaired. Almost always he minimises the exact amount of alcohol taken. Mood tends to fluctuate rapidly between an exaggerated cheerfulness and a shallow, self-pitying tearfulness. If he admits his habits elaborate promises to reform may be readily made, but commonly are just as readily broken.

At the same time, physical deterioration will often be present. **Cirrhosis** of the liver (with the possibility of ultimate liver failure) and **peripheral neuritis** are two of the commonest physical complications. In milder cases chronic **gastritis** leads to morning vomiting and a gross interference with appetite and digestion. The associated lack of vitamin B_1 (thiamin) may occasionally lead to **cardiac failure.**

The organic mental disorders which may be caused by prolonged alcoholic excess are described in Chapter 12 (p. 263).

Certain special aspects of the treatment of chronic alcoholism (uncomplicated by organic mental changes) are referred to on p. 373; the section later in this present chapter on the treatment of neurotic disorders is also relevant.

Dependence on Opiates

Dependence on morphine, heroin and other drugs of the opiate group used to be relatively rare in Western countries, being confined largely to those with easy access to such drugs, notably pharmacists, doctors and nurses—a group who are still at special risk. In more recent years illegal traffic in these drugs has become more extensive, to the point where they are not too difficult to obtain within the criminal subculture of most large cities, thus presenting a new and major public health problem. There is also a small group of addicts who have first been given opiates in the treatment of some painful, extended physical illness.

More than with any other drug, sudden cessation of a well-established opiate intake leads to profound mental and physical distress, the symptoms being referred to as **withdrawal symptoms** or as the **abstinence syndrome.** These are brought about by the sudden release of many bodily functions previously damped down by the constant presence of opiates; there is profuse lacrimation, sweating and sneezing, muscle twitching, pyrexia, vomiting and diarrhoea. Restlessness and mental anguish are usually very severe and in rare cases death may occur. For these reasons withdrawal of the drug is only undertaken in hospital and is always brought about gradually, the patient's distress being relieved by the simultaneous administration of large amounts of " Largactil " (chlorpromazine—p. 367) and /or barbiturates.

There are no sure signs of opiate addiction, many addicts remaining in apparently good physical and mental balance as long as they have uninterrupted supplies of the drug. Physical examination may show markedly contracted pupils and multiple small scars may be seen on the arms, abdomen and thighs as the end results of frequent, unsterile injections. Gradually a

NEUROTIC REACTIONS (CONTINUED)

moral deterioration ensues, probably not due so much to a direct effect of the drug as to the inevitable deception and perhaps criminality involved in securing steady supplies.

The basic neurotic character structure in opiate addiction seems essentially similar to, though perhaps even more severe than, the personality disorder of the alcoholic. For this reason the withdrawal of the drug is not even half the battle; many addicts will resume their former habits as soon as they are confronted with new stress and even the most efficient programme of rehabilitation and after-care will not always prevent this relapse, even though it should be attempted in every case and will at times be successful.

Dependence on Other Drugs

Barbiturates. Drugs of the barbiturate group, taken in sufficient quantities over a long period of time, can produce a true dependence in some individuals with unstable personalities. Symptoms and signs of dependence include severe and persistent fatigue, mild mental confusion and memory lapses, depression, emotional instability, unsteadiness of gait and muscular inco-ordination. If the patient is admitted to hospital and it is not known to the staff that he has been consuming excessive amounts of barbiturates, he may show sudden and severe withdrawal symptoms due to the abrupt cessation of his intake; a state of acute mental confusion may develop with extreme anxiety and restlessness. In such a state the occurrence of major epileptic seizures without any previous history of epilepsy is a point of particular importance.

Amphetamines. Drugs of the amphetamine group, notably " Dexedrine " and " Methedrine " (p. 371), are not uncommonly used by students and long-distance truck drivers, to keep themselves awake and in the quite mistaken belief that they will produce extra " pep " or increase their powers of concentration and memory (for which belief there is no evidence whatsoever, in fact the contrary has been clearly demonstrated).

As they produce an artificial elevation of mood which is found pleasant by some people, they are also fairly commonly used by some thrill-seeking youngsters (or neurotically bored housewives) as a first, usually fairly tentative experiment in drug-taking. In some instances, however, a genuine craving is developed, the dose is steadily increased (sometimes with resort to the intravenous route for greater speed of effect), so that with surprising rapidity a true dependence is established, sometimes with the intake of doses as large as 500 mgms. per day. Chronic insomnia, anorexia and restlessness are features of established dependence and heightened sexual excitability may occur. In such advanced cases it is not rare for a psychotic reaction to supervene, with vivid auditory and visual hallucinations and firmly held delusional beliefs, a clinical picture which may strikingly resemble that of an acute schizophrenic reaction, though without the classical thought disorder which characterises the latter illness (p. 219).

Amphetamines may also be taken, sometimes even on medical prescription, because they decrease appetite and may thus help in weight reduction, but the same risks and potentially serious consequences make this an undesirable procedure. For this reason a variety of alternative substances have been synthesised in an attempt to find a completely harmless appetite-depressant, but many of these are also likely to produce elevation of mood and thus drug dependence is still a real possibility with these preparations too. (So that the nurse who considers herself to be overweight should consult a doctor or a dietitian, *not* resort to an attempt at chemical control of her appetite!)

Marihuana. This drug (also known as **hashish, cannabis** and **hemp**) has become increasingly popular in recent years among (largely adolescent) drug-users in major Western cities, though its consumption has been widespread for centuries in many areas of Asia and Africa. Its main effect is to produce an elevated mood; tension is relaxed and social relationships easier for some unhappy, inhibited people while under its influence. Used regularly and in large doses it can certainly lead to a

NEUROTIC REACTIONS (CONTINUED)

psychotic illness, though a pronounced and intractable dependence seems only fairly rarely to be established, if at all. The particular danger in its use, as in the use of all such substances which profoundly distort reality, lies in its appeal to neurotic, often rather schizoid people, to whom it seems to offer the hope of a solution to personal difficulties by a route which does away with the need for personal effort; such a hope, one need hardly say, is doomed to cruel disappointment. There is also the real danger that individuals who have become dependent on marihuana may sooner or later experiment with far more dangerous drugs such as morphine and heroin, to which they are likely to be exposed in those circles where marihuana is used.

Lysergic Acid. This drug, the actions of which are described on p. 336), has also attained a certain popularity in drug-using subcultures. It seems that a true dependence is never established on this particular substance, but nevertheless its use has certain very real dangers. As with marihuana, it seems to exert a particular fascination for the individual with schizoid characteristics (p. 229), and in some of these young people it is undoubtedly capable of acting as the final precipitant of a frank schizophrenic illness which may require prolonged hospitalisation. There is also the risk that bizarre, unpredictable and out-of-character actions may be carried out while the person is under the influence of the drug, and in some instances these have caused serious harm either to the individual himself or to other people.

ANTISOCIAL CHARACTER DISORDERS

In some individuals with severe character neurosis the disorder takes the form of episodic or persistent actions directed against other people or against society and its laws. This behaviour may be of such severity as to involve them in police charges and a subsequent prison sentence; many criminals, though by no means all, have personality disorders of this kind. Others behave abnormally in a less spectacular fashion, their antisocial actions consisting of a chronic inability to adjust to the normal expectations of the society in which they live; they may drift from job to job without aim or purpose, refuse to accept any responsibility for their own lives or the welfare of their families, forming a series of short-lived and superficial relationships with others, many of them becoming the vagrants and hoboes of this world.

The essential feature of their disordered personality formation lies in a failure to develop adequate ego functions (p. 149). The normal child, as has been indicated in Chapter 5 (p. 82), gradually develops a system of controls over his basic, primitive, antisocial impulses; he learns to postpone satisfaction of his desires so that he will conform to the demands of his environment and he gradually becomes able to tolerate some degree of internal tension so that he does not have to translate all his wishes and impulses into immediate action. If circumstances are not such as to favour normal ego development, then these attributes will be to a greater or lesser extent absent from his personality. In some instances hereditary or organic factors are involved in this developmental failure; much more frequently early childhood experiences are of crucial significance, and in particular the nature and quality of the mother-child relationship, which has invariably been unsatisfactory for the child in these cases. The mother may have been a rejecting, aloof person; substantial periods of separation from mother may have occurred; through death or divorce there may have been one or more very early changes in mother-figures. Whatever the cause, the child grows up with inadequate controls over his basic instincts and with a poor capacity for real relationships with other people. Sometimes excessive amounts of aggressive feeling which cannot be handled by the ego arise as a consequence of extremely strict parental discipline.

In some of these individuals, but by no means in all, there is also inadequate superego formation (p. 84), so that they carry out their antisocial actions with little or no shame or guilt. Such patients are often referred to as **psychopathic personalities;** there is usually a history of aggressive, disturbed be-

NEUROTIC REACTIONS (CONTINUED)

haviour dating back to early childhood, gradually increasing in severity; they seem totally lacking in affection for others. Despite punishment for their misdeeds, they seem quite unable to learn from their experience, nor do they desire to do so. It must be stressed, however, that many or most character neurotics, in contrast to these "psychopathic" types, have relatively normal consciences and may suffer severely from remorse after they have temporarily given way to impulses which they were unable to control.

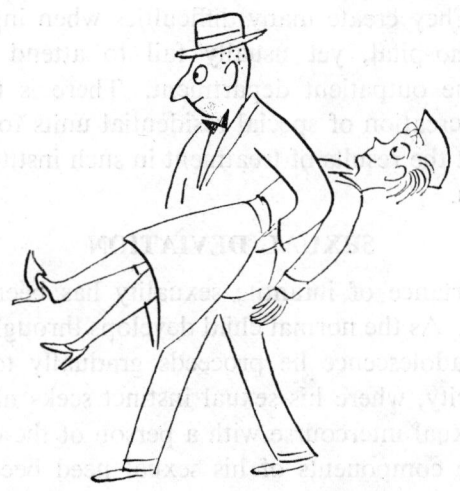

FIG. 16
Unconsciously trying to "steal" affection.

The variety of impulses which may be acted out by such patients is very extensive. Such clinical problems as impulsive fire-setting (pyromania) and impulsive stealing (kleptomania) come under this heading, as do most sexual offences (which are dealt with below). Much of the explosive aggression described in lurid detail in the evening papers is of this type. The particular behaviour often represents more than a simple escape of bottled up tension and may have a symbolic significance of its own; for example, the true kleptomaniac, who almost invariably steals articles for which he has no practical use, may be unconsciously trying to "steal" affection (Fig. 16).

Despite the community's desire to deal with these abnormalities of conduct as though they were purely moral problems, the nurse will learn through experience that these patients are without doubt suffering from serious emotional disturbance and personality immaturity. In adult offenders, at any rate, it is rare to find that punishment by itself significantly influences their behaviour for the better; nevertheless, they are usually also very unsatisfactory candidates for psychiatric treatment. They create many difficulties when inpatients of a psychiatric hospital, yet usually fail to attend regularly if treated in the outpatient department. There is now a move towards the creation of special residential units for patients of this type, but the results of treatment in such institutions are as yet uncertain.

SEXUAL DEVIATION

The importance of infantile sexuality has been considered in Chapter 7. As the normal child develops through the latency period and adolescence he proceeds gradually to a stage of sexual maturity, where his sexual instinct seeks ultimate satisfaction in sexual intercourse with a person of the opposite sex. The infantile components of his sexual need become increasingly unimportant; what remains is dealt with either by sublimation (for example, the toddler's pleasure in exhibiting his genitals becomes transformed into the normal adolescent's desire to show off his manliness in a socially acceptable way) or by becoming a small part of normal love-play (for example, the male's attraction to and interest in the female breast). If such transformations do not occur, then some part of infantile sexuality may remain of more importance to the adult than sexual intercourse itself and this condition is known as sexual deviation or sexual perversion.

Many patients apart from true sexual deviates, however, will be found to have persisting infantile sexual needs, even though these are unconscious and not openly expressed in a direct form; such tendencies have been dealt with by repression or a similar type of defence mechanism and may be the centre of major unconscious conflicts underlying neurotic or psychotic symptoms. Not a few neurotic patients, for example, develop their symptoms out of a need to defend themselves against the recognition of unconscious (latent) homosexual desires; for example, a male patient who developed acute feelings of panic if forced by circumstances to use a public toilet realised after lengthy treatment that this situation stimulated such unacceptable wishes. Many psychotic patients, as a consequence of the personality disintegration which may occur during the illness, manifest previously unsuspected deviant sexual trends. The difference between the sexual deviate and the symptom neurotic is often a difference primarily in the nature and quality of their ego defences; both groups of patients may have strong sexual urges of an infantile kind, but the sexual deviate periodically loses control of these impulses which then appear in open form, whereas the symptom neurotic represses them, only to have them appear later in a heavily disguised manner as phobias, compulsions and so on.

If the nurse grasps these principles she will see sexual deviation basically as a psychiatric problem and she should be able to separate herself very largely from the usual community attitude which tends to see such behaviour as " filthy ", " depraved " and so on. Many sexual deviates in fact have acutely sensitive consciences and suffer agonies of shame as a result of their behaviour.

The principal forms of sexual deviation are as follows:

Homosexuality: this term is used to describe sexual acts carried out with members of the same sex, usually as the individual's preferred or exclusive form of sexual activity. Despite the propaganda which is commonly put out by some homosexuals on their own behalf, it is without any doubt a form of sexual deviation, and is invariably accompanied by other evidence of neurotic character problems and not infrequently by frank neurotic symptoms, for example, disabling phobias. Some homosexuals are also capable of heterosexual intercourse, and a few may even participate in superficially adequate marital relationships; others avoid heterosexuality entirely. Many homosexuals lead relatively contented and often very productive lives (often in artistic fields) if they are not persecuted by the police or by their fellow citizens; others may enter into relatively lasting relationships with other homosexuals, towards whom they show a good deal of tenderness and loyalty, though these liaisons are almost invariably more tortured and abrasive than might appear on the surface.

Female homosexuality (Lesbianism) seems to be less common than the male form and meets, for some obscure reason, with slightly less social disapproval.

Contrary to popular belief, there is absolutely no evidence that biological factors play any part in the causation of homosexuality.

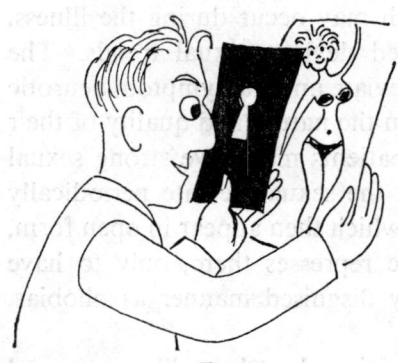

FIG. 17
Voyeurism . . . in slightly more acceptable form.

Exhibitionism: sexual pleasure derived from the open display of the genital organs; it is virtually seen only in males, who impulsively show the penis to women or young girls.

Voyeurism: the seeking of sexual pleasure through the witnessing of sexual scenes or through observing the naked body—the so-called " Peeping Tom ". It is again excessively rare in women. A large magazine trade caters for this deviant male interest in a slightly more socially acceptable form (Fig. 17).

Fetishism: in this condition sexual interest is excessively directed towards some part of the partner's body other than the genital areas or towards some inanimate object such as a slipper worn by another person. Sexual satisfaction is only possible in the presence of the fetish. Some cases of seemingly purposeless theft are based on a need to acquire objects which serve as fetishes, for example, handkerchiefs or female underwear.

Sadism: pleasure obtained through the infliction of pain, either physical or mental, on another person. This is basically a sexual pleasure though only in sexual assaults is its true nature directly apparent.

Masochism: pleasure derived from having pain inflicted on oneself. This is rare in a directly physical sense, but the association of pleasure with suffering is an extremely common complex in psychiatric patients; many individuals with symptom or character neuroses, and particularly depressed patients, derive a good deal of unconscious satisfaction from the distress caused to them by their own illness. Some physically ill persons are reluctant to abandon their illness for the same reason (p. 325).

Paedophilia: sexual desires directed towards children, either of the same or opposite sex. Such patients unconsciously feel that they are so immature sexually that they are incapable of managing sexual partners of the same age as themselves.

Transvestism and Transexualism: in these two related conditions the individual chooses to dress in the clothes of the opposite sex, episodically or continuously. In the former disorder this cross-dressing, as it is called, is associated with sexual arousal, but in the latter and more deep-seated condition the individual feels himself to be more properly a member of the opposite sex (although he is not truly delusional), and cross-dressing brings him a sense of calmness and serenity.

OTHER FORMS OF CHARACTER NEUROSIS

Some important varieties of neurotic character structure can best be considered in relation to the psychiatric illnesses with which they are commonly associated or prior to the onset of which they are of frequent occurrence. These are the **schizoid personality** (p. 229), the **paranoid personality** (p. 239), the **hysterical personality** (p. 187), the **cyclothymic personality** (p. 246) and the **compulsive personality** (p. 192).

Two other patterns which occur relatively frequently in hospital practice are:

The Passive-Aggressive Personality. This individual contains within him a great amount of latent aggression which is expressed by making life fairly constantly miserable for his fellows by techniques of passive opposition, stubbornness, crankiness and repeated dissatisfaction, all of which he may hide behind a smiling, seemingly agreeable exterior (p. 124). Occasionally under stress naked anger, sometimes in extreme form, may appear for a brief period. Even without such display, however, the aggressive meaning of his passive behaviour is not usually difficult to see if one looks below the surface.

The Emotionally Unstable Personality. Such personalities tend to react to relatively minor stresses with strong emotional outbursts of various kinds; their controlling mechanisms seem inadequate and they are easily moved to violence and destructiveness. There is often a history of repeated ineffectual suicidal attempts.

Such a list could be continued almost indefinitely; it could include, for example, people who have no apparent abnormality of character or conduct other than an extreme, morbid and all-consuming jealousy. Individuals with extreme shyness, or with severe inferiority feelings, can also be brought under this heading. The nurse must again be reminded that, especially with neurotic patients, the exact pinning of a diagnostic label is of little importance and is virtually of no assistance to her at all in planning her nursing care; what is important is a dynamic understanding of the meaning and origins of the patient's behaviour.

NEUROTIC REACTIONS (CONTINUED)

THE COURSE OF NEUROTIC ILLNESS

We have seen that the predisposition to neurotic illness is developed in infancy and early childhood and that in some instances actual neurotic symptoms may develop at this time (p. 178). Most neurotic reactions, however, first become apparent in late adolescence or in early adult life, most commonly between the ages of 15 and 35; if neurotic symptoms seem to develop for the first time after the age of 40 a full history usually reveals either previous episodes of neurotic illness or a long-lasting pattern of character neurosis. Sometimes organic brain disease in late life releases neurotic patterns of behaviour for the first time.

Once a **symptom neurosis** is clearly established, its subsequent course may be in one of five directions:

1. The symptoms subside again virtually completely and perhaps relatively quickly and do not occur again. This tends to happen particularly in those individuals whose childhood predisposition has not been very great and whose illness has been precipitated by unusually severe current stress, for example, neurotic reactions occurring during battle or after some very great personal crisis.

2. The illness largely or completely settles down but recurs in a similar form several times thereafter in response to further stress. Phobic and obsessive-compulsive reactions, for example, tend to follow a so-called phasic course, the phases of illness sometimes coinciding with pregnancy or the puerperium. Neurotic depressive reactions often recur whenever his life situation is felt by the patient to be unfavourable, as do episodes of dissociation.

3. The neurotic pattern subsides gradually in its original form but is replaced, after a shorter or longer period, by a neurotic reaction of a quite different type. It is not surprising that this should happen if nothing has occurred (either through treatment or from a change in the patient's life situation) to alter his underlying conflict. Close study of individual cases

will show many histories of this type, for example, the story of the heavy drinker who has "conquered" his alcoholism without in any way understanding it and who later develops episodes of depression or phobias.

4. The original episode fails to resolve or does so only in part and the patient continues, sometimes for many years, with fixed neurotic symptoms. This is particularly liable to occur with obsessions and compulsions, many phobias and some conversion symptoms. Some patients give a history of serious, sometimes almost total incapacitation due to neurotic symptoms for a period of 10 or more years prior to their first visit to a psychiatrist.

5. Rarely, neurotic symptoms increase in severity and are gradually or suddenly replaced by psychotic symptoms. The most common example of this is seen in the slow transformation of the obsessions of an obsessive-compulsive reaction into the delusions of a schizophrenic reaction. In other instances, what appears superficially to have been a neurotic disorder has been hiding an underlying psychotic process.

Patterns of **character neurosis,** because they involve large segments of the patient's personality, are by nature fairly stable and long-continued; the history usually extends back many years prior to his appearance for treatment. Many of these patients have little wish to alter the pattern of their lives and only seek specialist help to appease distressed relatives or in an attempt to modify the retribution of the law. Some may gradually develop more mature patterns of behaviour with the passing of the years; the adolescent antisocial delinquent not infrequently develops into a law-abiding citizen by the time he reaches 30. For others the course is steadily downhill and their entanglement with society becomes increasingly obvious and serious. For the schizoid, cyclothymic and paranoid personalities the development of later psychosis is a serious possibility, though it is by no means inevitable; similarly the hysterical and compulsive personalities are strongly predisposed to neurotic reactions of the appropriate type. But, generally speaking, if one has the opportunity to observe a patient with a character neurosis over a prolonged period of time, one finds that he changes little if at all, even though some particular form of impulsive behaviour may occur only at irregular intervals.

TREATMENT

In the previous chapter it was said that not all neurotic persons desire treatment. There may indeed be occasional instances in which the psychiatrist deliberately decides that the patient is best left with a neurotic symptom which he has learned to live with, rather than risk the possibility that the treatment may uncover deep conflicts which he is unable to handle in any other way.

The results of treatment in neurotic reactions are extremely difficult to measure with any accuracy. One of the reasons for this is the seemingly spontaneous disappearance of symptoms in many patients who are not receiving treatment at all, to which reference has already been made. Further, many neurotic patients are extremely sensitive to changes in their environment; individuals with great dependency needs, for example, may improve dramatically after only a few days in hospital, without special treatment of any kind. An even greater difficulty is to decide exactly what is meant by "improvement"; an unpleasant symptom such as a phobia may be lost, but this result may have been achieved at the price of his becoming a harder person with whom to live because his previously well-camouflaged aggressiveness is now more obvious. All treatment hopes in the long run to increase the maturity of the patient's behaviour, but this is itself a difficult concept to measure. In some cases the nurse, the psychiatrist, the patient himself and the patient's relatives may all have rather different ideas on just how effective treatment has been. Despite all these difficulties, however, there is a general understanding that the most desirable goals of treatment will be:

(i) to relieve the discomfort caused by the patient's symptoms, or to modify his antisocial acts;
(ii) to prevent a recurrence of the same or other neurotic symptoms through some alteration in his underlying conflicts and anxieties;
(iii) to assist him to behave in a more stable fashion and to lead a generally more contented and harmonious existence.

The treatment of neurotic reactions therefore involves either or both of the following approaches: (*a*) **symptomatic treatment,** aimed directly at the relief of his distress without regard to its origins; (*b*) **causal treatment,** aimed at some improvement in the basic pattern of conflict so that the symptom becomes no longer necessary.

Symptomatic Treatment. In a later section (p. 333) the principles of **supportive psychotherapy** are described. It has been abundantly demonstrated that many neurotic patients can experience a rapid and substantial alleviation of their distress if they meet regularly with a professional person who permits them to discuss their problems frankly, ventilate their feelings, and perhaps come to look at their conflicts in different ways and find some more appropriate solutions. For the hospitalised neurotic patient the support and protection provided by the hospital environment, together with the gratification derived from the relationships which he makes with professional staff and particularly with nurses, will be in themselves important factors in modifying his symptoms and behaviour. It is hardly surprising, however, that the available evidence suggests that long-standing character problems and personal difficulties are little affected in the great majority of cases by these relatively simple techniques.

In many instances (some would say too many instances) this supportive psychotherapy is coupled with the administration of drugs. If there is conspicuous anxiety and tension a sedative (or minor tranquilliser, which amounts to the same thing) may be given, though the dosage need only be small in most instances;

NEUROTIC REACTIONS (CONTINUED)

drugs frequently found useful are "Librium" (chlordiazepoxide) and "Valium" (diazepam), these usually being preferred to the short-acting barbiturates. If depression is a prominent feature one of the anti-depressant drugs (p. 371) may be employed. The excessive or long-continued use of drugs must, however, be strenuously avoided, for two reasons: firstly, they may abolish the patient's motivation to take constructive steps, with the psychiatrist's help, to deal with the problems in his life which are responsible for his painful emotions; secondly, in many of these patients the development of drug dependence is a real and serious possibility.

Occasionally modified insulin (p. 363) may be employed for patients showing intractable weight loss, anorexia, restlessness and tension. Very occasionally electrotherapy (p. 355) may temporarily lift a state of depression which has been unresponsive to other treatments.

Another method by which the patient's symptoms may be reduced is by one of the techniques of behaviour therapy (p. 340), though its supporters would argue that this is in fact a treatment directed at underlying causes, and thus should be considered in the following section.

Causal Treatment. Here an attempt is made to bring the patient to see something of the current conflicts and basic problems within his personality which are giving rise to his symptoms. In its most complete form, this involves the very extensive and radical procedure of psychoanalysis (p. 327), much more commonly, some type of psychological treatment is employed based on psychoanalytic principles but with substantial modifications. The various forms of such treatment, known as psychotherapy, are described in Chapter 16. Most prolonged psychotherapy is carried on at an outpatient level, though it may have been commenced in hospital; only a handful of extremely disturbed neurotic patients receive prolonged psychotherapy whilst inpatients on a psychiatric service.

Many patients with neurotic disorders will not however be receiving psychotherapy of this type. Sometimes the illness is felt to be too chronic for any success to be achieved, or the patient may be completely unable to accept the fact that he has feelings, conflicts and stresses which are related to his symptoms. Other patients are felt to be poor prospects by reason of limited intelligence or an apparently completely hopeless life situation. In yet other instances psychotherapy is regarded as desirable but the local psychiatric service simply lacks the trained persons necessary to provide it.

For one or more of these reasons symptomatic and supportive treatment is often all that can be offered to the neurotic patient; this however may be of considerable value to him and ease the almost unbearable burden of his existence.

NURSING PROBLEMS IN NEUROTIC REACTIONS

The nursing of patients with neurotic illnesses involves firstly a broad general understanding of the major principles of psychiatric nursing. Insight into the complexities of the nurse-patient relationship is a primary essential in each individual instance. Perhaps more so than with psychotic patients, whose major conflicts are often more obvious, the nurse requires frequent consultation with other members of the psychiatric team so that she can more fully understand the nature of the patient's anxieties and his defences, and in order that she can more adequately comprehend the goals of treatment and the most useful role for her to attempt to fill.

Even when in possession of adequate clinical information, however, many nurses express, directly or indirectly, a good deal of personal anxiety and discomfort concerning the nursing of neurotic patients. In an admission ward containing patients with a wide mixture of diagnoses it is common to find that those labelled as "neurotic" are the ones who present the greatest difficulty to the nurses, even those of wide experience, and they frequently create great tensions between staff members. There are several reasons for this:

(i) The typical patient with a neurotic reaction shows many areas of fairly healthy personality function; he is clearly less "sick" than the psychotic patients, and often gives the impression of being much more in command of his behaviour than in fact he is. It is, therefore, easier for the nurse to have moralistic and critical attitudes towards him, usually much harder in a personal sense for her to understand him.

(ii) The neurotic patient resembles much more closely the "normal", and therefore the nurse herself, than does the psychotic patient. The latter is usually so clearly different from herself, his behaviour often so peculiar and so obviously "mad", that he can comfortably be seen as somebody apart, whose problems bear no relation to her own. But the neurotic patient may show, although in a much more obvious and severe fashion, some of the same types of anxieties which she vaguely recognises within herself; she thus tends unwittingly to react defensively, for to face some of his problems might be equivalent to facing some of her own.

(iii) The neurotic patient is frequently treated by psychotherapy alone, often quite intensively; the nurse finds it difficult or impossible to know exactly what is going on between patient and psychiatrist and tends, therefore, to feel "shut out" and to lose interest. She may conclude, quite incorrectly, because his interviews with the psychiatrist loom so largely in the patient's life, that she herself is of no value to him. Because there is little or no opportunity for her to take up traditional nursing roles (for example, by giving medicines, assisting with physical treatment or in comforting a dependent, helpless bed patient), she tends to feel powerless in the treatment situation and to react with anger or indifference. The fact that none of these conclusions is correct is fully discussed in Chapter 16; the section entitled "The Role of the Nurse in Psychological Treatment" might well be read in conjunction with this present chapter.

(iv) Many neurotic patients, not only those with conversion reactions, show some or all of the features of the hysterical personality. The element of half-conscious "play-acting" in their behaviour is often irritating; there is a tendency to wonder whether they are in fact sick at all or whether they are simply acting a role in order to gain attention and sympathy. Their repeated demands for special care may prove aggravating to some nurses; others may find their shallow but noisy emotionality very wearing. It is vital to remember that, beneath these superficial characteristics which may seem so unlovable, there lies genuine anxiety which is being dealt with by these particular defence mechanisms.

(v) The secondary gain derived from his illness, while not apparent to the patient, may be readily obvious to the nurse. If she herself is experiencing difficulties with an unfavourable environment, and particularly if in addition she has her own extensive persisting needs for the gratification of dependent wishes, then she may well be handicapped in her care of such a patient by her unconscious resentment of the apparent solution he is finding for his problems.

Many other difficulties will be posed by special types of neurotic behaviour in individual cases; some nurses will find themselves unsympathetic towards the drug addict, others will find it difficult to establish a satisfactory relationship with the antisocial character, and so on. Through a critical evaluation of her own reactions, here as elsewhere, the nurse will learn important things about herself, and she will gradually develop an increasing capacity to understand, and therefore to work helpfully with, patients with neurotic illness. She will then find this to be an especially interesting segment of psychiatric nursing, far removed from the traditional medical concept of the nurse's role, but with its own very real satisfactions and rewards.

11

FUNCTIONAL PSYCHOTIC REACTIONS

THE disorders described in this chapter comprise all those reactions in which there develops a psychotic form of illness as previously defined (p. 158) without there being any evidence of brain disease, damage or poisoning. Taken together, they account for close to one-half of all the first admissions to a typical mental hospital, and make up an even larger proportion of the chronic, long-stay cases.

SCHIZOPHRENIC REACTIONS

The term schizophrenia literally means " split mind ", the name coming from one of the basic features of the reaction, the abnormal separation between the processes of thinking and feeling. It is a common illness, comprising more than 30 *per cent* of all first admissions to a mental hospital, and represents not only the greatest unsolved problem in psychiatry today but one of the biggest riddles in the entire field of medicine.

CLINICAL PICTURE

Those forms of reaction labelled as schizophrenic show a very wide variety in their clinical features, a variety which is so bewildering that the nurse has first to grasp the elements common to each case. These **basic symptoms and signs** are as follows:

Thought Disorder. Disturbance in the individual's capacity to form a normal linkage between the various ideas in his mind is highly characteristic of schizophrenic illnesses. This disorder in thinking, with its resultant disorder in speech, has been described on p. 111; it may produce an effect of mere "woolliness" and lack of clarity in the patient's ideas, but in more severe instances may lead to almost complete and occasionally total **incoherence** (p. 111). **Thought blocking** (p. 110) is common and **neologisms** (p. 111) may be employed. In a doubtful case the patient may be asked by the psychiatrist to interpret a common proverb; if he states, for example, that " a stitch in time saves nine " only means that " it's better to mend a rip in your shirt quickly because you will save yourself nine stitches later on ", then he demonstrates an inability to think in an abstract fashion, an important sign in early schizophrenic disorders. This replacement of **abstract** by **concrete** thinking, however, may also be seen in some patients with organic psychotic reactions and has no significance in any event in patients of below average intelligence.

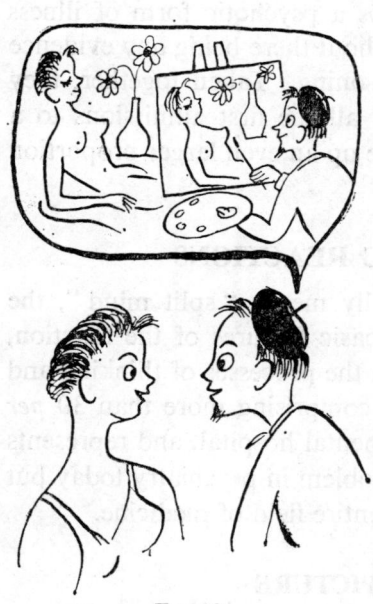

FIG. 18
Elaborate day-dreaming of a romantic and sexual kind.

Withdrawal from Reality. The schizophrenic patient progressively loses interest in relationships with other people, withdraws more and more into himself and substitutes increasing day-dreaming for involvement with the activities and objects of the real world. The content of his thought becomes much more determined by his own wishes and fantasies than by the demands and realities of everyday living, a type of thinking known as **autistic.** For example, instead of showing the normal young man's active interest in girls, the schizophrenic youth may indulge in elaborate day-dreaming of a romantic and sexual kind with less and less attempt to translate these wishes into reality. His own private, subjective world of fantasy becomes more important and more real to him than the external, objective world.

Disturbances of Ego Function. In Chapter 5 there has been described that part of our mental apparatus which is known as the ego (p. 83). Many of the basic and most characteristic symptoms of schizophrenic reactions can be understood as resulting from partial failure of ego functions, for example:

(*a*) Sudden outbursts of impulsive, perhaps violent, behaviour may indicate a deficiency of ego control over basic id drives.

(*b*) Complaints may be made of bodily disturbance which show clearly that the individual's perception of his own body has altered in a very serious and fundamental way. For example, a young woman with an early schizophrenic reaction complained that, during her recent confinement, her pelvic bones had been forced so far apart that they had not come together again; she stated that she could feel this separation quite distinctly. (See also section on delusions of bodily disease, p. 114). Other patients may suddenly complain of ugliness or attach a new significance to a long-standing minor deformity; sometimes they spend long periods gazing at themselves in the mirror.

(*c*) Outside events seem to have a direct impact on the patient as if no barrier existed between himself and the world. He may state that he is influenced or controlled by the actions or thoughts of others; conversely, he may believe his own thoughts or gestures to have extraordinary effects which are felt across the country or even throughout the world.

(*d*) There may be an absence of normal reticence and shame so that, in quite inappropriate circumstances, the patient talks with pathological frankness about intimate sexual matters or reveals without reserve grossly antisocial, obscene or destructive wishes.

Alterations in Affect. An important sign is a steadily increasing failure of normal emotional response to an event or situation. The affect may be **inappropriate** (p. 124), or in more advanced cases **apathy** (p. 124) and indifference may be noted. In early cases however mood can be quite appropriate to the complaints which the patient makes about himself and frank anxiety or depression are not uncommon at this stage. Distressing feelings of **depersonalisation** (p. 183) are not rare in such cases.

The development of further symptoms gives rise to a very great variety of clinical pictures. It is customary to describe several types of schizophrenic reaction, but the nurse should be clear, once again, that these types do not represent clear-cut disease patterns, but refer only to groupings of symptoms and signs which are seen together with sufficient frequency to warrant a label.

Types of Schizophrenic Reaction

Simple Type. The picture here is one of very gradual, at first barely noticeable, withdrawal from reality into fantasy, beginning almost invariably during the teenage period. There is a progressive failure of personal relationships and a decreasing capacity for appropriate emotional response. Thought disorder as previously defined may not be conspicuous though there is often excessive concentration on some extremely offbeat interest. Delusions, hallucinations and gross abnormalities of behaviour are not present. Many of these cases do not reach psychiatric care but lead progressively more disordered lives as petty criminals, tramps, vagrants, prostitutes and isolated eccentrics.

Hebephrenic Type. The most conspicuous change in this form is in the affect, which becomes fatuous and silly, the patient giggling inappropriately and joylessly as he expresses many foolish, often almost incoherent ideas. Thought disorder is usually very marked. Delusions and hallucinations are present in abundance; these may be extremely grotesque in their form but are not typically built up into a coherent system. **Mannerisms** (p. 106) and grimaces are common and there is a rapid decline in the patient's ability to care for himself; as contact with reality progressively dwindles he may become incontinent of both urine and faeces and show no concern for his appearance, though in other instances he may decorate himself in extraordinary ways. Habits may become extremely primitive and, in advanced cases, his shameless, noisy and randomly destructive behaviour may resemble very closely in many ways that seen in a small infant.

Catatonic Type. The onset here is usually acute. One manifestations is that of **catatonic stupor** (p. 108, in which the patient becomes completely withdrawn from outside stimulation, is mute and motionless, often lying in strange postures held with great muscular rigidity (**catatonia,** p. 106), or showing the sign of **waxy flexibility** (p. 106). He may be incontinent or may retain urine and faeces. It is most important for the nurse to understand that his isolation from his environment is only apparent and not real; though preoccupied with his own fantasies and delusional beliefs, he is often quite aware of all that is going on around him and every comment made in his presence must be carefully checked with this in mind.

Catatonic stupor may change very rapidly to a state of **catatonic excitement,** in which the patient is very restless, often extremely violent, showing behaviour which is impulsive and quite unpredictable because it is motivated by his own rapidly changing delusional and hallucinatory experiences. These patients are the most dangerous seen in a psychiatric hospital.

Other schizophrenic patients, whilst exhibiting neither clear-cut stupor nor excitement, may yet show some of the catatonic features of **negativism** (p. 108), **echolalia** and **echopraxia** (p. 109), peculiar **postures** and **mannerisms,** abnormalities of gait and **stereotypy** (p. 108).

Paranoid Type. In this form the predominant feature is the development of delusions and hallucinations, usually built up into a complex and elaborate system, often of an extremely fantastic kind. The illness may commence with **ideas of reference** (p. 113) and feelings of being influenced by others (**passivity feelings** (p. 113), and these may widen out into delusional beliefs of every conceivable variety. The most common are of **persecutory type,** but delusions of a **religious, erotic,** or **hypochondriacal** nature are also very frequent (p. 112). False beliefs may be expressed concerning the unfaithfulness of a marital partner, the most peculiar evidence being produced to support this idea. Other patients believe themselves to be in the possession of complex technical secrets and insist that they are inventors or scientific geniuses. When the delusions are of a persecutory nature, their increasing development may lead to the belief that a giant conspiracy, of which the patient is the victim, is being organised by the Queen or some foreign power. **Hallucinations** are prominent and may occur in all five senses, but are most commonly of an auditory kind (p. 117); voices of a threatening, accusing, sexual or religious nature may occupy the patient's awareness to the virtual exclusion of all else. Other symptoms and signs, at least in the early stages, may be less pronounced; thought disorder is less conspicuous and the affective response to the delusional material may at first be fairly appropriate, though as the reaction becomes chronic this usually flattens rapidly. In the well-developed case one finds gross inconsistency between the delusional belief and the accompanying mood and behaviour; the classic example is that of the mental hospital patient who firmly believes himself to be the Prime Minister, yet who is quite content with his daily task of cleaning the toilets. In very advanced cases one occasionally finds a profound deterioration in habits similar to that seen in the severe hebephrenic patient.

Schizo-affective Type. This label is useful to describe those cases in which there are present, as well as clear-cut schizophrenic features, some of the symptoms and signs of the affective disorders described later in this chapter. Such a patient may show, for example, definite thought disturbance and disorder of ego function to an extent that justifies a positive diagnosis of schizophrenic reaction, yet in addition be profoundly depressed or genuinely elated (in contrast to the fatuous silliness of some other schizophrenics).

Other Varieties of Schizophrenic Reaction. There will be many patients, clearly showing reactions of schizophrenic type, whose symptom patterns do not conform to any of the above groupings. In some instances one may be able to be no more precise than to label the illness **acute undifferentiated schizophrenic reaction** or **chronic undifferentiated schizophrenic reaction,** according to its duration. Other patients, even when first seen, have what can be described as a "burned out" schizophrenic process, without current florid symptoms, but with a history of having had a previous definite acute schizophrenic episode in the past which has largely subsided, leaving only a flatness of emotional response, some lack of drive and a few odd, irrational ideas. Such patients are diagnosed as suffering from a **schizophrenic reaction, residual type.**

In some early cases the basic symptoms, while discoverable after close observation and examination, are hidden behind other forms of abnormal thinking or behaviour which do not appear at first sight to be of schizophrenic nature. Some of these not uncommon camouflages for an underlying schizophrenic process include:

(*a*) multiple neurotic symptoms, especially phobic, obsessional and conversion symptoms;

(*b*) antisocial behaviour of any kind (especially if arising suddenly in adolescence);

(*c*) alcoholic excess, drug dependence or deviant sexual behaviour;

(*d*) acute mental confusion and bewilderment (of such an extent as to raise the possibility of an organic type of reaction), which may occur in the first week or so of a very acute schizophrenic illness.

Schizophrenic Reactions in Childhood. The clinical picture of childhood schizophrenia is in most instances totally unlike that of the adolescent or adult form of the disorder. There are characteristic disturbances of body movement, language development and personal relationships which are described in detail in Chapter 13 (p. 290).

CAUSATION

Even more obviously than in other forms of psychiatric illness there is no possibility of isolating one single cause for any schizophrenic reaction. Possible causative factors can be considered under three headings:

1. **Heredity.** The balance of evidence suggests that there is some hereditary predisposition towards the development of schizophrenic illnesses. Most studies reveal that if one examines identical twins, one of whom is schizophrenic, there is a higher chance that the other twin will also have a schizophrenic illness than if one makes the same study on twins who are non-identical. Even if twins are reared apart from birth, and thus exposed to different environmental conditions, the same sort of observation can still be made. Probably what is inherited is a tendency towards the schizoid type of personality (p. 229), that form of character neurosis which may break down under later stress into a frank schizophrenic illness; certainly psychological and environmental difficulties play an extremely important part in every case, but some people may have a partly inborn disposition to react to such stresses in a schizophrenic way, rather than becoming neurotic or depressed.

2. **Physical Factors.**

(*a*) BODY BUILD. 50 *per cent* of all cases occur in individuals whose body build is of the markedly angular, lean, flat-chested type (**asthenic** build). The presence of this body build usually suggests a poor outcome to the illness.

(*b*) ENDOCRINE GLANDS. Despite some suggestive findings which may at a later date be made more significant by further research, there is no conclusive evidence that endocrine abnormality plays any causal role in schizophrenia. Such alterations in thyroid and adrenal function which have been reported to date seem to be the result, rather than the cause, of the mental disturbance.

(c) BIOCHEMICAL FINDINGS. There are again as yet no consistent reports; abnormalities of uncertain significance can be demonstrated by complicated techniques in both blood and urine.

(d) BRAIN STRUCTURE. No changes of undoubted significance have been reported in the brain cells with any consistency; with present techniques the structure of the schizophrenic patient's brain appears to be identical with that of the normal person. There is a slightly higher percentage of abnormalities in the electroencephalographic (p. 278) tracings from schizophrenic patients, indicating a marked disturbance of the physiology of the brain in some instances; this is particularly common in catatonic cases.

3. Psychological Factors. There is a growing body of evidence to suggest that the development of faulty personal relationships from infancy and early childhood onwards is instrumental in setting the stage for the later development of schizophrenia. These patients seem with great frequency to have been reared in a family where husband and wife distrust, perhaps openly dislike, each other; their parents tend to have been inconsistent, unconsciously rejecting the child, yet often tying him to them by excessive over-protection. Some mothers of schizophrenics are unusually cold, aloof persons, incapable of expressing real emotional warmth towards the child. A striking feature in such a mother, which the alert nurse will quickly note in her contacts on visiting days, is her own capacity to distort reality, leading her to minimise the extent of her son or daughter's abnormality to a quite remarkable extent. These women show with great consistency a highly unhealthy and usually extremely critical attitude towards sexual matters, and in such an environment the child may have found it impossible to develop a completely satisfactory picture of himself or herself as truly male or truly female; this basic confusion may become very obvious during the overt illness, when ideas concerning change of sex are not uncommon. Put in another way, unsatisfactory, inconsistent and frustrating early childhood relationships may lead, especially in the presence of hereditary predisposition, to an ego which in times of later stress becomes incapable of adequate function (p. 149); the previously mentioned ego disturbances then appear, the patient fails to see himself as a completely separate, intact person and is unable to make adequate judgements about the real world.

Precipitating causes which set off a schizophrenic episode are not essentially different from the precipitating causes of psychiatric illness in general (p. 136).

ONSET AND COURSE

Schizophrenia is essentially an illness of young adults, the average age of onset being from 20 to 25 years, with the great majority of all cases arising between the ages of 14 and 40. The onset of schizophrenia in childhood is unusual, though such cases are serious and important. A small proportion of patients do not have their first episode until they are over the age of 40.

The onset is sometimes abrupt, either with or without some obvious preceding stress such as child-birth, this very acute presentation occurring most typically in catatonic and schizo-affective, and to a lesser extent in paranoid forms. Commonly however the illness comes on very gradually, its significance at first not realised by the patient's relatives, so that it may be difficult to state with any certainty at what precise point in time the actual psychotic reaction began. In roughly one-half of all cases a specific type of character neurosis has preceded the psychosis for many years; such patients have shown evidence of marked shyness, coldness, aloofness, seclusiveness, severe feelings of inferiority, unusually vivid and absorbing day-dreaming, sexual difficulties and eccentric behaviour of various kinds, these traits having sometimes been observable even in childhood. Such characteristics mark the **schizoid personality;** some individuals may have a personality disorder of this type without ever developing a definite schizophrenic reaction.

The outlook for the patient with a schizophrenic illness is usually very guarded, though there are some instances (particularly in the catatonic and schizo-affective forms) where the illness clears up relatively rapidly, with or without treatment, and does not recur for several years, if at all. Much more typically, however, the course is gradually or even rapidly downhill; even though moderate or marked improvement often occurs after the initial attack the patient may be left with some flattening of emotional response and some minor oddities of thinking and behaviour; a further acute episode may arise, or the patient may become increasingly out of touch with reality. These developments may be greatly modified, though probably not fully reversed, by adequate modern treatment, as will be seen. The picture of the so-called **deteriorated schizophrenic,** much as was described earlier in this chapter as a common end result of the hebephrenic form (p. 222), is sad indeed; it is still not quite clear, however, just how much of this deterioration is an essential part of the illness itself and how much is added by the extremely unfavourable environment provided by the average chronic mental hospital ward of recent times (p. 399). The chronic nature of the disorder in so many instances accounts for the fact that between 50 and 60 *per cent* of cases in a typical mental hospital will bear a schizophrenic diagnosis.

Factors usually associated with a better than average outlook are:

1. acute onset, especially if following some major stress situation;
2. previous history of adequate social and occupational adjustment, with few or none of the features of the schizoid personality;

3. some reasonable preservation of appropriate emotional response during the illness;
4. treatment begun early in the course of the illness;
5. diagnosis of a catatonic, schizo-affective or (to a lesser extent) paranoid type of reaction;
6. body build of the so-called **pyknic** type, *i.e.* short, stocky, well-rounded body with relatively short limbs;
7. onset relatively late in life—in general, the younger the patient the less likely is the chance of a favourable outcome.

TREATMENT

The treatment of schizophrenic reactions is at the present time highly unsatisfactory in many respects, even though it is much more adequate than it was 20 or even 10 years ago. There is a small group of patients, perhaps 10 *per cent*, who will improve rapidly with or without treatment; a much larger group, probably 50 to 60 *per cent* of the total, run a progressive course leading to chronic illness, a course which may be temporarily interrupted by treatment but probably in the long run not much influenced by it. In this group, however, treatment may be of very great value in modifying the illness in such a way that the patient and his relatives are less distressed by it; it may also enable him to live outside a mental hospital (certainly a worthwhile goal) and in some circumstances to earn his own living, even though the fundamental nature of his illness is not altered. In the remaining 30 to 40 *per cent* of cases early and effective treatment can substantially alter the subsequent course of the illness.

There are four principal therapeutic approaches employed —**physical, psychological, social** and **nursing** treatment; most patients will require and receive treatment of all four varieties.

Physical Treatment

Electrotherapy. An adequate course of electrotherapy (ECT)—at least 12 treatments—seems to influence favourably the immediate course of schizophrenia in slightly more than one-half of all cases if given within the first 12 months of the illness (p. 355). In some instances, notably in acute catatonic stupor or excitement and in schizo-affective cases, the beneficial result may be very dramatic. Little or no improvement occurs in the simple and hebephrenic forms. In a few instances ECT seems only to make the schizophrenic illness more obvious. Five years later there does not seem to be any fundamental difference between those patients who have received ECT and those patients who have not.

Insulin Coma Therapy. This form of treatment, which has now fallen almost completely into disuse, was once considered by many psychiatrists to be the treatment of choice for the patient with a well-established schizophrenic reaction. The aim was to induce, by the intramuscular injection of insulin, a coma of approximately one hour's duration each day, up to a total of 30 hours. It was a formidable procedure, with very real risks and potential complications, and most people now believe that there is nothing which can be achieved by insulin which cannot be achieved more easily and safely by electrotherapy and particularly by the tranquillising drugs. It is likely in retrospect that psychological factors played a substantial part in those instances where it was effective; certainly a strongly cohesive group tended to form in the insulin clinic which had many beneficial effects in its own right. Moreover, patients who might otherwise have had little close attention received " daily, devoted, personal care " (Bourne)[1] with its clear implications of a corrective " good mothering " experience.[1]

Tranquillising Drugs. Acute and distressing symptoms of schizophrenic reactions can in the majority of cases be controlled by an adequate dosage of one of the tranquillising drugs. Various types of disturbed behaviour in more chronic cases can also be substantially reduced; under their influence the patient comes into a more adequate contact with his

[1] Bourne, H. (1958). *Amer. J. Psychiat.* **114**, 1015.

environment, is an easier person to manage in the ward, and in not a few instances is able to lead a relatively trouble-free life outside the hospital while taking the drugs, a life which would have been quite impossible without them. There is no doubt that such drugs therefore have a secure place in the management of both acute and chronic schizophrenic reactions; nevertheless it is not believed that they produce any substantial, permanent modification in the underlying schizophrenic process.

A large number of drugs is available for this purpose, each having some advantages and disadvantages. Probably the most popular is still " Largactil ", but many other drugs have their advocates or are particularly valuable for certain types of patient, especially " Melleril " and " Stelazine ". These and several other tranquillising drugs are described in detail in Chapter 17.

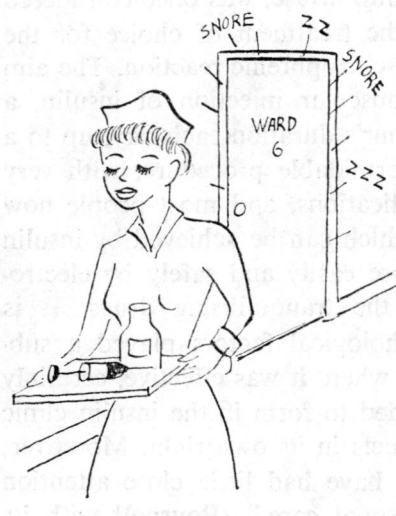

FIG. 19
A ward which is " easy " to run.

The grave danger of drug therapy in schizophrenia lies in the fact that it is so simple in many instances to abolish " difficult " behaviour and to produce a ward which is " easy " to run, but at the expense of any real understanding of the patient's needs and problems. Such patients, if they are tranquillised up to a point bordering on complete inertia, will be totally removed from real therapeutic influence.

Further details concerning the indications, contraindications, techniques and possible complications of these physical treatment procedures will be found in Chapter 17. Three general points, applicable to each procedure, must be made here:

1. There is no evidence that any physical treatment procedure in schizophrenia leads to a " cure ", nor that it changes in any fundamental way the abnormalities which form the basis of the illness.

2. Physical treatments may greatly modify the symptoms of schizophrenia in a desirable way. Not least important, the patient is usually brought into a better contact with his environment and is more likely to be able to derive benefit from nursing, social and recreational treatment programmes.

3. The important danger exists that, when physical treatment is being used, the nurse can so easily lose sight of the patient as anything other than a technical problem. If she reacts in this way, she will be failing to employ her most important weapon in treatment.

Psychological Treatment

In some hospitals a good deal of psychotherapy, either individually or in groups, is given by the psychiatrists to schizophrenic patients. More commonly, either through a shortage of staff time or through lack of conviction as to the effectiveness of psychotherapy in schizophrenia, little or no planned psychological treatment is available. Certainly the treatment of hospitalised schizophrenics by psychotherapy alone requires very many hours of extremely intensive work, and the results at present must be regarded as quite uncertain. Most of these patients, usually after receiving one of the varieties of physical treatment, will nevertheless benefit from a number of interviews with the psychiatrist aimed at sorting out their more obvious superficial problems and furthering their adaptation to the environment. Probably most people nowadays would see the psychological impact of the hospital's social structure and the nurse's relationship with her patient to be equally as significant as, and certainly much more practical than, direct psychological treatment in the vast majority of instances.

Social Treatment

Under this heading we include all the ways in which the hospital may provide an atmosphere best calculated to promote improvement. If schizophrenia is seen in part as the result of a breakdown in healthy personal relationships, then the patient must be able to find in the hospital a place where he can attempt to establish these relationships again in a setting of security and trust; he must be given the opportunity to discard gradually the unhealthy defences he has developed and to learn that withdrawal from other people into his own private world is not necessarily the only way of dealing with anxiety. The environment ideally must be one which accepts his behaviour, however disturbed, even whilst attempting to help him control and modify it.

Recreational and occupational activities, conducted in mixed-sex groups, are vital aspects of this programme (p. 466). Games, group activities, elementary industrial processes—all may be used to good effect. The more chronic and deteriorated schizophrenic patient will require, at least initially, to be given extremely simple tasks to perform. A sense of achievement must be fostered and an opportunity provided for the sublimation of unacceptable impulses, particularly aggressive ones. One must oppose at all times any tendency to see the occupation of patients as primarily for the benefit of the ward or the hospital (p. 462), nor must patients be allowed to shelter behind some routine, solitary activity which they unwittingly use to protect themselves from involvement with other people (p. 460). Creative activities such as art, music, dancing and journalism may each find a place in the programme of therapy. The principles and details of these therapeutic methods are discussed in Chapter 23.

The organisation of the hospital and of its individual wards is also of importance. In Chapter 19 we describe in detail some of the traditional practices of the older type of mental hospital which in fact made it harder, rather than easier, for patients to recover, and these effects were certainly felt most severely by the schizophrenic group. The steady deterioration of chronic schizophrenic patients which was so common within the " back wards " of large, poorly staffed hospitals was certainly, at least in large part, a result of the impersonal, tightly disciplined and charmless life which was so often led by patients in wards of this type. However humane and well-meaning the care in such a setting might have been, the lack of individual attention, the often complete failure to allow patients to show any initiative or to utilise what assets remained in their personality —these things tended to stamp the " chronic ", " deteriorated " label on a schizophrenic patient with a certain grim inevitability. Modern methods of care recognise this danger and have therefore given a great deal of attention to the environment in which a schizophrenic patient is treated. The development of a **therapeutic community** (p. 407) can therefore be seen from two viewpoints—the promotion of healthier and more mature personal relationships and the prevention of dreaded chronicity. The essential point is that each and every aspect of the patient's day must be regarded as liable to have some effect on him; the nurse's concern must be to ensure that as many as possible of these effects are beneficial.

Nursing Treatment

If the hospital is to meet the schizophrenic patient's needs and to deal with them as effectively as possible, then the responsibility for this will fall very largely on the nursing staff. The following are the basic principles which should be guiding the nurse in this situation:

1. The schizophrenic patient requires a substantial increase in his own self-esteem; nursing attitudes must at all times be such as to help develop and reinforce this.
2. He needs to be assisted to live in the real world, to emerge from his own preoccupation with fantasy and to do real things with real people. The nurse must be a constant representative of healthy reality, not arguing with him over

his delusional beliefs, but helping him when the occasion arises to see things in her own realistic terms rather than from his own distorted viewpoint.

3. He needs acceptance in the first place on his own terms; this involves the nurse in a constant, conscientious attempt to see his behaviour, however antisocial or " degraded ", as representing a pathetic and infantile attempt at communication rather than as evidence of his " badness ". The schizophrenic patient, for deep-seated psychological reasons, may *want* people in his environment to react to him with disgust; the nurse must be constantly alive to this trap which is being laid for her and must as often as possible prevent herself from falling into it. When his disturbed behaviour involves violence, open sexual practices, obscenity or shameless excretory habits, the nurse's tolerance may well be sorely tried, but the above principle still holds. She must at all times be attempting to convey the message, spoken or unspoken, that she sees him as a human being in distress; much as a normal parent does with a naughty child, unacceptable actions must be checked without conveying any sense of rejection to the individual responsible for the behaviour.

4. He needs to live a ward life which gives him the greatest possible chance to use his own initiative and judgement; it is undesirable for him to have to conform passively to the wishes of others except where this is absolutely unavoidable.

5. He needs patience and forbearance from staff members; experience suggests that he can never be forced or hurried into more mature patterns of behaviour or new relationships, usually first requiring to test them out in small ways over a long period.

6. He needs warmth and friendliness, even though in the early period of his hospitalisation he may recoil from this, frightened of being close to other people—partly for fear that they may go away again and leave him worse off than before, partly because closeness makes him afraid of his own anger and destructiveness. Friendliness towards him must be con-

sistent; he will be angry, and his worst fears about human relationships will be confirmed, if the nurse withdraws from him after a period of warm interest.

7. He needs human contacts, even when his outward behaviour suggests that he wants exactly the opposite; his activity needs to be stimulated, his chances of complete withdrawal made as few as possible. He may well react with further isolation if he senses that the nurse, consciously or unconsciously, is avoiding him. Any activity, however small, is better than complete and solitary idleness.

8. He needs to find in the nurse a stable, consistent model on which he can commence to pattern himself in the way that the growing infant patterns himself on his parents. Any identification (p. 49) of the patient with the nurse is a good sign; he may begin to copy her tasks and wish to be of assistance to her, behaviour that should be met by her with warm approval.

9. Severely ill patients may require human contacts of a quite basic and elementary kind, maternal or paternal in nature —though to force these on an unwilling person may only increase his anger and withdrawal. Clearly anything which might be construed by a suspicious patient as a sexually seductive approach must be carefully avoided. Opportunities to establish a basic, warm relationship often exist at meal and bath times, periods which are of special importance to this type of patient.

10. He needs in many cases reassurance as to his own personal identity; this will be helped by allowing him, whenever possible, to wear his own clothes, to keep them in a private place and to retain some personal possessions which the nurse treats with respect.

These general principles have some degree of application in the nursing of every schizophrenic patient and in our view are the foundation of his proper care in hospital. Special problems may require special techniques, which are described in detail in Chapter 22; the sections on the aggressive patient

(p. 451) and on those who need long-term care (p. 439) are of particular importance.

PARANOID REACTIONS

Clinical Picture

The clinical picture of the paranoid state is one of the development of delusions, often accompanied by hallucinations, without any other significant disorganisation of the patient's personality. The patient, usually aged 40 or over and never under the age of 30, shows few or no outward signs of abnormality. He can give a coherent account of his delusional beliefs and retains an appropriate emotional response to them; for example, a middle-aged school-teacher who believed that his next-door neighbour was pumping poisonous gases into his flat complained repeatedly and bitterly to the police about this and threatened legal action to stop his persecution. Delusions of this persecutory kind are the most common, but beliefs of a grandiose, religious or erotic nature are not infrequent. The hallucinations may affect any of the five senses, but are most commonly of the auditory variety. Some psychiatrists (and text-books) still use the term **paraphrenia** to describe this condition.

The term **paranoia** is used to describe an extremely rare form of mental disturbance, rather similar to the more common paranoid state, but in which the delusions are of such a kind, and are talked about so convincingly, that there may be real difficulty in deciding whether these beliefs are evidence of a psychiatric illness or not. Hallucinations do not occur, nor is there any other indication that the patient is mentally disturbed.

The difference between a patient with paranoid schizophrenia and a patient with a paranoid state may be one of degree only, and there are some cases in which it is difficult

or impossible to be certain which label to apply. The points in favour of a diagnosis of paranoid state are, in summary:
1. Older age of onset.
2. Illness always commences gradually, never acutely.
4. No thought disorder of a schizophrenic kind (p. 111).
4. Appropriate emotional response to the delusional and hallucinatory experiences; also, because he senses people's response to his delusions, he is more likely to attempt to hide them.
5. Little or no external evidence of psychiatric illness—patients are not infrequently able to carry on their normal occupation even when the delusional process is fully developed; many can be supported indefinitely at an outpatient level.
6. No deterioration of the personality.
7. Course only very gradually progressive, if at all; the patient's mental condition may stay essentially the same over 10 or 20 years.

Causation

There is no evidence that organic factors play any part in the causation of paranoid states. Usually there is evidence that for many years the patient has shown signs of that form of character neurosis known as the **paranoid personality**; such people are suspicious, very ready to take offence and to feel slighted, usually irritable, sarcastic and cynical, trusting other people so little that they do not enter into close personal relationships, often sullen and obstinate. The transition from this long-standing, highly sensitive state into that of definite delusion formation may be so very gradual that it is quite impossible to say exactly when the change took place. In some instances the presence of a hearing defect favours this deterioration.

The mechanism of **projection** (p. 100) plays a large part in the development of a paranoid state; unwanted aspects of the patient's personality and certain basic drives which are unacceptable to him have been disowned or the blame for them placed on to others. This tendency extends far back into early life and arises out of unfavourable childhood experiences, as a result of which these patients thereafter are unwittingly struggling to control enormously strong destructive impulses. Unconscious sexual wishes, particularly of a homosexual kind, are also of great importance in paranoid conditions; a big proportion of these patients is unmarried.

Treatment

Paranoid states are the most fixed of all psychiatric illnesses with the exception of some of those which accompany structural damage to the brain. The usual **physical treatments** have little or no effect; occasionally some psychiatrists use very intensive electrotherapy but the results are, to say the least, very doubtful. Tranquillising drugs may diminish tension and assist the patient in controlling his behaviour. Patients with paranoid beliefs, however, are very apt to see the use of physical treatments as further evidence of persecution.

The very occasional paranoid patient is highly dangerous; completely under the influence of his delusions he may make an attack on those persons whom he believes to be harming him. The great majority, however, while irritable, difficult and constantly complaining in the ward, are only aggressive at a verbal level. It is not reasonable to hope that such patients' attitudes can be radically changed by nursing care, but certain important principles in the **nursing of the paranoid patient** may greatly ease his distress and will add to the comfort of the nurse's own task.

1. Give him as much freedom of action as is compatible with the doctor's estimate of his potential for danger. The more he is required to experience petty restrictions and interference with his freedom and privacy, the more irritable and difficult he will become. Paranoid patients are more likely to attempt to escape from closed wards than from open ones.

FUNCTIONAL PSYCHOTIC REACTIONS

2. Always be completely truthful in dealings with him; his capacity to sense other people's motives is so acute that it is better that no attempt be made to deceive him.

3. Avoid being drawn into any argument with him over his delusional beliefs; no benefit can come from this, only an increase in his (and probably the nurse's own) irritability.

4. If forced into a situation where some comment on his beliefs cannot be avoided, the nurse should try to convey the impression that, while she accepts the fact that they are real to him, she cannot herself agree that things are exactly as he says they are. It is not in the long run helpful to him for her to indicate that she shares his delusions and it may in some circumstances be harmful and even dangerous.

5. No attempt should be made to force him into group activities, although the availability of these should be made clear to him; his temperament may be such that it will have to be accepted that he is less disturbed (and causes less disturbance to others) if he works alone.

6. The possibility must always be kept in mind that delusional beliefs involving other patients or staff may lead to violence directed towards them.

7. Avoid any possible suggestion of prying into the patient's background or even into his current activities, unless these seem likely to be harmful to himself or to others.

8. Some of these patients function more adequately if granted positions of minor responsibility within the ward or hospital; any move in this direction should be encouraged if the psychiatrist is in agreement.

Many psychiatric patients show strongly paranoid attitudes without warranting the diagnosis of a fully developed paranoid state; the nursing principles just listed are equally applicable in these cases.

AFFECTIVE REACTIONS

Under this heading are included all those disorders in which the primary change is in the patient's affect or mood, all other features of the illness being secondary to this change. There are two principal forms of this disorder, the **manic reaction** and the **depressive reaction;** because some patients show episodes of each type during their lifetime the illness is known as the **manic-depressive reaction.**

MANIC REACTION

The chief symptoms and signs of this disorder are:

Elevated Mood. The patient's affect is one of **euphoria** (p. 122) in mild cases, progressing to **elation** and even **ecstasy** if the illness is more severe. The mood is one of genuine cheerfulness (in contrast to the joyless laughter of some schizophrenic patients) and often will provoke responsive amusement in the nurse herself. The patient is over-optimistic, supremely confident of his own powers and full of grandiose and quite unrealistic plans for his future. However, it is common for the mood to change rapidly to one of irritability and even gross hostility if obstacles are placed in his path.

Acceleration of Speech. The rate of speech may be mildly increased (**pressure of talk**) or may be of such rapidity that the patient's train of thought is difficult or almost impossible to follow (**flight of ideas**). Silly puns, juvenile witticisms, rhyming and **clang assocations** (p. 110) may be observed. He may declaim loudly as if on a stage and in the most acute cases may be extremely noisy indeed. Lessening of normal social restraints may lead to very direct and personal comments about staff members and other patients, often accompanied by remarks of a frankly sexual nature and by obscene or blasphemous jokes.

Accelerated Motor Activity. The manic patient is invariably **overactive;** this in milder cases may be at the level of busy, meddlesome interference in the affairs of others, in more severely ill patients resulting in violent and destructive behaviour. Clothes may be discarded and frank sexual advances made by patients of either sex. There is usually little need

FUNCTIONAL PSYCHOTIC REACTIONS

felt for sleep, and in the most acute cases the patient may be too active to pause long enough to take adequate food.

The fully developed form of the manic reaction is termed **acute mania;** less severe cases are said to be suffering from **hypomania.** In neither illness are delusions or hallucinations important signs, though in the most acute cases the patient's ideas of his own power and importance may for a brief period be of delusional quality. If delusions and hallucinations do appear as prominent and persistent features of the illness then the psychosis, despite the elevation of mood, is probably of schizophrenic type.

DEPRESSIVE REACTION

The only unvarying sign of this reaction is the **depressed mood** itself. This ranges in intensity from moderate gloom and pessimism up to, in severe cases, an overpowering sense of hopelessness and despair. In typical cases the mood is not influenced to any appreciable extent by pleasant happenings in the environment but shows a spontaneous fluctuation during the day, being most severe in the early morning and least distressing in the late afternoon and evening. In these patients the possibility of **suicide** is very real, even when the depression does not on the surface appear to be of great intensity.

Level of Activity. In the majority of cases the patient is strikingly **retarded** (p. 108); he complains of tiredness, disinterest and feelings of bodily heaviness, and to the outside observer he may appear slowed in all his movements. In rare, extremely severe cases this may progress to a condition of **stupor** (p. 108). Bodily functions are also slowed down—anorexia, weight loss, constipation and amenorrhoea are usually conspicuous symptoms. Sometimes the physical complaints, which may be very variable and include vague aches in any region, are almost more prominent than the depression itself, and some of these patients are at first considered to be suffering from a bodily illness.

Other patients with depressive reactions, particularly those over 40, may show marked **agitation**. They are extremely restless, pacing incessantly up and down, wringing their hands and moaning constantly about their suffering and perhaps their guilt. Constant picking at the face may lead to multiple small scars, or there may be destructiveness of clothing, nails or hair.

Speech. The patient is usually slowed down in thought and speech, in extreme cases not speaking at all (**mutism**, p. 110). More typically he speaks little, what does emerge being obviously the product of great effort, and he may trail off halfway through a sentence. Agitated patients may talk a good deal, but very commonly only repeat over and over again a few phrases indicating their despair.

Delusions. These are common in severe depressions, being most typically of a guilty nature, occasionally of nihilistic and hypochondriacal types (p. 112). The patient may believe that he is about to be killed because of all his past wickedness. Hallucinations are unusual and are rarely prominent; when present, they take the form of threatening, accusing voices.

Other Symptoms. Insomnia is always a problem in severe depressions, the patient typically waking very early in the morning, perhaps even at 2 or 3 a.m. Depersonalisation (p. 183) is a distressing complaint in some cases. There is no interest in social contacts and patients left to their own devices tend to withdraw completely from company. Sexual drive is usually greatly reduced.

Causation

There is good evidence to suggest that an hereditary predisposing factor is important both in manic illnesses and in the psychotic forms of depression. This statement however fails to justify the frequently expressed opinion that these severe affective illnesses are determined entirely by biological and constitutional factors, personality dynamics and environmental events being quite irrelevant. Such a notion is usually inherent in the use of the word **endogenous,** a term which means so many different things to different people that it is wise to regard it with considerable suspicion. Certainly there is a good deal of evidence to show that severe depressive illnesses are associated with certain biochemical and physiological changes, such as reduced salivary secretion, a measurable alteration in the excitability of the nervous system, and alterations in the blood and urine levels of adrenal cortical hormones. It remains an open question, however, whether these changes are responsible for the depressed mood in a causal sense, whether they occur as a consequence of the depression, or whether they reflect two related aspects of the one central phenomenon. It is now certain that, whatever the importance of biological predisposition may be, depressive illnesses (even those of the most severe kind) are preceded by alterations in the patient's life circumstances, usually those which are likely to have been perceived by him as threatening him and lowering his self-esteem for one of many possible reasons. The clinical situation is often made even more complicated because the depressive patient, always prone to use denial mechanisms (p. 93), may refute any suggestion that his illness is related to any aspect of his life situation.

Onset and Course

Though a manic or depressive episode may occur in late adolescence the great majority of first attacks develop between the ages of 20 and 40. Frequently, especially in depressive cases, the illness arises with quite dramatic suddenness; it may be in some instances that the patient shows no outward signs of disturbance prior to a suicidal attempt being made. The outlook for recovery in each episode is good, particularly with modern treatment, but even prior to this time patients tended towards a gradual, spontaneous improvement over a period of some months. A further attack, either of the same or of the opposite kind (for example, a manic reaction followed by a later depressive one), is almost the rule, and some patients may have such episodes almost yearly or even more frequently;

however, in other instances 20 or more years elapse between episodes. Between these attacks the patient's personality returns to its basic state; there is no personality deterioration such as is so common after schizophrenic illnesses, and almost all patients carry on their usual occupation after recovery. Some patients have repeated depressive illnesses of this type without ever showing manic features; the opposite situation is much less common.

Some patients who subsequently develop manic or depressive illnesses have shown for many years a character neurosis of the type known as the **cyclothymic personality.** Such patients are prone to quite marked, apparently spontaneous variations of mood, both in the direction of elation and of gloom, but without reaching the extremes of definite mania or depression. Others show extremely dependent attitudes in their basic personality (often well-hidden behind a superficial independence and efficiency), others again have chronic problems connected with aggression.

Depressions occurring for the first time after the age of 45 (known as **involutional melancholia**) are of a somewhat different nature. The previous character neurosis has been of the compulsive type (p. 192); the patient, more commonly female than male, has been for years a chronic, pessimistic worrier, extremely fussy and over-conscientious, narrow-minded, intolerant, and accepting nothing less than perfection in herself and in others. In this form of depression the prospect of recovery from each attack is also good, but again there is a strong probability of recurrence and in this instance each attack may respond less fully to treatment than the previous one.

The Diagnosis of States of Depression

Depression is probably the commonest single symptom seen in psychiatric patients; it is in fact one of the most common complaints in the whole field of medicine. By no means all

FUNCTIONAL PSYCHOTIC REACTIONS

Psychotic Depression	Neurotic Depression
1. Depression not much affected, if at all, by pleasant environment.	1. Depression may lift markedly in cheerful company.
2. Sleep disturbance invariably severe, usually wakes early.	2. Sleep disturbance may or may not be severe, usually has major difficulty in getting off to sleep.
3. Physical symptoms marked: amenorrhoea, impotence, constipation, anorexia and weight loss.	3. Physical symptoms, if present, not accompanied by obvious changes in body function such as amenorrhoea, constipation.
4. True retardation common.	4. Never retarded in the true sense, but may complain bitterly of fatigue.
5. Speech commonly slowed, or patient mute.	5. Usually talkative, anxious to discuss symptoms, complains a great deal.
6. Delusions commonly present.	6. Delusions never present.
7. Patient tends to blame himself for his troubles.	7. Patient usually blames other people or his environment for his troubles.
8. Patient may not realise he is ill.	8. Patient acknowledges fact of illness.

patients who complain of feeling depressed are suffering from a depressive reaction in the sense just described. Depression may be a prominent symptom in early schizophrenic reactions and in early cases of organic brain disease; also many patients with neurotic illness show genuine depression as an important symptom and in the neurotic depressive reaction the depressed mood is the most outstanding feature (p. 193).

The major differences between the psychotic varieties of depression as described in this present chapter and the neurotic depressive reactions are shown in the table on page 247.

The value to the nurse of these distinctions, which it should be stressed may be difficult or impossible to make in some instances, is shown in the following section.

Treatment of Depressive Reactions

States of severe depression are almost invariably treated by physical means in the first instance. An adequate course of **electrotherapy** (p. 355) produces a substantial lifting of the depressive mood in from 60-80 *per cent* of those cases with the features listed above under " psychotic depression " although, as in other illnesses, it does nothing to prevent or delay subsequent recurrence. A striking response may be observed in some instances after only two or three treatments. It may also be of benefit, though less spectacularly so, in those cases showing the features of a neurotic depressive reaction. Increasing use is being made of the newer **anti-depressant drugs** (p. 371) but the delay before they produce their effect may be as long as three weeks, so that in severely ill patients ECT is still usually employed. In some depressive patients who have substantially improved but who are still tense, restless and considerably underweight, **modified insulin therapy** may be of value (p. 363). The very rare patient who fails to respond to an adequate trial of all other methods of treatment may be submitted to **cerebral surgery,** sometimes with strikingly beneficial results.

Occupational and recreational therapy have an important role in the management of depressed patients. Occupational tasks should, at least in the first instance, be simple in nature, with no possibility of failure which would only deepen the patient's sense of unworthiness and dissatisfaction with himself. Any element of competition in his activities must be avoided at this stage. The nurse should remember also that he will certainly only be capable of sustaining interest in the one task for a fairly brief period and may in fact be difficult to get started on any assignment at all. Occupied he should be, however, if at all possible, as solitary meditation about his condition will be certain to worsen it.

Nursing Care. The most vital role of the nurse in dealing with any substantially depressed person is in the **prevention of suicide.** This topic is fully dealt with in Chapter 22 (p. 447), where detailed practical advice is offered concerning this problem. Though it may be unpleasant for the nurse to have to maintain a constant, unobtrusive watch over every segment of a patient's life, such precautions are at times inevitable if unnecessary deaths are to be avoided. The more experienced the nurse, the more she will be able to exercise such unremitting attention in the most tactful and least objectionable way. She must be aware that a few patients, deeply determined on a course of self-destruction, will deliberately hide their intentions from the nursing and medical staff; in the early stages of one's acquaintance with a depressed person too much reliance should not be placed on his " promises " in this connection, nor on such statements as " I would never do it because of my children " or " because of my religion ". Special attention should be given to the patient who expresses complete pessimism about the outcome of his illness. Patients showing features of the psychotic depressive reaction tend to be much more serious risks than the neurotic cases, but the possibility is by no means absent in the latter group.

Other important nursing problems with depressed patients are the securing of adequate sleep and the maintenance of a satisfactory food intake. Weight, bowel function and menstrual periods need to be charted with special care; weight gain, disappearance of constipation and the return of menstruation will all be important signs of improvement. In the agitated depressed patient special care may need to be taken to prevent self-mutilation.

The nurse's attitude and behaviour towards the patient will be all-important in some instances. In the very severe case an atmosphere of noisy optimism and enthusiasm created by the nurse will almost certainly tend to make the patient only more acutely aware of his own gloom and tend to deepen his despair. Rather she must try to be patiently and quietly encouraging, suggesting in small ways the possibility of participation in ward and recreational activities. Subtle influences in the ward —pleasant flowers, agreeable music, attractive presentation of food—plus her own quiet, persisting personal interest may all help to turn him to some extent from his preoccupation with himself. No attempt should be made to enter into conversation with the patient about his depressing thoughts or delusions and argument must certainly be avoided about what he believes to be the facts of his life, as should any attempt to discover more about his background, unless actively and obviously welcomed by the patient. An earnest attempt to understand him through personal conversation, as has been suggested in this book in relation to some other types of psychiatric illness, may well be capable in this instance of doing further harm.

When there is a clear-cut picture of the neurotic type of reaction, the nurse can usually afford to be more active in her dealings with the patient, more openly encouraging, more positive in providing a stimulating environment and more ready to engage in conversation about his present symptoms and life situation. This type of patient will not be helped by providing too special an environment and should be actively drawn into every aspect of ward routine; tendencies for him to regard himself as an invalid should be patiently but firmly resisted.

Because of the difficulty involved in the accurate assessment of the various types of depression, the nurse should, at least until she has had considerable personal experience, be guided by psychiatrists and senior nursing colleagues in deciding the correct method of approach.

Treatment of Manic Reactions

In a case of any severity physical treatment will be used from the beginning to bring the disordered mood and behaviour under control. **Tranquillising drugs,** for example " Largactil " (p. 367), are very useful agents in symptomatic management, though the dose may need to be extremely high and there is little to suggest that they fundamentally change the basic course of the disorder, even though the patient becomes much more tractable under their influence. There is now a large body of research which indicates that the use of **lithium** compounds has a quite specific effect on the manic syndrome, and these substances are commonly prescribed early in the course of an episode, sometimes right at the beginning; note also their even better documented value as a prophylactic agent in preventing further recurrences (p. 370). It is now uncommon for **electrotherapy** (p. 355) to be used in this illness, although it may on rare occasions be life-saving where the very existence of a severely ill patient is threatened by the severity and constancy of his excitement.

Nursing Care. These patients are usually very trying nursing problems; the patient with hypomania in particular, less obviously " sick " than the full-blown manic case, tends to be a recurring source of irritation to the nurse because of his constant interference in her own and other patients' routines, his incessant activity and conversation and seemingly limitless energy, his repeated criticisms of patients and staff and his readiness to take offence. If she finds herself reacting to these provocations with anger his own behaviour will almost certainly be worsened, so that this situation demands from her the utmost in self-control and understanding. Limits to his behaviour must nevertheless be set, and consistent firmness is an invaluable tool in management.

The most difficult nursing problem arises from his excessive

PSYCHIATRIC NURSING

energy and enthusiasm, which will certainly be troublesome if not directed into harmless and, if possible, useful channels. The nurse will need to use considerable ingenuity in finding suitable tasks for him and must be prepared for the fact that he will almost certainly want to change his occupations with great rapidity. The more physical exercise he can be given, the easier will be his ward management.

In more severe cases special nursing problems will be presented. Sleeplessness and refusal of food may both reach serious proportions and will need to be handled with great tact and skill; hypnotic drugs will almost certainly be employed at night, but the provision of a non-stimulating environment is equally as important. Violent behaviour may easily be provoked in those patients whose elation turns rapidly to a suspicious irritability; the greatest possible forethought is required in the handling of such a patient and the nurse must keep a careful check on her own behaviour and conversation in an attempt to avoid any action or remark which could arouse hostility. Comment on his usually fleeting delusions should be avoided.

The behaviour of the manic (or hypomanic) person is such as to be a repeated source of irritation to other patients; the experienced nurse will learn how to move quietly and quickly to avoid or minimise disturbance, distracting him wherever possible and directing his interest into other channels. She will soon find that direct commands or threats will get her nowhere save into further trouble; much more will be accomplished by the subtle, perhaps even unspoken, provision of alternative outlets into which the patient's energies can be diverted.

12

ORGANIC REACTIONS

IN this chapter there are described those forms of psychiatric illness which are brought about by some physical change in the brain substance. This change may be the result of a wide variety of conditions, ranging from the acute and temporary poisoning of the neurones due to acute alcoholic intoxication up to the permanent mental changes induced by the degeneration of brain substance in old age. These illnesses are common and many may lead to a state requiring permanent hospital care. Some of the acute forms, however, recover within a few days or even hours in the ordinary wards of a general hospital.

Organic reactions are divided into two main types, which vary in their duration, their onset and their manifestations. The **acute organic reaction,** sometimes called a **delirium,** a **confusional state** or **toxic-confusional psychosis,** begins relatively acutely and tends to settle down rapidly if the cause can be discovered and proper treatment given. The **chronic organic reaction,** sometimes called a **dementia,** usually begins slowly and insidiously and, though it may be capable of considerable modification by proper medical and nursing care, cannot except in rare instances be reversed by treatment.

In North America in particular the terms **acute brain syndrome** and **chronic brain syndrome** are often used to label these two groups of illnesses.

ACUTE ORGANIC REACTIONS
CLINICAL FEATURES

The clinical picture of the acute organic reaction is substantially the same whatever its cause. It is most common—and most serious—at the extremes of life, that is, in infants and

253

young children and in the elderly. Though only rarely fatal in itself, it may be a serious complication for a patient who is for any reason in poor physical condition.

The outstanding aspects of the clinical picture are:

Confusion. There is always some alteration in the patient's state of consciousness so that he loses touch with his surroundings to a greater or lesser extent (p. 128). In the milder cases it may simply be that he is unable to follow what is going on around him and he becomes bewildered and perplexed by what seem to him to be strange and meaningless events. This may progress rapidly to a state of **disorientation** (p. 129). He is unable to give the correct date or time of day, he cannot say where he is and frequently does not recognise even familiar people in his environment. He may say, for example, that he is in court or in prison and may believe that his nurses and doctors are policemen or gaolers. In severe cases his speech becomes rambling and disorganised.

It is a striking feature of such reactions that the confusion is almost invariably much worse during the hours of night; in fact in some instances gross mental disorganisation by night may go hand in hand with complete or almost complete clarity by day. Even during the daytime the level of consciousness may fluctuate quite widely over a short space of time. This fact has important implications for nursing care, as will be seen later.

Apprehension. The mood in a well-developed acute organic reaction is almost invariably one of great fearfulness, sometimes leading to noisy panic. Patients with **delirium tremens** (" D.T.'s "), a state of confusion brought about by alcoholic excess, are often said to be in " the horrors ".

Hallucinations and Illusions. The apprehension is connected with the nature of the hallucinations and illusions, which are usually unpleasant, often disgusting and horrifying. Patients commonly see hordes of small insects coming towards them across the floor or pouring through the ventilators; unpleasant

ORGANIC REACTIONS

animals of all kinds may be seen on the bed or felt crawling on the skin. At the same time ordinary noises are misinterpreted in keeping with the mood of fear; a quiet conversation outside the door of his room becomes in the patient's mind the whispering of enemies plotting to destroy him. Sometimes he is made even more terrified by accusing hallucinatory voices threatening or abusing him.

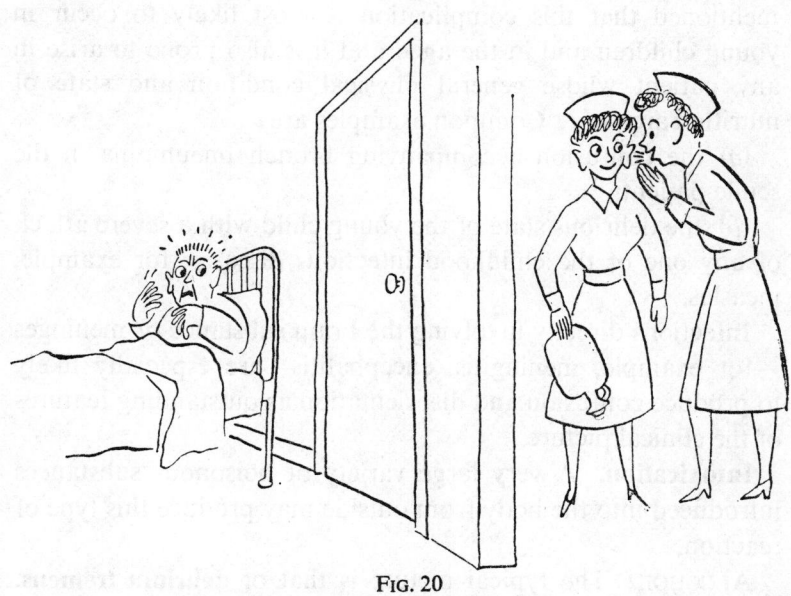

FIG. 20
The whispering of enemies plotting to destroy him.

Restlessness. Such patients, not surprisingly, are agitated and restless, often to an extreme degree. They may easily become violent in an attempt to ward off their imagined enemies, lashing out at whoever comes near or attempting to leap from a window. This overactivity may have serious consequences in that it may further weaken an already gravely ill person. If such a patient passes into a partial or complete state of stupor, the so-called " muttering delirium ", matters are then critical indeed.

In many patients with an acute organic reaction there will be found physical signs of the illness responsible for the disorder. Some of these are mentioned in the following section.

CAUSES

Infection. Mental confusion may develop as an accompaniment of any severe infection in association with other signs of infection such as fever and tachycardia. It was previously mentioned that this complication is most likely to occur in young children and in the aged and it is also prone to arise in any patient whose general physical condition and state of nutrition are poor. Common examples are:

(*a*) the confusion accompanying bronchopneumonia in the senile patient;

(*b*) the delirious state of the young child with a severe attack of any one of the childhood infectious diseases, for example, measles.

Infections directly involving the brain substance or meninges —for example, meningitis, encephalitis—are especially likely to produce confusion and disorientation as outstanding features of the clinical picture.

Intoxication. A very large variety of poisonous substances introduced into the body from outside may produce this type of reaction.

ALCOHOL: The typical picture is that of **delirium tremens.** This may follow a prolonged alcoholic orgy, or arise after a sudden, enforced interruption in the intake of alcohol (for example, as a result of admission to hospital). Probably the patient's extremely poor diet during the drinking bout contributes to this state. The name is derived from the severe tremor of hands and tongue which is seen in these cases. Pulse is rapid and temperature elevated, even without accompanying infection. Insomnia is very severe. In the most serious cases symptoms and signs of cardiac failure may develop (dyspnoea, oedema and so on) and pneumonia is a not uncommon complication.

ORGANIC REACTIONS

BROMIDES AND BARBITURATES: Excessive intake of these sedatives may lead in time to an acute organic reaction. As the patient becomes restless and apprehensive he frequently, not realising the nature or cause of his condition, increases the dose of the mixture which is already causing him such harm.

AMPHETAMINES: The occasional person who has become dependent on amphetamine drugs will develop a psychotic illness characterised by vivid hallucinations and excitement; though mentioned for the sake of completeness under this heading, true confusion is not, however, a feature of this disorder.

OTHER DRUGS: Many other drugs and poisons may cause an acute mental disturbance, which usually but not invariably has the classical features of an acute organic reaction. A wide variety of agents used in industrial processes can occasionally produce this effect (for example, lead), as well as substances used in medical treatment such as digitalis, penicillin, atropine and belladonna, cortisone and corticotrophin (ACTH).

Head Injury. Following severe injury to the head a typical acute organic reaction may occur; commonly this has been preceded by a period of concussion or of complete unconsciousness.

Bodily Illnesses (other than Infection). The most important conditions here are:

CARDIAC FAILURE: Interference with the function of the heart from any cause may lead to an impaired supply of blood and therefore of oxygen to the neurones. In these circumstances their normal function is impaired and confusion is the result.

DIABETES MELLITUS: States of **hyperglycaemia** and **hypoglycaemia** (high and low blood sugar respectively) may each produce a picture of acute organic mental change.

LIVER FAILURE: Advanced states of liver disease may be responsible for a confusional state.

RENAL FAILURE: The state of uraemia developing as a late manifestation of urinary tract disease is typically accompanied by a disturbance of consciousness. (It therefore is doubly important to carry out routine urine testing on any confused patient.)

POST-OPERATIVE STATES: Following any major surgical procedure a state of mental confusion may occur. Many factors may play a part in causing this: infection, loss of blood, toxic effects of the anaesthetic, excessive post-operative sedation and so on. From the nurse's point of view it is important to remember that the effect of all these factors will be magnified many times if the patient is in pain and in an emotional state of fear and bewilderment.

PUERPERIUM: Rarely an acute organic reaction may occur immediately following child-birth. More commonly, psychiatric illnesses which arise at this time and which appear superficially to be of this type are found on closer observation to be of schizophrenic nature.

TREATMENT

The psychiatrist will order specific investigations and treatment depending on his assessment of the underlying cause. Investigations may include blood count, X-rays of chest or skull, lumbar puncture and electroencephalography (EEG). Special treatment plans will be carried out by the nurse at the same time as she employs certain general nursing measures which are applicable in each instance.

Some Specific Treatments

Infections. Antibiotics will certainly be prescribed by the psychiatrist according to the nature of the infecting organism. Prompt and careful administration of these will be a vital part of the nurse's role.

Delirium Tremens. Unless cardiac failure is present as a complication a high fluid intake is essential; constant nursing attention will probably be required to achieve this. Tube feeding may be necessary and in some cases resort will be had to slow intravenous drip therapy with glucose in saline solution. To this infusion thiamin and nicotinic acid may be added because, due to the almost invariable presence of chronic gastritis, digestion and absorption from the gastrointestinal tract may be severely hampered. Some psychiatrists also add corticotrophin (ACTH) to the intravenous infusion. Small doses of insulin (5-15 units by hypodermic injection prior to meals) may be used to increase appetite.

Bromide Delirium. Careful, tactful check should be made of the patient's possessions to ensure that he is not still, unwittingly or deliberately, consuming preparations containing bromide. Sodium chloride (common salt) aids the excretion of bromide from the body and may be prescribed in tablet form in a dosage as high as 12 gms./day. Copious fluids also assist the process of bromide excretion.

Nursing Care

Rest. The physical condition of some of these patients will be grave and the nurse may have serious difficulty in controlling the restlessness which is a feature of their psychiatric illness and which is posing a further threat to their lives. Sedation will certainly have been prescribed and its proper timing should be a matter of frequent consultation between psychiatrist and nurse. Tranquillising drugs (p. 366) are of special value, and may in very acute cases be given by the parenteral route. Any reasonable request from the patient which appears likely to exert a calming effect on him should be granted if the psychiatrist permits.

Environment. The less stimulation available for the patient to misinterpret the less agitated will he be. Single-room nursing is essential and should be in the quietest part of the ward compatible with efficient observation. It is desirable for him to have as few changes in nursing attendants as practicable. If the presence of one member of his immediate family reassures and relaxes him this should be encouraged—but the doctor should be asked to forbid visiting if this obviously distresses him. Quietness and gentleness in the nurse's movements are essential; soft, repeated reassurance may be found in some instances to be the best " tranquilliser " available.

Night-nursing. Almost all these patients tend to be worse during the hours of darkness. A simple night light, clearly but softly illuminating the whole room, reduces the possibility of misinterpretation of shadows and of objects tucked away in corners.

Protection. Under the influence of his fear-producing hallucinations the patient may make impulsive attempts to injure himself; particularly he may try to escape from his room through the door or window in an effort to evade his imagined pursuers. Constant supervision will be necessary to guard against harm occurring to him in this way.

Nutrition. These patients need an easily digestible, highly nourishing diet; protein supplements are of value. Frequent small meals are usually desirable. Extra vitamins, particularly of the B group, will usually be prescribed by the doctor, and are a vital part of his treatment.

Fluid Intake. This should be carefully watched and a fluid balance chart maintained in any case where the slightest doubt exists about the adequacy of his fluid intake.

General Physical Care. Oral hygiene may lapse, attention to which may greatly increase the patient's comfort. Frequent sponging may be soothing and help to induce rest. Bowel and bladder function should be carefully noted and inadequate excretion promptly reported. Temperature, pulse and respiration charts need to be maintained with special care.

Prevention

Acute episodes of confusion at times occur in a psychiatric hospital in patients under treatment for some other condition; they are also common in the ordinary medical and surgical wards of a general hospital. The nurse is frequently in the best position to forestall their full-blown development by noting any early signs indicating that the patient is not fully in touch with his environment. Even minor degrees of disorientation in time (p. 129) may be of significance, as are any pieces of evidence that his judgement is disturbed or that he is failing to understand simple instructions. Any deviation from what is known to be the patient's typical behaviour should be at once reported, as this may be an important pointer to the beginning of some degree of clouding of his consciousness.

CHRONIC ORGANIC REACTIONS
CLINICAL FEATURES

As with the acute states, the picture of the chronic organic reaction tends to have certain common features whatever its cause. In addition certain aspects of the behaviour which appear are typical, not of the cause, but of the patient's own individual personality and reflect his customary defence mechanisms. It is a matter of common observation, for example, that in extreme old age the person's pattern of behaviour tends to be an exaggeration of the personality features he has shown early in life—the friendless adult tends to become the withdrawn and secretive old man; the somewhat suspicious middle-aged lady may, with the development of senility, become the victim of frank delusions of persecution.

What happens here is that the cerebral cortex, which is the area most likely to suffer from any disease process affecting the brain, normally keeps control over our more primitive and antisocial desires and feelings. Interference with this controlling function leads therefore to some degree of uninhibited behaviour, the nature of which depends on the person's deeper personality structure. When the elderly man with brain damage of whatever cause begins, for example, to behave in an overaffectionate or seductive manner towards children, the damage to his brain has not *caused* this form of behaviour but has *released* such tendencies from control; these have long been a part of him but have until this time been kept hidden and possibly out of his own awareness by the normal functioning of his cerebral cortex. Other aspects of the brain-damaged person's behaviour are the result of defensive attempts at compensation for the mental or physical functions lost or hampered by the disease process; declining mental ability, for example, is a very real stress to many individuals and any of the ego defences previously described may unconsciously come into action in an effort to cope with the resultant anxiety.

The major symptoms and signs of the chronic organic reaction are:

Deterioration of Intellectual Functions. Some degree of decline in the individual's mental capacity is usually the first noticeable sign.

(*a*) Judgement suffers; the person begins to make foolish and inappropriate decisions quite out of keeping with his previous record. He has difficulty in grasping ideas expressed by others, especially if these are new to him; his patterns of thinking become more set and less capable of change.

(*b*) Memory disturbance may be severe. Typically it involves recent memories long before there is loss of memory for past events; he forgets the incidents of the preceding day yet can still give a very detailed account of some happenings in his childhood. He may speak of persons long since dead as though they were still alive.

(*c*) Orientation is progressively disturbed; in advanced cases orientation for time, place and person are all affected.

(*d*) Superimposed on the background of chronic mental deterioration acute episodes of confusion may occur (as described earlier in this chapter).

Deterioration in Habits. Due to reduced cortical control primitive, less civilised behaviour may be noted or reported by others. Less care is taken of personal appearance; clothes appeared uncared for and hygiene suffers—the occurrence of " gravy stains on the waistcoat " is a minor but typical example frequently noted in senile men. In advanced cases control lapses over bowel and bladder functions, at first by night only, later during the day as well. Language may coarsen and inappropriate sexual behaviour make its appearance.

Emotional Lability. This is a special aspect of the failure of the controlling mechanisms. The patient weeps readily and profusely in response to a minor set-back, but is found only minutes later in a state of uproarious hilarity over some equally trivial incident. The phrase " emotional incontinence " is sometimes used to describe this behaviour. In some cases acute spells of overwhelming anxiety occur, partly in response to a realisation by the patient of the decline in his mental capacities.

CAUSES

Infection. Syphilis is the only important infection leading to chronic organic psychiatric illness. Some five to 30 years after the initial syphilitic infection the organism in some instances invades the brain and leads to the destruction of some neurones, resulting in an organic reaction without special psychiatric features. Certain typical physical signs may be found by the doctor in examining the nervous system and as the disease advances paralysis, coarse tremors, slurring of speech and seizures of epileptic type may develop. The older name for this condition was **general paralysis of the insane.**

Blood and cerebro-spinal fluid will be examined and will show positive evidence of syphilitic infection.

Encephalitis, particularly in childhood, is an occasional cause of later psychiatric illness which is not however of typical organic type. Some affected children become very serious behaviour problems, frequently being cruel, destructive and untruthful and showing open sexual and antisocial misbehaviour. Intelligence is often unimpaired.

Intoxication. The most important poison giving rise to chronic organic states is **alcohol.** The patient, most commonly a male, has usually been a chronic alcoholic for many years (p. 198), though due to memory defect he may not be able to give an adequate history of this or he may deny his behaviour. Episodes of acute confusion in the past, including frank delirium tremens, may be reported by his relatives or friends. As chronic alcoholics so often lead socially isolated lives it is in many instances impossible to find out how long he has been mentally deteriorating prior to his admission to hospital.

The clinical picture shows the typical features of the chronic organic reaction. These patients are commonly very cheerful and talkative and often produce copious untrue anecdotes to fill in the great gaps in their memory (**confabulation,** p. 126). Physical complications of alcoholism are frequently present such as cirrhosis of the liver. There may be damage to the peripheral nerves, particularly in the legs, with resultant pain and tenderness in the calves and weakness of the muscles of the feet. This combination of mental changes and peripheral neuritis is known as **Korsakow's psychosis** after the Russian psychiatrist who first described this in 1877.

Head Injury. Mental deterioration occasionally develops following severe head injury. Physical signs of damage to the brain are usually present (for example, paralyses or aphasia) and epileptic fits may occur.

However by no means all the psychiatric disturbances which arise following head injury are due to actual brain damage (p. 136). If the injured person has a high degree of neurotic predisposition an accident of this type can act as a powerful precipitant of frank neurotic illness; headache, giddiness, a feeling of confusion and interference with concentration and mental alertness are common symptoms. Even psychotic reactions of functional type (for example, schizophrenia) may be precipitated in this way. Head injuries, even very minor ones, are often the starting point for a compensation neurosis (p. 186).

Cerebral Arteriosclerosis. Narrowing of the arteries which supply blood to the brain tissue (commonly called " hardening of the arteries ") interferes with the proper function of the neurones and sooner or later will lead to their death. A chronic

ORGANIC REACTIONS

organic reaction develops, usually between the ages of 50 and 70, which has all the characteristics previously described. There are in addition certain other features often noted in this condition:

(a) The onset is often sudden following a small or large " stroke " (a cerebral thrombosis), after which the deterioration tends to progress in a somewhat jerky manner if further little strokes occur. Relatives may report that the patient was quite normal until one day he suddenly became confused and had difficulty in speaking; when these symptoms cleared up after a few hours his mental impairment was first noted.

(b) More than in other conditions of this type patients tend to retain a substantial awareness of their failing mental capacity. Because of this awareness they tend to be rather more tragic figures than some patients whose deterioration may be far greater but who seem almost totally indifferent to their handicap.

(c) There is a marked tendency for the degree of mental impairment and confusion to fluctuate from day to day.

(d) Headache and giddiness are common complaints and may be severe.

Epilepsy. The psychiatric disorders associated with epilepsy are considered separately at the end of this chapter.

Senility. There is a steady increase in the number of persons being admitted to mental hospitals with organic mental disturbances due to old age. Largely if not completely this increase can be explained by the fact that modern medical treatment of physical illnesses is making people live longer, without providing their brain tissues with any greater resistance to the ordinary processes of ageing. There are also many personal and social problems associated with growing old in our society (p. 72). Partly because of heredity, partly perhaps because of more regular mental activity, some people retain full mental powers until a late age—Sir Winston Churchill is a recent famous example of this. Others show a substantial decline in mental powers in their late 60's and have a fully developed **senile dementia** shortly afterwards. Rarely, similar changes in the brain and similar mental symptoms may occur before the age of 65, which is the usual time accepted as the commencement of old age; if these are not due to arteriosclerosis or other special causes the patient is said to be suffering from **presenile dementia**.

To the basic chronic organic picture there are often added marked depressive and/or paranoid features, at least until the disease process is far advanced. Misplacing some personal possession due to forgetfulness the suspicious senile patient may accuse the nurse or other patients of stealing his belongings. The behaviour, perhaps even more obviously than in other organic states, is a caricature of the previous personality.

As the condition progresses the physical changes of senility become increasingly marked. The skin becomes dry and wrinkled, the posture stooped and the gait shuffling. Much weight is lost, speech becomes quavering and tremor of the hand very apparent.

Brain Tumour and other Brain Disease. Mental changes of organic type are common in patients with brain tumours. The mental symptoms in some instances develop before any physical signs of brain disease can be detected, particularly in those cases where the tumour involves the frontal lobes. Epileptic seizures may occur. Headache and vomiting are common associated symptoms and are due to the growth of the tumour causing increased pressure inside the skull.

Huntington's Chorea is a very rare hereditary form of psychiatric disorder confined entirely to certain families. Usually in early middle age, the patient develops a chronic organic reaction associated with irregular, constant, jerking movements of the face and limbs. 50 *per cent* of the patient's children will develop the disease.

Parkinson's Disease (paralysis agitans), a degeneration of the brain occurring in late middle life characterised by rigidity and tremor in the face and limbs, is in some cases accompanied by organic mental changes. A similar physical picture may be produced by some of the drugs at present commonly employed in psychiatric hospitals, for example, " Largactil " and "Stelazine " (p. 369).

Other Bodily Illnesses. In rare instances disease processes involving other systems of the body may have direct effects on brain tissue leading to a chronic organic reaction.

CARDIAC ARREST. Cases are occasionally seen in which chronic mental changes result from complete temporary cessation of the heart's action, either occurring during anaesthesia or from some other cause such as drowning. Interruption of the blood supply to the brain has been so severe as to lead to the death of vital neurones.

CARDIAC FAILURE. It has already been mentioned that inefficient cardiac function due to heart disease may cause mental confusion because of the resulting inadequacy of oxygen supply to the brain. If long-continued this may lead to permanent mental change.

SEVERE ANAEMIA. Organic mental changes are occasionally noted in patients with profound anaemia, especially of the pernicious type.

PELLAGRA. Chronic deficiency of nicotinic acid, an essential substance, may lead to the easily remembered symptoms of *d*ermatitis, *d*iarrhoea, and *d*ementia.

Many other physical illnesses may have psychiatric complications in which the typical organic features are not prominent, even though the mental symptoms are brought about by some variety of toxic effect on the brain. These diseases include endocrine abnormalities such as myxoedema and Cushing's syndrome, also porphyria, disseminated lupus erythematosus and other collagen diseases.

TREATMENT

Once a patient has been diagnosed as suffering from a chronic organic form of mental impairment it is often too readily assumed that there is little or nothing that the psychiatric nurse can do. Such cases are frequently dismissed as "hopeless" before any real assessment is made, yet systematic nursing principles applied to their care may be extremely rewarding and may lead to real improvement in mental and physical function. It is true that brain cells, once damaged, can never be replaced. What is even more true, however, is that the patient's behaviour and mental state can be vastly influenced by the efficiency or otherwise with which his surviving brain tissue continues to function. This efficiency is a direct measure of the quality of his environment and therefore of his nursing care.

Consider, for example, the not uncommon instance of an elderly man admitted to a surgical ward of a general hospital for some operative procedure. His relatives report no evidence of mental disturbance whilst in his own home, yet he may be confused and disorientated within 48 hours of entering hospital, before any toxic factors such as drugs or anaesthesia have been brought into the picture. The brain damage responsible for the confusion must have been present for some time, yet it gave rise to no symptoms while his surviving neurones functioned smoothly in the contentment and familiar surroundings of his home environment. Admission to hospital leads to anxiety, which may be very severe; the surroundings are unfamiliar, the faces strange, the ward procedures and routine all too often mechanical and impersonal leading to a sense of isolation and insignificance. All these factors, adding to his anxiety over the separation from his family and over the imminent operation, decrease the capacity of his surviving neurones to deal adequately and intelligently with his experiences; the organic defect, present for some time, now becomes obvious.

The nursing care of the patient with a chronic organic reaction has **four basic and interlocking aims:**

(i) to ensure that the patient has the greatest possible contact with and participation in his environment, by decreasing anxiety and other disorganising emotions;

(ii) to achieve this by any specific treatment prescribed and through general nursing principles;

(iii) to make the last years of such patients as comfortable and as pleasant as possible;

(iv) to achieve for the nurse herself, by a combination of the above aims, a more smoothly running ward through the lessening of confused and disturbed behaviour.

Specific Treatment

Syphilis. The use of penicillin in high dosage has completely replaced all other treatments previously employed for syphilitic brain disease. Treatment procedures vary very widely; a dosage of 1,000,000 units per day for 10 to 20 days is one of many routines. Early and thorough treatment leads to striking improvement in many cases and probably one-half of the early treated patients will be able to return to work; unfortunately many sufferers do not come under notice until relatively late in the course of their disease when little or no improvement can be expected.

Korsakow's Psychosis (alcoholic dementia). The patient must obviously be prevented from consuming further alcohol. High protein, high vitamin diet is essential and large doses of vitamin B complex will be added. Bed rest and physiotherapy will be prescribed for peripheral neuritis; a plaster back-slab may be used for a lengthy period in an effort to prevent permanent footdrop. Even with intensive treatment, however, it is rare for such patients to show substantial recovery of mental function.

Brain Tumour. Some tumours are removable by neurosurgical procedures. In other instances radiotherapy (deep X-ray) may be the only available treatment. Treatment of the tumour, even its complete removal, does not lead in all instances to a total recovery of normal mental function.

Drug Treatment in Chronic Organic Reactions. In the great majority of illnesses of this type drug treatment can only be used to control certain specific symptoms, rather than radically alter the basic disease process. **Restlessness** and agitation, which may be extreme, are usually best controlled by one of the tranquillising drugs (p. 366); barbiturates usually only increase the patient's confusion. **Destructiveness** also frequently responds well to tranquillisers. Barbiturates, especially of the long-acting variety, are also poor drugs for the management of **insomnia** in these cases; older drugs such as paraldehyde and chloral hydrate are safer and more reliable, as are some of the newer synthetic preparations.

Various drugs are available for relief of the rigidity and tremor of Parkinson's disease, and are equally effective when similar symptoms result from the use of tranquillising drugs (p. 369). Of these probably the most widely employed is "Artane" (trihexyphenidyl) in a dosage of 2-6 mgms./day. " Cogentin " (benztropine) and " Kemadrin " (procyclidine) are other drugs with similar action.

Nursing Care

The general aims of nursing care in chronic organic psychiatric illness have already been outlined. Translation of these principles into practice will be found in Chapter 22 in those sections entitled "Aims for Those Who Need Long-Term Hospital Care " and " Habit Training ". These topics have been grouped together in that chapter because many of the important nursing techniques are relevant, not only to the care of chronic organic reactions, but to the management of any patient suffering from a psychiatric disorder requiring prolonged or permanent hospitalisation.

EPILEPSY

This is a common disorder in which periodic abnormal electrical discharges in the brain substance lead to episodes of altered mental and bodily function, always with some type of seizure or " fit ". The majority of epileptic patients require only medical care and do not come into psychiatric hands, but a certain number present mental and emotional disorders, some of which are mild but others very serious. In these individuals any of the following factors may be involved:

(i) Epileptic seizures may be arising as the result of major organic brain damage. This is the case in some mental defectives and in some of the organic reactions of later life such as cerebral arteriosclerosis, cerebral tumour and syphilitic brain disease.

(ii) Epileptic seizures arising as a result of disease of the temporal lobe of the brain are especially liable to be associated with a major behaviour disorder, as described below.

(iii) Epilepsy, especially if severe and if arising in early life, can be a substantial handicap to the individual's personality development. Primitive superstitions about the nature of epilepsy may cause other people to shun him to some extent, serious job difficulties may be encountered and major problems tend to occur in his social and sexual life.

(iv) If an epileptic patient experiences the type of childhood environment which would be likely to lead in any event to later neurotic or psychotic problems, the presence of even minor degrees of brain damage associated with epilepsy may allow abnormal behaviour to become apparent because the mechanisms of control are less adequate.

TYPES OF SEIZURE

Epileptic seizures are classified in the following way:

(i) **Generalised seizures,** of which there are three principal varieties—(a) *grand mal* convulsions; (b) *petit mal* attacks; (c) myoclonic jerks.

(ii) **Partial** or **focal seizures,** such as Jacksonian seizures and the abnormalities associated with temporal lobe disease.

This division is not, however, a watertight one, for many attacks may have focal features at the beginning, depending on the particular part of the brain which is the site of disease or abnormality, the abnormal electrical discharge then spreading throughout the deeper structures of the brain to produce a generalised convulsion of *grand mal* type. In such a case the earliest symptoms or signs, preceding the generalised seizure, are known as the **aura** and give a warning to such patients that a convulsion is imminent; usually the aura takes the same form on each occasion, and may consist of a twitching in one or more muscles, a feeling of numbness or tingling in some particular region of the body, flashes of light, definite hallucinations involving any sensation, strange alterations in mental state, and so on.

The principal types of seizure are now described in more detail:

Grand Mal. The sequence of events follows a standard pattern, whether or not there has been a preceding aura as just described:

(i) *The cry*: sudden contraction of the muscles involved in respiration forces air through the larynx, producing a typical loud shout known as the **epileptic cry.**

(ii) *Tonic phase*: at the same time all the muscles of the body contract and remain in spasm for some 15-30 seconds. The patient falls to the ground and may sustain minor or even serious injury. Due to the temporary interruption of respiration the face becomes cyanosed. The tongue may be bitten either in this or in the subsequent phase. Urine and faeces are commonly passed involuntarily.

(iii) *Clonic phase*: the tonic phase passes gradually into a period of intermittent, usually violent, generalised muscle contraction—this is the phase recognised as a "fit" by the untrained observer. It lasts for 30-60 seconds, before the contractions die away gradually. Blood-stained saliva may appear on the lips.

(iv) *Recovery phase*: some patients sleep for an hour or more following the seizure and still feel confused and distressed on awakening. Others are mentally alert and active within a short space of time. In other instances the patient may be unable to speak for a brief period, or may have a temporary paralysis of some part of the body, facts which should be very carefully noted by the nurse. Sometimes the patient behaves in a confused, repetitive fashion, clearly without being aware that he is doing so, this state being known as an **automatism.** Rarely this brief period of confusion passes into a longer and more serious confusional episode which may last for hours or even days. In this condition, known as the **epileptic twilight state,** the patient is grossly disorientated and is typically extremely restless, often suspicious and at times violent. He may wander around purposelessly and in rare instances may commit acts of violence which he later does not recall.

Petit Mal. In its typical form the patient suffers a very brief loss or disturbance of consciousness lasting from five to 20 seconds. He suddenly stops what he is doing, stares vacantly ahead of him, and may drop any article held in the hand. Consciousness returns just as abruptly as it was interrupted and the patient carries on his activity where he left off. Occasionally the seizure may be so short that the patient himself does not recognise that it has occurred.

Myoclonic Jerks. These consist of rapid muscular contractions, without warning, usually causing flexion of both arms but occasionally involving all four limbs, in which case the patient falls to the ground.

Jacksonian Seizure. This is a type of focal epilepsy, named after a famous neurologist, Hughlings Jackson, who was the first person to describe it. The focus is in the motor cortex of the brain, and the fit consists of muscular contractions beginning in a localised area of the body, for example, in one hand or one side of the face, but spreading in an orderly sequence to involve other muscle groups and commonly ending in a *grand mal* seizure.

Temporal Lobe Epilepsy. This is a special variety of partial or focal seizure in which the epileptic process begins in the anterior portion of the temporal lobe of the brain. The seizure may have any of the following manifestations, alone or in combination:

(i) Sudden attacks of fear or anxiety, feelings of strangeness and alteration in the outside world or in the patient's own body, *déjà vu* sensations (p. 127), unpleasant thoughts "forcing" their way into the mind or hallucinations of an auditory, visual or olfactory nature.

(ii) Clouding of consciousness with confusion and automatic motor activity; the patient's behaviour may not even attract the attention of the casual onlooker, but his movements are aimless and he is definitely out of contact with his environment. Speech is muttering and often incomprehensible, or the patient is unable to speak at all. Attacks of this type are sometimes described as **psychomotor epilepsy.**

(iii) Especially in the presence of olfactory hallucinations, the patient may show very typical smacking movements of the lips accompanied by chewing and swallowing.

(iv) The fit may consist of extremely violent and destructive behaviour, with sudden wild activity in which in extreme cases crimes may be committed. This is the so-called **epileptic furor.**

(v) Occasionally the patient wanders away during the seizure, in a disturbed state of consciousness, this being known as an **epileptic fugue.** This state may be very difficult to differentiate from similar episodes in neurotic patients brought about by the mechanism of dissociation (p. 182).

As is the case in any patient with focal epilepsy, any of these manifestations of temporal lobe involvement may be immediately followed by a typical *grand mal* seizure.

Status Epilepticus

This term refers to a series of epileptic seizures, of either *grand mal* or focal type, following one another in quick succession without the patient regaining consciousness between the fits. It is a serious emergency which may in rare instances be fatal.

CAUSE

There are two great classes of epileptic patients, those in whom the fits arise as a result of some definite disease of the

ORGANIC REACTIONS

brain or elsewhere (**symptomatic epilepsy**), and those in whom there is no particular disease process in evidence, only an abnormal liability to sudden, explosive electrical discharges in the brain (**idiopathic epilepsy**).

Symptomatic Epilepsy. Practically any disease process affecting the brain substance may give rise to an epileptic seizure as one of its manifestations. The list includes cerebral tumour, cerebral syphilis, cerebral arteriosclerosis, head injury and the various congenital abnormalities of the brain found in childhood which may be associated with mental retardation. In addition certain bodily disturbances such as hypoglycaemia and other situations such as sudden cessation of barbiturate drugs (p. 201) or withdrawal of alcohol may give rise to fits. When epilepsy arises for the first time in middle or late life a definite underlying cause will usually be discovered. It is particularly important, therefore, for the nurse to report accurately and in detail any seizure occurring in an adult patient not previously known to be epileptic.

Idiopathic Epilepsy. The use of the term "idiopathic" means that the condition has no known origin in disease of the brain structure. Such cases commonly have an hereditary basis and the incidence of epilepsy in other members of the family is high. If the seizures are of *grand mal* type they most commonly first show themselves during the teenage period, though they may commence in childhood. *Petit mal* seizures begin invariably in very early life, occur classically between the ages of five and 15, and are relatively uncommon in adults.

In all epileptics, whatever the basic cause, certain factors will tend to act as **precipitants of fits**. These include **emotional stress, fever, hypoglycaemia, alcoholic excess,** sudden **cessation of a heavy alcohol intake,** any **excessive fluid intake** and **mental idleness.** Epileptic seizures in females tend to be more common around the time of menstruation.

PSYCHIATRIC COMPLICATIONS

1. Some temporal lobe seizures, consisting largely or entirely of peculiar behaviour, may appear at first sight to be

purely psychiatric problems and their epileptic nature may not be realised.

2. Many epileptic patients become markedly irritable, depressed and perhaps suspicious for a few hours or even a few days prior to a seizure. The experienced nurse, when familiar with the individual patient, will learn to know his typical pattern of behaviour at this time, during which he may be extremely argumentative and even violent. Typically these changes disappear after the fit and many nurses (and patients' relatives) will describe a happier disposition in epileptics who have occasional seizures, in contrast to the not infrequent report of difficult and demanding behaviour in the same patient if his seizures are being completely abolished by drugs. (This fact explains the occasional use of electrotherapy (p. 357) in epileptic patients showing disordered behaviour; even one fit artificially brought about by electricity may lead to a striking improvement in such a patient's mood.)

3. Some epileptic patients have episodes of grossly psychotic behaviour, most typically showing symptoms resembling a schizophrenic reaction but occasionally with chiefly depressive or paranoid features. Such patients usually have temporal lobe epilepsy. The abnormality shown by others consists of chronically unstable, unpredictable, even antisocial behaviour.

4. **The " Epileptic Personality ".** Some of these patients show certain personality characteristics with great frequency. They tend to be slow in their mental reactions, very fixed in their opinions and often extremely self-centred and excessively concerned about their bodily functions. They may be fairly constantly irritable and even violent on slight provocation. Many experienced psychiatric nurses would say that, as a group, epileptic patients are the most difficult in their wards. A few will deteriorate to a state resembling a chronic organic reaction **(epileptic dementia).** These changes seem only to be found in patients with underlying brain damage; the long-continued administration of sedative drugs may also play some part in their causation.

ORGANIC REACTIONS

It must be stressed that all the above mental changes, while common in those epileptic patients found in a psychiatric hospital, are far from being inevitable complications of epilepsy. The majority, particularly those of the idiopathic variety, are able to lead almost normal lives in the outside world without significant mental abnormality.

DIAGNOSIS

The nurse has a very important role to play in the diagnosis of epileptic disorders, particularly in those patients who are admitted to hospital in order that a decision can be reached concerning the true nature of their fits. As only rarely does the doctor himself witness a seizure great emphasis will be placed on the nurse's report and she must learn to provide an accurate, detailed description of any fit which takes place in her presence. The following matters will need to be noted:

1. Time of occurrence.
2. Any particular external circumstances existing at the time.
3. Patient's mental condition prior to the seizure.
4. Presence or absence of onlookers.
5. Nature of onset, whether sudden or gradual.
6. Any complaint made by the patient just prior to the seizure which may indicate the presence of an aura (p. 272).
7. Presence or absence of the epileptic cry (p. 272).
8. State of consciousness during the seizure—whether completely out of contact, partially in contact or completely in contact with surroundings.
9. Muscular movements during the seizure—presence or absence of well-defined tonic or clonic phases (p. 272), movements of head, lips and tongue, violent thrashing movements of the limbs or entire body. It is especially important to observe whether the movements of each side of the body are symmetrical; the convulsive movements may be unilateral, or only one limb or muscle

group may be involved, and in such cases a careful note must be made of the part or area affected. Note whether there is any turning of the head and eyes to one side.
10. Presence or absence of cyanosis, pallor or flushing.
11. Presence or absence of incontinence of urine and/or faeces.
12. Presence or absence of tongue-biting and frothing at the mouth.
13. Presence or absence of other bodily injury.
14. Mental and physical state at the completion of the seizure.
15. Total duration of the seizure and of subsequent unconsciousness (if any).
16. Patient's subsequent ability to recall any part of the attack.
17. Any unusual behaviour following the seizure, *e.g.* automatism.
18. The occurrence of any temporary paralysis following the seizure, the area affected being carefully recorded.

Armed with this information, plus the history from the patient and his relatives, the findings on physical examination and special tests, the psychiatrist will then be in a position to determine the nature and cause of the seizure. Attacks closely resembling epilepsy occur in some patients with conversion reactions (" hysterical fits ") but the differentiation of these two conditions may be very difficult and the nurse must refrain from passing hasty judgements (even in her own mind) on whether the seizure is " epileptic " or " hysterical " (p. 184). Some genuine epileptics have seizures which show additional conversion hysterical features.

Electroencephalography (EEG)

All patients suspected of having an epileptic disorder will be investigated by means of the electroencephalograph (EEG). This is a machine which records the electrical currents of the brain by means of small electrodes placed on the scalp and which gives a great deal of information to the doctor concerning the patient's brain function.

EEG recordings are also of value in the diagnosis of other brain disorders such as cerebral tumour and are frequently employed in the investigation of psychiatric illnesses of uncertain causation.

TREATMENT

Management of the Convulsion. During a *grand mal* seizure the less that is done by the nurse the better. The only exception to this is the possibility that a mouth gag or any large soft object *may* be able to be inserted between the teeth to prevent injury to the tongue, but no force must be used to achieve this and the attempt should be abandoned if not easily successful. No effort should be made to move or to restrain the patient during the convulsion. After its termination any tight clothing should be loosened and the head turned to one side to allow saliva to drain out of the throat rather than be inhaled. The patient should be supervised until fully conscious and any injury sustained should be noted and immediately reported. Where doubt exists as to the nature of the attack a full account should be written up as soon as possible.

Status Epilepticus. Heavy sedation will be given by the doctor either intramuscularly or intravenously and appropriate trays should be prepared immediately this condition is realised to exist. Continuous oxygen administration by intranasal catheter is advisable. Maintenance of fluid balance may be a problem.

Drug Treatment. Modern drugs greatly reduce the number and severity of epileptic seizures. Patients with *grand mal* convulsions and temporal lobe epilepsy are usually treated with two or more of the following drugs: " Dilantin " (diphenylhydantoin sodium), " Mesantoin " (methoin), phenobarbitone (phenobarbital sodium), " Prominal " (methylphenobarbitone) and " Mysoline " (primidone). *Petit mal* seizures usually respond to " Tridione ", " Paradione " (paramethadione), "Zarontin" (ethosuximide) or "Milontin" (methylphenylsuccinimide). To counteract the sedative effects of the barbiturate drugs quite large doses of "Dexedrine" may be given in addition. Because retention of fluid may increase the number of seizures a diuretic drug such as "Diamox" (acetazolamide) is used by some doctors.

With any of these drugs, watch must be kept for toxic effects such as unsteadiness of gait, undue drowsiness, sore throat, skin rashes, slurred speech and fever; the occurrence of any of these signs should be at once reported. Occasional patients receiving "Dilantin" develop an overgrowth of the gums around the teeth; oral hygiene is particularly important in the prevention of this complication.

Surgery. In a very few cases where a brain tissue scar is known to be the cause of the seizures surgical removal of this may be successful if treatment by drugs is ineffective. In suitable cases of temporal lobe epilepsy surgical removal of the anterior portion of the temporal lobe on the affected side may produce very satisfactory results, not only the frequency of seizures but also the personality disturbance being substantially improved in some instances.

Nursing Care. In the known epileptic certain factors tend to increase the frequency of seizures (p. 275). Nursing care will aim in the first instance at avoidance of these situations wherever possible. Care will be taken to avoid hypoglycaemia by the provision of adequate food at regular intervals and by ensuring that the patient does not miss meals. In those epileptic patients who have the majority of their seizures in the very early morning a light but nourishing snack during the night, together with a sweetened drink, may have some preventive value. Any tendency to excessive fluid intake should be controlled if possible.

Avoidance of emotional stress and mental conflict are of great importance and the nurse will learn to recognise those patients under her care in whom seizures are likely to be precipitated by anger or anxiety. With hospitalised epileptics

ORGANIC REACTIONS

elimination where possible of friction between patients and patients and between patients and staff will pay substantial dividends. Some epileptic patients who have major neurotic conflicts may consciously or unconsciously sabotage their own treatment, sometimes up to the point of omitting to take their anti-epileptic drugs; this must be considered as a possible explanation for an apparent failure to respond to therapy, or for a sudden increase in the number of seizures reported. In some cases an organised programme of psychotherapy (p. 331), either individual or group, may be prescribed by the psychiatrist.

As mental inactivity increases the frequency of seizures, the importance of an adequate occupational and recreational programme is obvious.

With the epileptic patient encountered in the general hospital or the outpatient clinic the nurse must by her attitude avoid any possible suggestion that she is handling him as a special " afflicted " person. Certain restrictions on his activity will be imposed by the doctor—avoidance of certain occupations, of car-driving, of swimming without a trusted friend—and the nurse may be placed in situations where she is required to use her influence to emphasise these. This however can be done realistically and without raising undue anxiety. If the opportunity presents itself she may also reinforce, both with the patient and his relatives, the necessity for regular, uninterrupted taking of the various tablets prescribed.

In most instances the doctor will require, both with in-patients and outpatients, a record to be kept of the number of seizures occurring, their nature and the time of day at which they occur. In a psychiatric hospital special charts will be available for this purpose which must be maintained conscientiously by the nurse—at the time when the fits occur, not using her memory a day or two later. She should also be able to guide the outpatient or, better still, his closest relative, in the way in which they can most simply provide the information sought by the psychiatrist.

CONCLUSION

Epilepsy is a disorder of brain function without any magical significance. The nurse, both on and off duty, should by her example be helping to create an atmosphere of tolerance for the epileptic patient, trying whenever she can to counteract any tendency to set him apart from the rest of society and assisting in the creation of a supportive, sensible atmosphere in which he can be treated. There is no place for out of date superstitions in the management of this disease.

13

CHILD PSYCHIATRY

EVEN though children and adolescents grow up to become adults, so that there is continuity of personality development from infancy onwards, there are nevertheless certain aspects of psychiatric disorder in childhood which make it very different from adult psychiatry. Certain matters become more important—others are less so.

1. Because the child is immature and still has a considerable potential for later development, there is a greater accent on altering the child's environment and on his general management, rather than on physical and drug treatment.

2. Situations that may be extremely harmful to a child often have little effect on an adult. An obvious example of this is that the infant or young child parted from his mother for a substantial period of time may suffer serious consequences (p. 40), whereas an adolescent or an adult should not be significantly harmed by such a separation.

3. A child's environment is largely determined by his parents' attitudes. Any modification of his environment must therefore involve some sort of approach to his parents and a child psychiatric unit is always staffed in such a way that it can work effectively with a family. In such a setting social workers usually see the parents while the psychiatrist is treating the child.

4. In child psychiatry the complaint about the patient is more likely to come from the child's parents than from the child himself; in other instances the child patient is recommended for treatment by his school, the Child Welfare Department or the Children's Court. The child patient, although he may be upsetting others, may not be suffering from his symptoms and there may therefore be little co-operation from

him. Because of the varied sources of referral, the treatment programme may involve the school, a Child Welfare Officer, or some voluntary agency.

5. Many symptoms for which children are treated appear to be quite minor in comparison with the complaints of adult psychiatric patients. This is because in childhood our efforts are directed much more towards prevention and early treatment, for it is hoped that early attention to symptoms will prevent their being " built in " to the personality. In children we aim to improve their mental health, rather than simply treat their mental illnesses.

6. The symptoms of emotional disturbance in children vary from those seen in adults. Gross symptoms such as hallucinations and delusions are extremely rare and the child's illness is more likely to be indicated by disturbance in his relationship with others.

7. Because the child's personality is still in the process of development, even severe symptoms may have a less ominous significance than an equivalent amount of disturbance in adults. For example, some children are brought to a clinic because at the thought of going to school they dissolve into tears, have tantrums or become panicky; they are said to be suffering from **school phobia**. They may make a good and quick response to a suitable management programme, whereas an adult distressed to the same extent by the thought of going to work would be much more severely disturbed and the outlook would be much more doubtful. Even symptoms with a great nuisance value do not necessarily indicate an extremely severe underlying disturbance; in fact, some less noticeable symptoms such as severe shyness and withdrawal may have a more serious significance.

THE FORMS OF PSYCHIATRIC ILLNESS IN CHILDHOOD

In Chapter 8 it was said that children may show various types of **adjustment reaction** to the stresses which they encounter and these reactions were divided up into three groups —Habit Disturbance, Conduct Disturbance and Neurotic Traits (p. 162). This classification must now be expanded to include the wide variety of symptoms which may be shown by the disturbed child.

Nervous Disorders (that is, in the popular sense). Included here are such symptoms as anxiety, temper tantrums, fearfulness, shyness, excessive restlessness and excitability. Children often present with a generalised form of anxiety, that is to say, situations which cause a normal child a small amount of anxiety give these child patients a very great deal of distress. They may be unusually frightened of the dark, of strange places, of animals, of being hurt and so on. In the older child, particularly when he passes into adolescence, the picture of anxiety resembles more and more closely that which is seen in the adult anxiety reaction (p. 179). In the adolescent, as has been indicated in Chaper 5 (p. 88), anxiety may stem from a variety of problems connected with dependence, sexual feelings and so on, whereas in the very young child anxiety is more likely to be a direct response to his relationship with his parents, such a child seeming almost to " catch " (like the measles) the tension which exists in his family circle.

Habit Disturbances. There are two types:

(1) PRIMARY HABIT DISTURBANCES. These are connected with those functions that normally develop an habitual pattern at a fairly early age, in particular eating, sleeping and excretion. **Feeding disorders** are common between the ages of one and five, especially at 18 months or thereabouts when the child's first moves towards independence may lead him to refuse food as part of his generally negativistic behaviour. An anxious child may have little appetite, or he may be restless and therefore difficult to feed; in some of these circumstances the table becomes a veritable battle-ground between mother and child. On the other hand, some children who are hungry for affection may overeat, whereas others again persistently

eat dirt and rubbish, incidentally running the risk of serious poisoning.

Other children show **disturbance in sleeping habits,** settling at no routine time or else frequently waking with nightmares. In later childhood, most commonly between the ages of nine and 12, **night terrors** may occur, often at the same hour each night; the child wakes in a state of great fear and may walk in his sleep and seem to be quite out of touch with his environment.

A very common disturbance is that of bed-wetting, known as **enuresis.** This is not usually considered a symptom in a child under six; after this age about one child in five will wet the bed occasionally, though in the majority of these it disappears spontaneously. Some of these children are extremely tense, anxious and ambitious; others seem to wet the bed largely as a result of poor training, or because they at one time developed the symptom to attract attention and it now persists although the need for attention has largely passed. In some children it will be found that bed-wetting has an aggressive quality about it and is retained as a symptom because of the annoyance it causes the parents; in others again it seems to represent a desire to cling to infantile behaviour. Similar mechanisms underlie the development of **encopresis,** the involuntary passing of faeces, sometimes known as " soiling ".

(2) SECONDARY HABIT DISTURBANCES. These represent more than a simple failure to establish the habit patterns of the normal child. Many of them are obviously pleasurable to the child and are known as **gratification habits;** these include thumb-sucking and other pleasurable manipulations of the body, particularly masturbation. Children who are bored and lonely and who are not getting the affection they need are more likely to indulge in these habits to excess, although to a lesser extent they occur normally as part of the process of development. Masturbation in particular is a universal practice at some stage in childhood; as the child develops an increasing awareness of his body he becomes interested in his

genitals and finds that he can produce pleasurable sensations from touching them. In itself masturbation is of little importance if the child's condition is otherwise satisfactory; there is nothing to indicate that it causes any physical or mental harm, although this threat is often used by parents (and even, regrettably, by some nurses) in an attempt to stop the habit. These threats, of course, create an additional problem for the child by increasing guilt and worry and by causing him to lose self-respect. In the child or adolescent in whom masturbation becomes excessive it is necessary to discover why he is failing to gain satisfaction from other activities. One looks at the environment to see if there are defects in it which might be remedied and one tries to help his general adjustment and to build up his self-esteem.

Some degree of sexual play in childhood is not uncommon. When it is brought to light the child should be made to understand that it is considered to be unsuitable behaviour, yet at the same time he must be reassured that no harm has been done and that it can now be forgotten. Occasionally a child is markedly upset by involvement in sexual play and requires reassurance and support. Certainly more harm is created by the guilt and anxiety which can so easily come to surround sexual activity in childhood than is caused by the sexual behaviour itself.

Other habits found in childhood are known as **tension habits;** these include such practices as nail-biting, head-banging, pulling out of hair and other types of self-mutilation. They are seen in the tense child who is directing his aggression towards himself. Occasionally in some children with behaviour disturbances associated with brain damage (for example, due to encephalitis), or in some mental defectives, head-banging can be so severe as to become an actual threat to the child's life.

Conduct Disturbances. In this group are included thieving, lying, cruelty and truancy from school. In older children and in adolescents various forms of behaviour of this type, with or without sexual misdemeanours, are described under the general heading of **delinquency**. A wide range of conditions, both inside the child and in his environment, may contribute to the development of such disordered behaviour, though in each individual case one set of factors commonly dominates the situation. Not all problem behaviour develops as a result of mental ill-health; some arises from a combination of immature judgement, poor company and lack of adequate supervision. More commonly, however, there appears to be a definite relationship between persistent antisocial conduct and a past history of deprivation in the child's emotional life. Frequently it will be found that there has been a substantial deficiency in the quality of the parental care received by the child, especially in his very early years. Though it is true that many children from inadequate homes do not develop problem behaviour, generally it is found that antisocial conduct is more common in such circumstances than in children from stable, harmonious homes. Delinquents very commonly have been reared in families where there has been little understanding, affection, stability or moral fibre, and frequently their parents have shown themselves unfit to be effective guides or protectors. The child, as was seen in Chapter 5 (p. 83), develops his superego by building into his personality the morals and standards of his parent figures; if the standards of his parents are themselves antisocial the child's conscience is likely to be one which permits him to indulge in antisocial acts.

One extreme example is the so-called **separation syndrome** (p. 40), in which deprivation in the mother-child relationship has produced what Bowlby has called an affectionless character. These are the children who have had prolonged separation from mother, without the provision of an adequate substitute, during the period from 18 months to three years of age. They tend to become emotionally shallow children, careless of the rights of others and overcompensating for feelings of inadequacy by persistent attention-seeking behaviour. Other children, reared by perfectionistic parents, may respond with chronic rebellion to all demands made on them, whether by the family or by society.

Physical factors may also contribute to behaviour disorders. About 60 *per cent* of these children show abnormal electroencephalographic (EEG) records (p. 278), though some of these improve as the child grows older; the patients in this particular group may simply be maturing and developing controls over their behaviour at a later age than the normal child. Brain damage may also play a part in behaviour disorders, as it is often associated with impulsive, aggressive and destructive conduct (see below).

Neurotic Reactions. Here the symptoms result from emotional conflict that has in some way been built into the personality. Most of the neurotic symptoms found in adults are rare in childhood or occur only in a mild form. Obsessions and compulsions are, for example, frequent in early childhood but are nearly always minor and certainly are not necessarily pathological in children from four to six years old. At this age many children's games have an obsessional quality; they may also get upset if there is any disturbance in the fixed routines which they have worked out in regard to clothes or in the order of going to bed. On the other hand, from nine to 15 years of age some obsessional and phobic states can be serious and difficult to help.

Excessive concern about bodily health (hypochondriasis— p. 120) may be a problem in some children. Parental handling, and sometimes the attitudes of doctors and nurses, may encourage a child to concentrate too much upon his own body and this concern may become a real barrier to his adjustment. Exaggerated tiredness, tummy pains and headache are common symptoms. Conversion reactions are rare before puberty. Anorexia is also relatively uncommon; on the contrary, overeating is more likely to be a problem.

Psychosomatic Reactions (p. 313). Childhood patterns of psychosomatic illness include migraine, asthma and eczema.

Migraine may appear in the form of abdominal pain and nausea rather than as the headache which is the more usual adult manifestation. There is also a condition of **psychogenic fever** which is rare in adults but may occur in young children, particularly if they are away from their normal environment; they run a temperature which cannot be explained on any physical basis, which clears up on their return home and which seems to have been a reaction to stress.

Organic Reactions. Brain damage in a child, however caused, may lead to a variety of symptoms. The behaviour of the brain-damaged child may be quite unpredictable, with his mood fluctuating rapidly for no apparent reason. Often he is overactive, restless, running about and shouting and quite unable to relax. Attention and concentration are poor and he is easily distracted from any task. Impulsiveness and irritability may lead to severe temper tantrums, the child responding explosively to quite minor irritations. There may be a high degree of anxiety and an obvious emotional immaturity. Many of these children become negativistic and stubborn; they may be unpleasant bullies or indulge in uncontrolled sexual behaviour.

Psychotic Reactions. Because doctors were looking for the same type of symptoms as occur in adults, childhood psychosis was considered rare until about 1930. But **schizophrenia in childhood,** arising in a developing personality, presents a picture very different from any of the adult varieties. Some children who are found on close study to be schizophrenic appear on the surface to be mentally retarded, presenting as extremely inhibited and withdrawn, perhaps mute and incapable of social relationships; in others there is a wide range of anxiety symptoms, phobias, obsessions, compulsions and disturbances of the child's picture of his own body. Yet others, usually in the older age group, present with a largely antisocial picture, indulging in aggressive actions without apparent guilt and expressing many feelings of persecution.

One particular form of childhood schizophrenic reaction is called **early infantile autism**. This condition is characterised by the child's inability, right from the beginning of life, to develop ordinary relationships to people and to situations. They may as infants appear to be good babies, undemanding and happy by themselves, but by six months of age are seen to be unresponsive and may be thought to be deaf or mentally retarded. They do not respond well to nursing and prefer to take the bottle in the cot; though they do not seem to desire contact with human beings, they usually take great interest in certain objects and may have a high degree of muscular co-ordination. They are not unaware of people but seem to be unaffected by them, remaining in a state of extreme self-isolation. They like to maintain a sameness in their environment and are grossly lacking in spontaneity, being very much dependent on ritual and routine. Though many appear to have an unusually good memory, they may lack the ability to speak or may speak in a highly unusual way. Gratification habits such as rocking are common.

The causation of childhood schizophrenia is as yet uncertain. With regard to early infantile autism it has often been observed that such infants have emotionally cold parents and the disorder is said to be a response to the total lack of warmth in the family setting. As in adult varieties of schizophrenic reaction it is probable that hereditary factors are of importance, the child inheriting an inadequate capacity to develop normal ego functions. Presumably both hereditary and environmental factors are involved.

Educational Difficulties. Though any of the symptom patterns previously described may well interfere with the child's adjustment to schooling, in other children this inability to progress at school is the major symptom. Some children respond to stress by functioning persistently below their capacity and their intellectual functions may for this reason be so handicapped as to lead to a severe limitation of their school performance.

CAUSATION

As in adult psychiatry, there are very few examples of a simple relationship between cause and effect in the disturbances shown by children. Almost invariably, even though one factor has a dominant role, the illness is the result of many stresses which add up until a symptom is produced. Moreover, the same sort of cause will tend to produce different symptoms at different ages—for example, severe frustration in the infant may lead to breath-holding attacks, in young children to temper tantrums and in older children to sullenness and withdrawal. Anxiety in the very young child tends to lead to bodily restlessness; in the older child it appears more commonly as mental restlessness and lack of concentration.

It has been frequently suggested in the previous pages that the child's symptoms are often his response to the conflicts of his parents, which have been reflected in their attitudes towards him and in their handling of him. Many parents, who are themselves emotionally disturbed or immature, are unable to a greater or lesser extent to provide a loving, supportive and therefore healthy atmosphere in which their children can develop (p. 68). Many show some degree of hostility towards the child, though the parents themselves are almost invariably unaware of this. In particular, a woman who has never developed any real satisfaction or contentment in her relationship with her own mother will find it difficult to fulfil adequately the role of mother to a young child.

These various disturbances of parental attitude are described collectively as **parental rejection**; because in the early years the mother tends to be the more significant parent in the child's eyes one commonly talks of **maternal rejection,** though father is far from being unimportant, as has been seen (p. 46). This rejection is rarely shown openly, though one does see occasional instances of children being obviously ill-treated or neglected or in some cases deliberately and literally abandoned. Far more commonly rejecting attitudes are hidden in various ways, usually hidden even from the parents themselves. Some children, though cared for efficiently from a material point of view, are grossly **deprived of mothering,** either being left with relatives or in day nurseries, or failing to receive any warmth and emotional stimulation even though in their own home.

Rejection may be cloaked by what is described as **perfectionism;** the parents justify their hostility towards the child on the grounds that he does not come up to imaginary and usually quite impossible standards. Whatever the reason given, whether it be a physical failing or some alleged abnormality of behaviour, they are not satisfied with him the way he is. Such children often have serious feelings of guilt and inferiority and may tend to develop obsessional characteristics, often associated with a good deal of rebellion. Sometimes they are brought to a child psychiatrist by parents who are dissatisfied with some quite minor defect which they have magnified into a major problem.

In yet other instances the unconscious rejection is masked by **overprotection;** the mother's behaviour proclaims to the world and to herself " it couldn't be said that I have any aggression towards this child—look how much care I take of him ". Such a child is over-mothered and the resultant " spoiling " is likely to delay his progress to maturity; he is not allowed to face difficulties for himself and tends to cling to mother long past the normal age. (Not all overprotected children are unconsciously rejected; overprotection of a more normal kind can occur in any situation where a child has become particularly precious, as in the case of an only child of elderly parents who can have no more children, or when parents have lost one child and have understandable anxiety for the well-being of the remaining one.)

Such deficiencies in the mother-child relationship may have long-lasting effects. Emotional instability tends to be handed down from one generation to the next, because deprived children who have come from broken and unhappy homes frequently reproduce similar conditions when they become parents themselves. The potentially harmful effects of separation have already been stressed. For this reason it is usually advisable for an infant who has lost his parents to be cared for in a foster-home or to be adopted, rather than to be brought up in an institution. For the same reason some hospitals provide flats in order that a mother can live in and care for her own child if he requires hospital treatment (p. 386).

In other cases the child's basic handicap is an organic one. His primary disability may be due to brain damage or mild mental retardation, or to some defect in hearing, vision or motor skills. In many cases the child's disturbance is the result of a combination of organic and psychological factors, often with the additional presence of some social problem.

Whatever the cause, symptoms are usually exaggerations or distortions of normal behaviour and frequently indicate a persistence of, or a regression to, immature levels of development. Because of the child's dependence and his position in the family he may achieve substantial secondary gains (p. 185) from his disturbance, even in obscure ways—for example, an attention-seeking child may find that punishment from his parents is better than no attention at all. More commonly it will be found that the symptom, which is caused by anxiety and represents an attempt to deal with it, attracts criticism or punishment, which create further anxiety and therefore a greater need for the symptom, with the result that a vicious circle is set up.

TREATMENT

Treatment must be adapted to each individual child. In the mildest cases nothing more may be required than advice and reassurance to the parent; at the other end of the scale, hospitalisation or placement in an institution is recommended if the condition is particularly severe. The following are the **general principles of treatment:**

1. Attempts are made to improve the **psychological environment** of the child by interviewing the parents in an effort to

modify their attitudes and patterns of child care. (This is often the task of the psychiatric social worker.) In physical medicine, for example, it would not be possible to treat the undernourished child's frequent infections and fevers without paying attention to his basic state of malnutrition—similarly, a child starved of a good psychological environment is more susceptible to emotional disturbance and behaviour disorders. But it is seldom a simple matter for parents to change their attitudes, for it has already been pointed out that these reflect their own unresolved childhood problems carried over into adult life. In not a few instances the parent or parents are recommended for long-term psychotherapy (p. 327).

2. Any **physical defects** and handicaps are recognised and modified where possible; this includes the improvement of general physical health and the correction of abnormalities of vision and hearing.

3. Severe anxiety and overactivity may be modified by **drug treatment;** a wide variety of sedatives and tranquillisers (p. 364) can be employed. " Dexedrine " (p. 371) is of value in certain behaviour disorders. Children who are brain-damaged or epileptic may be particularly helped by a programme of treatment which includes drugs.

4. In some instances **retraining programmes** can be effective. These include special types of education, such as is required for the stammerer or the child with a reading disability, or may consist of deliberate training in new habits as in some cases of bed-wetting, when a management programme involving charts and rewards may help to abolish the symptom.

5. Management programmes may require the co-operation of significant people in the child's environment. He may be helped, for example, by a transfer to a more suitable class in his school or by the arrangement of social activities.

6. **Psychotherapy.** It is often surprising how effective simple advice can be if a good relationship has been made with the child and if he feels he is getting a sympathetic hearing and being understood. Psychotherapy, as with adults (see Chapter

16), varies from suggestion and reassurance up to a detailed examination of his conflicts with explanation and interpretation. Obviously psychotherapy in its ordinary form can only be helpful when a good contact can be made between the therapist and the patient and this may be difficult for a variety of reasons. Particularly in young children, who have only a limited ability to talk about their problems, treatment may take the form of **play therapy**. Through play, including drawing, the child is encouraged to express himself and his feelings and can often get rid of important inner tensions. Through observation of the sort of play situation which he constructs valuable information can be obtained about his unconscious mental life, just as dreams in adults may reveal their buried wishes.

7. If the child's environmental difficulties cannot be relieved then consideration is given to his removal from this environment and his **placement** in a more suitable one. This may involve moving from one home to another, for example to the house of a relative, or to a foster-home, or to a children's hostel or institution. Obviously such a transfer must always have advantages and disadvantages; if he is removed from his own unsatisfactory home it may sometimes be later found that it is worse for him to have no home at all. Delinquent children may be required to appear before a Children's Court, and if the Magistrate is satisfied that the child is uncontrollable or neglected he may order that he be removed from his own home and committed to the care of an approved person or to an institution (training school).

8. In the most severe cases a child may have to be admitted to a **specialised psychiatric unit.** Here he will usually receive individual psychotherapy, some type of retraining programme and drug treatment where necessary. At the same time intensive efforts will be made to modify his parents' attitudes. But all this treatment will be of little value unless the environment of the unit is more beneficial to him than the environment in which he was situated at home; the creation of this therapeutic

atmosphere is largely the responsibility, under medical supervision, of the psychiatric nurse.

THE ROLE OF THE NURSE IN CHILD PSYCHIATRY

Much of what has been written in this chapter will be seen to have application to the work of the nurse in the medical and surgical units of a children's hospital. Any nurse working in a situation which involves child care will quickly encounter one or other of the various common disorders described and, though she herself may not be directly involved in their treatment, her understanding of the factors responsible for such disturbances should assist her in their general management and nursing. More particularly in this section we are concerned with the role of the nurse in a residential child psychiatric unit, dealing with the most severe forms of childhood disturbance; her task in this situation is an absolutely vital one and she will be instrumental in determining the success or failure of the unit's treatment programme. In most units of this type she will participate actively in discussions with senior staff concerning the individualised programme for each child, but certain **general principles** are of great importance.

1. To a much greater extent than is customary she will be required to tolerate behaviour of an antisocial kind. Punishment has almost always been tried by the parents prior to the child's admission and will have been found to have no value. The nurse's primary task is to understand the child and to realise that his symptoms represent the result of underlying conflicts and handicaps.

2. Wherever possible, she aims to give the children some share in the running of the group life of the ward so that they can experience for themselves the effects of undesirable behaviour.

3. It is necessary to create a regular pattern of ward life, for consistent handling of the disturbed child is even more important than for his normal counterpart.

4. In the early stages, and in special circumstances, some " bad " behaviour will be tolerated, but as increasing contacts are made with the children and stronger relationships are established they will be corrected for wrong-doing in a firm but kindly way.

5. Contact with parents will be maintained as much as possible and no effort will be spared to prevent their feeling excluded from the treatment programme.

6. Despite the importance of consistency, treatment programmes in a children's ward need to be flexible and will need considerable modification as the child improves. There is no place for attitudes determined by how the child *should* respond, only for those determined by how the child actually *does* respond.

With the most severely disturbed children, including the psychotic ones, a very special type of relationship may need to be established between the nurse and the child. Here the nurse becomes, more than ever, a kind of mother-substitute and permits the child to go back to a quite infantile level of behaviour in order to encourage the establishment of contact with her. This regression, always under a psychiatrist's supervision, might permit a child of six or eight years of age to go back to bottle-feeding and to being cared for in napkins. In such a regressed state good emotional contact may be made for the first time, following which the ordinary pressures will be brought to bear on him towards domestic socialisation, toilet-training, good eating and sleeping habits, but skilfully and in such a way as not to interfere with the relationship between nurse and child. This specialised kind of nursing programme with severely disturbed children is a very exacting task and some nurses, however adequate in other areas, will find that their personalities do not enable them to carry out this type of work with any degree of comfort. Others will find in this form of nursing therapy a particular challenge, demanding exceptional patience and tolerance, yet bringing its own very special rewards.

14

MENTAL RETARDATION

In recent years there has been an increasing interest in the problems of the mentally retarded child and adult. In the past the subject has been seriously neglected, partly because there seemed to be so little that could be done by way of treatment; even more than this, the mentally retarded person was presented as a grave threat to society and was blamed indiscriminately for many social evils. It was feared that their number was increasing, so much so that serious writers felt that they might multiply to such an extent as to threaten our society with disaster. **Binet,** a French psychologist who in 1910 developed very valuable methods of measuring intelligence, was nevertheless extremely pessimistic about the possibilities of improving the life of the mentally retarded child through training and education. Because there were no specific medical cures, because the liability to crime was felt to be so great, and because the community did not wish to be reminded of the problem, large isolated hospitals were built for the mentally retarded, effectively excluding the majority of these patients from society.

Recent advances in knowledge have corrected many of these ideas. It has been found, for example, that those who are seriously mentally retarded do not in fact reproduce their kind. We now know that all but the most profoundly retarded can show some improvement if given the right sort of training. Increasing research and technical skills are producing different kinds of special education, the results of which are often surprising and rewarding. The development of hostels for the retarded in the community, and in particular the development of sheltered workshops, have clarified the goals of early training and have indicated that the mentally retarded person *can* contribute to society, even though in a limited way.

WHAT IS MENTAL RETARDATION?

The term mental retardation refers to a group of conditions in which the intellectual functions are markedly below the average range, the social adjustment is inadequate, there is a reduction of the capacity to learn and ordinary skills are acquired slowly or not at all, these characteristics being present from birth or from a very early age.

Though the term mental retardation is used throughout this book for the sake of consistency, precise terminology varies from one country to another. Following the Mental Health Act of 1959, the term **mental subnormality** is used in the United Kingdom, with two subcategories of degree, **subnormality** and **severe subnormality**. In other English speaking countries the terms **mentally defective** person or **intellectually handicapped** person may be employed, and it is usual to describe four degrees of defect—**mild, moderate, severe** and **profound**.

Those suffering from a **profound** degree of mental retardation are *totally dependent*; they are unable to protect themselves from ordinary physical dangers and require constant care and supervision. Those with a **severe** degree of retardation can respond to a very limited extent to a training programme and can achieve only an elementary degree of socialisation and habit training and a minimum standard of personal care; they too require unremitting care and supervision. Profound and severe degrees of retardation are almost invariably due to underlying brain damage or defect, and the failure in intellectual development is only one aspect of the total problem in these individuals; as well as a low level of drive, limited ability to form relationships and an absence of speech there may be fits, poor motor development, sensory defects and behaviour disorders.

Those with **moderate** retardation are less handicapped, are *trainable* and may achieve a semi-independent state in adult life. As children, though unable to benefit from formal education, they may respond to specialised education and training programmes.

When retardation is **mild** the child will still need supervision and guidance; though he will be incapable of receiving the proper benefit from normal education he will respond to a modified formal educational programme, conducted either in a special school or in a special class in a normal school.

THE FREQUENCY OF MENTAL RETARDATION

Many surveys have shown that the average community contains approximately 1 *per cent* of mentally retarded individuals. Roughly 75 *per cent* of these will be mildly retarded, 20 *per cent* will be moderately retarded and 5 *per cent* will be in the severely or profoundly retarded groups. A further 1 *per cent* of the community, while not retarded in the true sense, will be of borderline or dull-normal intelligence (p. 306) and will require special educational facilities. The ratio of children to adults in each of these groups will be higher than for the community as a whole, partly because the mentally retarded have a substantially lower life expectancy than that of the general population, this being particularly marked for those who are severely handicapped. Many who are mildly retarded are unrecognised before they commence to attend school, or fade away into the community after completing their education, so that it is during the period of schooling, particularly at the secondary level, that the problem shows up most clearly. Figures indicate that the period between the ages of 10 and 16 is probably the most testing time for the mildly retarded.

CAUSATION

Just as in every community there are some people who are tall and others who are short, so there are some with a better intellectual endowment than others. Every community also has some extremely short people, much smaller than the average, whose lack of height is due to the fact that they are at one extreme of the range of variation and has not been brought about by any bodily disease. Similarly there is a substantial number of people who have no disease of their brain tissue but who have an intelligence much lower than the community average. These people comprise a significant percentage of the mentally retarded group, although their retardation is always of mild degree.

Other extremely short people have failed to grow because of some disease process affecting their bodily structures. Similarly many mentally retarded persons are abnormal because of a definite defect in the development of the brain, which may have been brought about in a wide variety of ways. These **pathological cases** of retardation are divided into two large groups.

A. Conditions Determined by Genes. Every cell in the body contains 46 **chromosomes** with the exception of the sex cells (produced by the ovaries and testes) which contain 23 and which unite in the process of fertilisation to produce the full number of 46 again. These chromosomes carry the **genes** which contain the basis of our inherited characteristics. Some abnormal genes, responsible for a particular physical or mental abnormality, may pass directly from one parent to the child, who will then be affected by the disease; these are known as **dominant genes.** Some rare conditions of this type which lead to disturbance in the developing brain tissue are **epiloia** (tuberous sclerosis), **acrocephaly** (oxycephaly) and **Huntington's chorea** (though this last does not produce mental retardation but leads to a chronic organic reaction later in life —p. 266).

In other instances the abnormal genes need to be present in both of the chromosomes which unite at fertilisation in order to produce a pathological condition; these are known as **recessive genes.** If marriage occurs between two persons, each of whom carries the abnormal recessive gene, then there is one chance in four that an offspring of their union will contain both recessives, and only in this instance does the particular abnormality develop. An example of this type of situation causing retardation is found in **phenylketonuria**. This is an inherited condition in which an abnormality of metabolism leads to brain damage and to the appearance of an abnormal substance in the urine from the time the child is six weeks old. These children, who are usually fair-haired and blue-eyed, are very rare but are of great interest as they have one of the few forms of mental retardation which can be corrected by early treatment. If the abnormal substance is detected in the urine at an early enough stage (and the test is a very simple one), it has recently been found that with special dietary treatment the development of mental retardation can be prevented.

Another abnormality connected with the chromosomes is found in the condition known as **Down's syndrome** (mongolism). Recent research has established that the cells of such an individual contain 47 chromosomes and not the usual 46; how this situation comes about is not at all clear but there appears to be some definite connection with the mother's age, as the average age of the mother of a mongol baby is 36 years compared with an average for all births of 28 years. Other factors, as yet unknown, are probably important. Down's syndrome, which accounts for about 10 *per cent* of all forms of mental retardation, is a condition characterised by a round skull (rather flattened at the back), a small mouth, large tongue, eyes which slope downwards and inwards with a fold of skin at their medial border, scanty hair, simple ears and square and pudgy hands with characteristic markings and from which the fingers stick out in a distinctive way. Congenital heart disease is frequently associated with this condition and there is a flabby muscular system. Retardation is most commonly of moderate degree, though about one-third are severely affected; only very few are mildly handicapped. They are usually placid and easily managed, though they are very susceptible to infection; before the development of modern chemotherapy it was unusual for them to reach adult life.

B. Mental Retardation Caused by Damage to the Brain.
Mental retardation can be brought about by a wide range of conditions which affect the brain and which may act either during pregnancy, during birth or in the early months or years of life.

PRENATAL FACTORS. Virus diseases such as German measles, mumps and possibly chickenpox occurring in the mother during the first three months of her pregnancy may cause damage to the nervous system of the foetus. X-rays in pregnancy may be a potential danger. Anything which reduces the supply of oxygen to the baby, such as a threatened miscarriage, may damage the nervous tissue, because this is the part of the body which is most susceptible to oxygen lack. Occasionally brain damage occurs in the child of a woman with a special blood group known as " Rh negative " who is married to a man of the " Rh positive " blood group.

FACTORS OPERATING AT BIRTH. A difficult, precipitate or prolonged labour may cause brain damage either directly, through deprivation of oxygen, or through haemorrhage into the brain tissue.

FACTORS IN EARLY CHILDHOOD. Brain damage in early life may be due to infections such as encephalitis, meningitis, congenital syphilis or brain abscess. Various poisons may produce the same effect, as may any direct physical injury to the brain. A very small percentage of mentally retarded children have a defective development of the thyroid gland; they are known as **cretins** and if given early treatment with thyroid tablets or thyroxine they will frequently achieve normal physical and mental growth.

A further group of cases is described under the heading of **secondary mental retardation.** The personality, including the intellectual functions, cannot develop in isolation but will mature only in response to appropriate conditions in the environment. If the child is for any reason cut off from his environment, his intelligence cannot develop adequately and this situation leads to what is known as secondary retardation.

For example, if a child is deaf from birth and is not given a special education and training to overcome this handicap, his intellectual development must inevitably be limited. Similarly, if he is handicapped by some speech disorder through which he is unable to express himself, or if he is kept in a very limited environment due to some other type of physical disability, then again he will be deprived of many of the situations which normally promote intellectual growth. A child who is severely emotionally disturbed, perhaps suffering from a psychiatric illness from early infancy onwards, will be similarly cut off from his environment and the same sort of result would be anticipated. Other children are not actually isolated from their environment but are reared in an emotional climate which is so poor that it fails to promote the normal development of personality. One writer found that 10 *per cent* of cases in a hospital for the mentally retarded had no physical abnormality and considered that the cause of the mental backwardness in these individuals lay in grossly inadequate mothering.[1]

It should be noted that many cases of mental retardation are not brought about by one factor alone but are the end result of a combination of two or more of the factors considered in this chapter.

DIAGNOSIS AND TREATMENT

The greater the variation of the child from the normal, the earlier will his defect be diagnosed. Once it is established that the child is mentally retarded then the psychiatrist attempts to ascertain a cause for the condition, though this is not possible in every case. A search for causes not infrequently reveals factors which can be corrected; for example, the child may be found to be deaf or to have marked emotional disturbance. We must however face the unfortunate fact that there are very few forms of mental retardation which respond to specific medical treatment; phenylketonuria and cretinism are two important exceptions.

[1] Bourne, H. (1955). *Lancet* 2, 1156.

What can be done is to reduce to a minimum the degree of handicap which the child experiences as a result of his retardation. There will be need for a suitable training programme for him and a good deal of guidance and support for the family, for the discovery that a child is mentally backward invariably causes parents a good deal of stress, often associated with guilt, and they need the opportunity to discuss their feelings to help them to come to grips with the situation.

It is obviously important, when considering training, to assess the degree of mental retardation which is present and **intelligence tests** have been devised to assist in this regard. If a child can carry out a variety of tests which have been found to be at the level of capacity of a normal eight-year-old, then we say that this child has a **mental age** of eight, whatever his true age. If his true age (known as his **chronological age**) is 12, then we can derive from these figures an estimate of his intelligence known as the **intelligence quotient** (I.Q.) which is measured as follows:

$$\frac{\text{Mental Age (M.A.)}}{\text{Chronological Age (C.A.)}} \times 100 = \text{Intelligence Quotient (I.Q.)}.$$

For the above-mentioned child the intelligence quotient is 66 (*i.e.*, $\frac{8}{12} \times 100 = 66$).

Normal intelligence quotients range from 90 to 110, but we do not label a person as mentally retarded unless his I.Q. is below 70. Those individuals with an I.Q. of between 80 and 90 are said to have **dull-normal intelligence,** while those with an I.Q. of between 70 and 80 are described as **borderline.** In measuring the degree of retardation described earlier in this chapter it will be found that those of mild degree have an I.Q. range of approximately 55 to 70, the moderately retarded have an I.Q. between 35 and 55, the severely retarded between 20 and 35, while those whose retardation is profound have an I.Q. of less than 20, their mental age not developing beyond two years or thereabouts. The mild group, as previously mentioned, are capable of benefiting from a modified programme of formal schooling, but the moderately and severely retarded, while not responsive to formal education, can usually be trained in many domestic, social and practical situations.

From a psychological point of view the mentally retarded child has all the ordinary needs of a normal child plus additional requirements created by his handicap. Like the normal child he requires affection, acceptance, consistency and the right amount of stimulation at the right time; even more than the normal child he will be at a disadvantage if rejected or overprotected or if forced beyond his capacities.

HOME OR INSTITUTION?

The parents of a mentally retarded child often face a major decision as to whether the child should be cared for at home or in an institution. This decision is influenced by many factors—the actual condition of the child, the personalities and financial resources of the parents, the likely effects on other children in the home and the services available in the neighbourhood. The problem posed by a mentally handicapped child who is accepted by his parents and who lives in a neighbourhood where there is a special school and good community resources is a very different problem from that which exists where a child, equally retarded, is poorly tolerated at home and where there are no community services. The position is particularly complicated in the case of illegitimate children, who might normally be adopted but who cannot be treated in this way if they show obvious signs of mental retardation.

Though as a general rule home care is to be preferred, at least during the earliest years, it may in individual cases be very difficult to decide whether a child should be placed in an institution, or when this placement should take place. Severely retarded children usually get placed in institutions early and have little likelihood of getting out. A child with Down's syndrome, because of the distinctive physical signs, can usually be recognised at birth. Many mentally retarded children in the moderate range, but without distinctive physical signs, do not have their condition diagnosed until the age of 12 months or even later, when much has happened to establish the child in his family and by which time the parents may have come to love him and the child to respond to them.

The modern management of the mentally retarded child tends more and more towards the provision of services to help the family keep him at home where this is possible, to assist them with their difficult burden and to arrange training and day care at centres in the community. Nevertheless, for a variety of reasons, a large number of retarded children will require long-term residential care.

RESIDENTIAL CARE

It is important that institutions should never be regarded merely as places for permanent isolation of the mentally retarded. Every effort should be made to develop living conditions which approximate the normal as closely as possible. A child who is placed away from home should not have his ties with his family severed. If there is any possibility of his rehabilitation into the community then his training and education should be directed towards this end. Like any psychiatric patient it is desirable for him to be occupied in satisfying and useful ways, though the danger is always present that the institution may come to rely on his work and that he will become so valuable to it that he will have less chance of leaving.

For children in institutions an especially important matter will be their training in personal care, cleanliness and social independence. This training, though directed by a psychiatrist or educationalist, will ultimately be the responsibility of the nurse.

Training Programmes[1]

Effective training requires the use of skilled and keenly interested staff and is best carried out with small groups of

[1] The principles in this section have been slightly adapted from Schonell, F. J., Richardson, J. A. & McConnell, Thelma S. (1958). *The Subnormal Child At Home*. London: Macmillan & Co.

patients who do not differ widely in their degree of retardation. All the following points will need consideration in the establishment of an adequate training programme:

1. Because of their handicap, most of these children can only be expected to acquire simple habits and will do so at a slow rate.

2. The task to be learned should be divided into a succession of very simple steps to be taken one at a time.

3. They become frustrated very easily when they do not know exactly what it is they are required to do.

4. Training must provide these children with activities which are within their understanding and which will give them the experience of success, however limited the actual achievement may be.

5. The question of timing is therefore important; it is desirable that a child be taught a certain skill when he really needs it and only when it seems possible that he will achieve some degree of mastery.

6. A substantial number of repetitions will usually be necessary to produce a new piece of behaviour.

7. It will be found that a small amount of teaching at frequent intervals is much more satisfactory than long periods of instruction.

8. It is desirable wherever possible to relate the learning process to the child's everyday life, when he will have a much better chance to understand what is really required.

9. Group experiences are important, because some of their emotional needs will be best met if they have the opportunity to mix with other children and take part in group play; such activities may also help to stabilise their behaviour.

10. Even though training is best carried out in groups, the level of teaching must however be graded to the capacities and needs of each individual child.

11. These children tend to be afraid of new situations, in confronting which they need a good deal of extra support.

PSYCHIATRIC NURSING

12. Discipline needs to be consistent, even more so than with normal children, yet without diminishing emphasis on the fact that the child is loved and wanted.

13. It is important that incontinent children should be kept dry as far as possible, so that dryness becomes the more usual condition and the more pleasant and desirable one.

Special Problems

Many mentally retarded children, especially where the condition is due to brain damage, will show behaviour problems in addition to their retardation and may display all the features of the brain-damaged child set out in the previous chapter (p. 290). Epileptic seizures are not infrequent and require the usual nursing care (p. 280). In addition the presence of mental retardation, together with other contributing causes, may lead to emotional problems which will require the same sort of understanding as they do when they occur in a child who is not retarded. Very common personality difficulties in these children are temper tantrums, sulking, babyish behaviour, stubbornness, vague feelings of persecution, cruelty and destructiveness. At times such a child may pretend to be physically ill in order to gain attention; in fact attention-seeking behaviour of various kinds is often a major problem. It should be within the nurse's power to find out what is causing some of these reactions; they may be a response to failure, to a sense of isolation or to boredom.

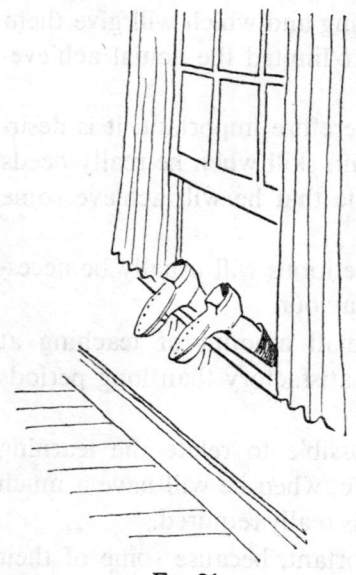

Fig. 21
Attention-seeking behaviour may be a major problem

The management of behaviour problems in the retarded, however, tends to be restricted in its effectiveness because of their limited ability in the areas of verbal communication, concept formation and abstract thought. For this reason behaviour therapy (p. 340) may be one of the more rewarding approaches to the reduction of behaviour problems in the moderately, severely and profoundly retarded. The diagnostic process must include a careful assessment of the patient's areas of good function and malfunction so that a " precision " training programme may be prescribed.

THE RETARDED CHILD IN THE COMMUNITY

The child who remains at home will still require special education and training, preferably in a small class and with teaching particularly directed towards personal development and social adjustment. Temporary relief for the mother should always be available. Recently there has been considerable development in the provision of special education for this group, with an increasing availability of special schools and classes and day attendance programmes.

When the handicapped child leaves school it may be unrealistic to attempt to place him in open employment, and it may be desirable for him to attend a sheltered workshop, either a terminal or a training workshop. In a **terminal workshop** a moderately or severely retarded youth or adult can do useful and remunerative work under supervision, tasks such as assembly jobs, folding cardboard boxes and paper-bags, packaging and dismantling—in fact the kind of work that most people would consider tedious and uninteresting. These workshops also provide a focal point for some kind of social life for the retarded adult who lives at home. Mildly retarded persons, who are unable to enter open employment on leaving school, may be able to do so after a period of attendance at a **training workshop,** where they develop simple skills, a work routine and a higher measure of social independence.

CONCLUSION

A firm diagnosis of mental retardation means that, except in rare instances, we are dealing with an individual whose intellectual and social handicap will be lifelong and for whom ordinary medical treatment is of no avail. The problem then becomes one of making the most of such a person's assets, and modern educational and training programmes are beginning to dispel the pessimism which previously surrounded the whole subject. Though these programmes are best undertaken in the community wherever possible, there will always be a substantial demand for hospital care to meet the needs of a limited group, and in this setting the skills and enthusiasm of the psychiatric nurse are of crucial importance.

15

PSYCHOSOMATIC REACTIONS

THE term psychosomatic comes from two Greek words meaning **mind** and **body**. Though it is by now firmly established as part of the language of doctors and nurses it is basically an unfortunate word, because it quite incorrectly suggests that mind and body are two separate and distinct things, each of which is capable of functioning independently of the other. The use of the word " mind ", however, is only a shorthand way of describing various functions of one part of the body, namely the brain. The thoughts, feelings and drives which make up mental life are products of the function of the brain, just as blood cells are the products of bone marrow and bile the result of liver function. A useful definition of mind, in fact, is " brain in action ". So that, when we use the word " psychosomatic ", we are simply describing the ways in which the activity of one particular part of the body, the brain, can affect the function of other bodily organs and systems.

MIND-BODY RELATIONSHIPS

It is nevertheless vital to consider the various ways in which one's feelings can affect the functioning of bodily organs. (Note that it is feelings, rather than thoughts, which are of major concern.) Also later in this chapter there will be noted some of the ways in which disease in the bodily structures may alter the state of a person's feelings. Both of these processes are common knowledge—it has been recognised for centuries that various emotions produce certain physical sensations. We speak in everyday language of people being " sick with anxiety ", " hoarse with rage ", or " trembling with fear "; a person's heart may " race with excitement " or a situation may be described as "so disgusting that it made me want to vomit". Many completely normal individuals find that a period of marked anxiety can produce headache, indigestion, diarrhoea (" pre-examination diarrhoea "), frequency of urination and so on. On the other hand, quite minor physical ailments, a persistently sore toe or a severe cold, can create a mood of irritability and depression. Even the normal bodily changes of the menstrual cycle will be found by many women to affect their mental outlook, a mood of anxiety, irritability or pessimism being extremely common in the few days before the menstrual flow begins. (Some bodily illnesses cause a *physical* effect on the brain by depriving it of oxygen or through a toxic process—for example, congestive cardiac failure or pneumonia—but these are regarded as organic, not psychosomatic reactions, and have been described in Chapter 12.)

Some of the most common effects which emotions can produce on bodily organs are shown in the following paragraphs.

Cardiovascular System: Alteration in heart rate (usually faster, occasionally slower); alteration in skin colour (blushing or pallor produced by changes in the small blood vessels in the skin); rise or fall in blood pressure.

Respiratory System: Increased respiratory rate; contraction of small bronchioles.

Gastrointestinal System: Alteration in gastric activity and the secretion of the stomach's glands (each may be either increased or decreased); increased peristalsis and rapid evacuation of the intestines, or interference with intestinal activity.

Blood: Blood clotting hastened, increased red blood cell count and blood volume (due to contraction of the spleen).

Endocrine System: Increased activity of various endocrine glands, particularly the thyroid and adrenal glands.

Urinary System: Frequency of urination; alteration in the amount of salt and water excreted by the kidney.

Reproductive System: Increase or decrease of menstrual flow (which may cease entirely during severe emotional stress); drying of secretions.

Locomotor System: Increased muscle tension—less commonly, muscular weakness.

It is also probable that different emotions have different effects on the body. Probably the most famous stomach ever known belonged to a man named Tom who, following an illness in childhood, underwent an operation which left part of the lining of his stomach lying outside the wall of his abdomen, so that changes in it could be clearly seen. He worked for two American doctors and allowed them to record the effect on his stomach of various situations, findings which proved to be so important that an entire book was written about them.[1] Among many other things it was noted that feelings of fear or depression caused his gastric mucous membrane to turn pale and led to reduced activity of the stomach. But on occasions when he was angry or resentful the stomach lining became red and engorged with blood, gastric activity was increased and there was much more secretion of gastric juice.

Another experiment, carried out on a group of normal American college students, suggested that the effect of anger on the heart and blood pressure depended on whether the students were angry with themselves or angry with other people.

THE CAUSES OF PSYCHOSOMATIC REACTIONS

All the effects of emotion so far described can be observed in quite normal people. A particular state of feeling produces some temporary alteration in the function of one of the body systems and then, when the emotion subsides, the bodily change also settles down and no harm has been done. But the term psychosomatic reaction is used to describe those

---

[1] Wolf, S. & Wolff, H. G. (1947). *Human Gastric Function*. London: Oxford University Press.

conditions in which emotion, usually long-continued, creates a bodily change which does *not* subside. The end result is a definite physical change in the organs concerned which cannot easily be reversed. The patient has developed a physical illness as a result, at least partly, of emotional disturbance.

Other factors enter into causation in most instances. Many psychosomatic illnesses run in families, the patient seemingly having an inherited tendency to respond to stress by a reaction in one particular organ or system. Causes of a directly physical kind are often of substantial importance, though they play a greater part in some cases than others. In asthma, for example, both infection in the respiratory passages and allergy to some particular substance may contribute towards the development of an asthmatic attack, yet in many patients the symptoms only appear when emotional disturbance is finally added to the other two factors.

Why emotions have such a serious effect on some people and not others is not fully understood. The additional hereditary and physical factors may be vital in some instances, but the way in which the individual deals with emotion seems also to be of great importance. If a man should encounter a situation which causes him to feel angry, certain changes—in stomach, or blood vessels, or intestines—occur in his body; if he can *be* angry, " blow off " his emotion, as it were, then the feeling passes and the condition of his organs returns to normal. But he may not be able to show his anger (he may, for instance, be angry with the boss on whom he depends for his livelihood, or with his invalid wife) so that the feeling may persist, with the result that the bodily changes also persist. Alternatively, it may be that he is a chronically angry person, always full of resentment towards the people and things around him; it may even be that he is fairly regularly angry without being aware of this, for unconscious long-continued emotional states may produce the same effects on his body as conscious ones. Yet another possibility is that he is aware of his anger but, because of certain deep conflicts about angry feelings (p. 145), he cannot allow himself to express them even though the external situation would not prevent it. It may be, for example, that his conscience is so strict that he cannot allow himself to acknowledge angry feelings as part of his personality. In all these situations bodily changes are occurring which are not being adequately reversed and a pathological alteration in the organs may be the result.

Similarly, arousal of sexual feelings normally leads to an increased flow of blood to the sexual organs; this persists until the excitement culminates in the sexual climax or orgasm, after which the organs return to their basic state. If this climax does not occur, then the increased blood flow may to some extent persist, leading after a period of time to chronic congestion in the pelvis which gives rise to pain, tenderness and excessive menstruation. An unsatisfying sexual life, with repeated sexual arousal short of orgasm, may therefore lead directly to common gynaecological symptoms.

The deeper psychological factors involved in the causation of psychosomatic reactions seem to be very similar to those found in the study of neurotic and psychotic illnesses. Here again we find emotional conflicts, usually repressed, with their origins in childhood experience and leading to major difficulties concerning sex, aggression and so on. Why it is that some individuals develop psychosomatic reactions, and not neurotic symptoms or character problems as the end result of these conflicts, is not yet clearly known. The mechanism by which the bodily changes are brought about is however quite definite. Most of the alterations described, it will be noted, are in those organs whose nerve supply is through the involuntary or autonomic nervous system, chronic emotional stress leading to overactivity of either the sympathetic or parasympathetic divisions of this system, or to a lack of balance between the actions of these two divisions. In other instances the bodily changes are the result of alterations in the function of endocrine glands, the primary effect being on the anterior part of the pituitary and the adrenal cortex. Both these mechanisms are dependent upon the activity of the hypothalamus which is in turn influenced by the cerebral cortex.

There are many diseases or specific symptom complexes in which emotional conflicts play a significant causative role. In some instances the psychomatic factor seems to be the predominant one, in other patients it is but one of several factors which combine to make the illness manifest or which trigger bouts of illness in those which run an intermittent course, such as migraine or bronchial asthma. Yet another possibility is that the psychosomatic factor is partly responsible for the instability of the disease or its failure to respond to treatment; some adolescent diabetics, for example, show this very clearly.

As far as the **cardiovascular system** is concerned, important psychosomatic issues arise in diseases as diverse as essential hypertension, myocardial infaction and migraine, but chronic conflict and underlying neurotic problems may also lead to pain in the region of the heart, palpitation, breathlessness and weakness without any evidence of structural heart disease.

In the **respiratory system** the most serious example is bronchial asthma, but many patients with chronic anxiety may present with rapid, shallow breathing, feelings of faintness and tingling in the hands (the hyperventilation syndrome). Emotionally induced disturbances of the **gastrointestinal system** may appear as chronic constipation or diarrhoea without structural change, but there is also a good deal of evidence to show that both duodenal ulcer and ulcerative colitis are significantly related to personality problems. Emotional conflict may also result in major disturbances of appetite, leading either to obesity or to the very important syndrome of **anorexia nervosa,** a disorder chiefly seen in adolescent girls which is characterised by refusal of food, amenorrhoea, restlessness and a degree of weight loss which may reach life-threatening proportions.

Disturbances of the **endocrine system** which fall into this category are thyrotoxicosis and diabetes mellitus. In the **repro-**

ductive system emotional problems may manifest themselves in a number of ways: any of the common disturbances of menstruation may be induced in this manner, and many patients with chronic pelvic pain represent examples of psychosomatic problems. Moreover, some of the most common and troublesome disturbances in sexual life, such as impotence and premature ejaculation in the male, or painful intercourse in the female, are nearly always due to psychological causes. The **skin** is one of the most obvious and common areas affected, as in many patients with neurodermatitis and eczema, pruritus (itching)—particularly when involving the genital or anal areas —and some forms of urticaria (" hives "). Finally, the psychosomatic disturbances of the **locomotor system** make up a large proportion of those patients who seek relief from general practitioners and specialists, complaining of various types of muscular pain, commonly but not exclusively in the lower region of the back or in the head (" tension headache "). Emotional conflict also plays a role in the causation or precipitation of at least some cases of rheumatoid arthritis.

It must also be mentioned that a large number of disease processes which are not caused by psychosomatic mechanisms are nevertheless aggravated or prolonged by emotional factors. In chronic cardiac disease of whatever type, for example, emotional conflict may, through a variety of mechanisms, act as the last straw which tips the patient into frank cardiac failure. Psychological conflicts are in some instances responsible for the development or the continuance of much of the abdominal distress and discomfort which may follow gastrectomy operations. Moving into still wider fields there is some evidence, far from satisfactory as yet, that personality factors play some part in the predisposition to such diseases as pulmonary tuberculosis and even cancer.

The influence of mental processes on bodily states is even more extensive than the above discussion implies, even though it is only when emotional conflict directly causes disturbed function in internal organs that we label this process " psychosomatic" in the strict sense. A disease such as cirrhosis of the liver is often brought about by prolonged alcoholic excess and malnutrition, yet these two causal factors are themselves the result of personality problems. The man who is brought to the casualty ward with a fractured skull following a vehicle accident has in not a few instances sustained this physical damage as a consequence of dangerous driving, itself the expression of his extremely aggressive personality. Cancer of the lung is now known to have a definite link with heavy cigarette smoking, but this habit is at least in part psychologically determined. The more one pursues the subject the more one realises, as was stated in the opening paragraph of this chapter, that the distinction between mind and body is an extremely artificial, even if convenient one and that a very large segment of human illness results from an interplay between those events we call "mental" and those events we call "physical".

MANAGEMENT

The proper management of the patient with a psychosomatic illness ideally involves close and careful co-operation between the psychiatric service and the general medical service of a hospital. Unfortunately in most general hospitals today, still sadly short of psychiatrically trained personnel, the psychological aspects of these conditions tend in all too many instances to be completely ignored or to be handled extremely superficially.

First-class nursing care for these patients involves detailed attention to the physical nursing procedures ordered by the physician; in such diseases as duodenal ulcer, ulcerative colitis or severe asthma these may be extremely complex and their proper employment may be literally life-saving in some instances. A proper understanding of the psychological factors leading up to the illness does not make these physical treatment procedures any less important.

Awareness of the significance of emotional factors does not

justify any probing, by the nurse or any other individual, into the patient's personal life. Some aspects of this may be spontaneously revealed by him in discussion with the nurse, but in psychosomatic reactions energetic efforts to discover his emotional conflicts may be positively harmful. Even if the psychiatrist is called in consultation and takes the patient into psychotherapy, he too will only with great caution utilise the " uncovering " type of approach which is frequently used in the management of neurotic reactions (p. 330).

Nevertheless, psychological aspects of nursing care may be of profound importance in these disorders. First and foremost, many or most of these patients have deep, often very guilt-laden regressive tendencies, that is, they have at an unconscious level profound wishes to be completely taken care of, but hesitate to abandon themselves to these because of the guilty feelings which would result. Part of the care of psychosomatic reactions may involve gratification of these wishes; in the hospitalised patient with peptic ulcer it is without doubt the complete dependence permitted by the hospital, as much or more than the rigid diet of milk and soft foods (which in itself may have the symbolic meaning of regression to infancy), which is an important part of the healing process. Many ulcer patients, symptom-free in hospital, experience pain immediately after discharge, even though they maintain their medical and dietary treatment. An important part of nursing care, therefore, is the provision of an environment in which the patient can give himself up for a time to his dependent wishes without anxiety or guilt. Measures of this kind are of great importance in such diverse diseases as duodenal ulcer, thyrotoxicosis and diabetes mellitus. The nurse need have no fear that she is making the patient's problem more difficult in the long run by temporarily giving in to his wish for total dependence.

The other important aspect of nursing care is the tactful provision of an emotional climate in which the patient can feel free to express his feelings. It is often thought that, because feelings are responsible for the illness, correct management should therefore involve the damping down of these feelings, either by the prescription of a sedative drug or by well-meant but useless advice to "stop worrying". In actual fact, as the earlier part of this chapter has shown, it is not simply the presence of feelings which creates difficulty, but the existence of *hidden* feelings which, for one reason or another, are unable to be expressed. It has often been reported, for instance, that a severe attack of asthma ceased abruptly when the patient gave vent to his feelings by crying, or by expressing anger in a strong and direct fashion. Many sufferers from migraine report that an attack will subside, or may even be forestalled, if an opportunity exists to express angry feelings. It follows that, without any suspicion of prying, the nurse may be of great assistance to her patient if he can use her for an informal, frank discussion of his feelings. If she has time to let him talk these out, this is a far better approach than advising him not to feel angry or not to feel worried.

Many patients with psychosomatic disorders need to be taken into long-term psychotherapy and indeed, in some instances, into psychoanalytic treatment (p. 327). Several studies suggest that adequate, long-continued psychological treatment helps to produce a remission of symptoms and may prevent or minimise the possibility of relapse in later years.

The physical treatments of psychiatry are rarely if ever employed in these conditions, except for the symptomatic use of sedatives and tranquillisers.

PSYCHOLOGICAL ASPECTS OF MEDICAL AND SURGICAL ILLNESSES

Every episode of physical illness has some degree of emotional significance for the patient. In Chapter 7 it was noted that certain aspects of illness might seriously threaten the individual's adjustment and act as the direct precipitants of a psychiatric disturbance (p. 137). Also, in Chapter 18, certain conflicts associated with illness and hospitalisation are referred to, and many of the principles set forth in that chapter are relevant to medical as well as psychiatric illnesses. We deal briefly at this point with the ordinary patient on the medical and surgical wards of a general hospital who, without being psychiatrically ill in any definable way, may yet by reason of his illness pose certain psychological problems of which the general hospital nurse should be aware.

Even the well-adjusted person undergoes certain changes in his mental life as a result of sickness, for all mentally healthy people take a certain degree of interest in the appearance and well-being of their own bodies. In physical illness much more attention is focussed on the diseased organs, the patient's other interests and relationships tending to be relatively lacking in genuine emotional participation. Particularly when surgical procedures are contemplated or imminent, this tendency will be greatly heightened. Even though some patients are more successful than others in concealing the extent of their concern about an operation, psychological tests show clearly that a great deal of anxiety, as might be expected, is always present at this time, although the patient's defence mechanisms may in some circumstances be so rigid that he is not even aware of it himself.

This anxiety is not harmful to the patient, being a perfectly healthy response to a very real stress. It is desirable that these feelings should be freely ventilated; many nurses and doctors find themselves too busy, or are themselves too anxious, to allow the patient to talk about his fears. Such talk is essential for many people to prevent their anxieties getting out of hand. The patient's questions need to be answered as frankly as possible at this time and, within reasonable limits, he should be aware of what is going to happen to him. This applies as much to children as to adults; experience shows that, although he may be openly anxious when first informed, it is better for a child to have an idea, within the limits of his understanding, of what is likely to take place in hospital, rather than be kept in ignorance until the very last minute.

Obviously any circumstances which create unnecessary anxiety must be strenuously avoided. A nurse, however junior, must realise that a patient sets great store by what she says, and careless remarks in his hearing may cause quite needless worry. Nurses, as well as doctors, are also apt at times to use unnecessarily complicated technical terms when explaining matters to a patient; these words, unfamiliar to him, can again be a powerful source of increased apprehension.

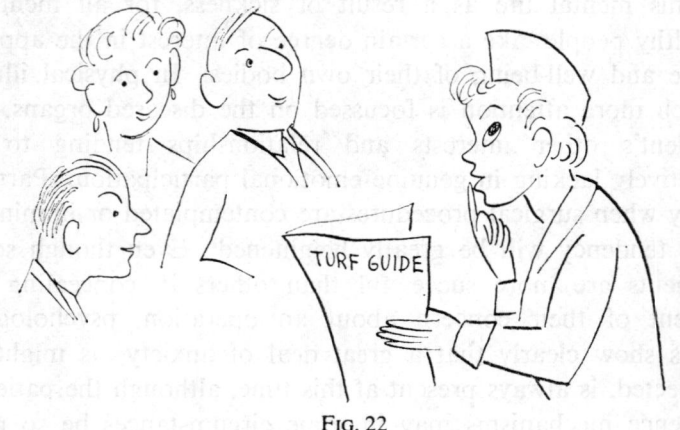

Fig. 22
A patient sets great store by what the nurse says.

When physical illness has been present for some substantial period of time, it has come to play a very significant role in the patient's mental life, and forms a part of his total adjustment to the world about him. If he has, for example, progressive heart disease, he develops a certain status as a "cardiac patient", both in his own eyes and in his contacts with his own family and wider community. The normal person can make the necessary psychological adjustments to this long-continued situation, but to the individual with latent or overt neurotic tendencies such a state of illness may be unconsciously used by him as an alibi for all sorts of failures and difficulties in his life. That is to say, physical illness may provide the opportunity for a socially acceptable avoidance of some of the individual's problems.

A brief case report may clarify this matter. A girl in early adolescence was correctly diagnosed as having mitral stenosis and over the next 10 years became increasingly disabled by progressive breathlessness and weakness. At the age of 20 she married but, because of her status as a cardiac invalid, she lived with her husband's relations, her mother-in-law running the home and caring for the patient's child. She had had an extremely disturbed childhood development and this had led to a variety of fears and anxieties concerning sexual matters; she was therefore secretly glad that her heart disease gave her a watertight excuse for avoiding, almost completely, an active sexual life. At the age of 23 she underwent a heart operation with very successful results at a physical level—yet, unexpectedly in the surgeon's eyes, she made little progress and her symptoms were as bad as ever before. What had happened was that her alibi had gone; new responsibilities were expected of her in all areas, pressure was put on her to move into a new house where she would be required to take full care of her family, her husband made normal sexual demands on her and wanted further children. The result in this case was a frank neurotic illness, with the development of psychogenic symptoms of a somatic kind which closely mimicked her pre-operative complaints. She had grown so accustomed to her role as a cardiac patient that she felt unable to face life without this shield, although in fact she later did quite well with psychiatric treatment.

In other patients unconscious needs for self-punishment, known as masochistic needs, may substantially interfere with recovery from physical illness. The patient consciously wishes to get well, but unconsciously wants his illness to continue. Other patients with hysterical personalities unwittingly prolong or exaggerate physical disabilities in order to maintain the attention-seeking relationship with other persons which is part of their way of getting by in the world (p. 187).

Special problems arise when physical illness develops in the older person; here again illnesses which involve surgical procedures appear to be especially threatening. There is an added difficulty at this time of life in that the old person is likely to be disturbed by hospitalisation and may even in some circumstances develop mental confusion as a result of separation from familiar surroundings (p. 268). Also, persons over the age of 65 are particularly liable to develop organic reactions following surgical procedures; the brain of such a person is more susceptible to the effects of anaesthesia and even small degrees of blood loss (p. 258). Even more commonly than these organic forms of reaction there may develop in the aged person a pessimistic, bitter depression as a result of his illness; the "will to live" is often weak or absent and this may be especially noticeable following the death of another patient in the ward. Many factors within the hospital may exaggerate this type of reaction. If hospital wards can be made more cheerful and less barren places than they so often are, and if the nurses can be more patient with the old person's slow reactions and fixed habits, then his overall adjustment to his illness will be greatly improved.

Convalescence and subsequent rehabilitation may pose further problems for some patients with physical illness. Much of Chapter 24, which deals in detail with this topic, will be found to have application to the care of the medical and surgical patient.

CONCLUSION

"Body" and "mind" are two aspects of the one person. Any significant interference with one aspect of the individual will have some type of effect upon the other. In some instances prolonged emotional disturbance, conscious or unconscious, may lead to serious physical changes in certain organs of the body, usually those supplied with nerve fibres by the autonomic nervous system. On the other hand, any significant degree of physical illness will affect the patient's emotional state and an adequate programme of medical and nursing care must recognise the significance to him of his disease.

16

PSYCHIATRIC TREATMENT
A: PSYCHOLOGICAL METHODS

It is customary to describe the treatments used in psychiatry under two broad headings—the **psychological forms** of treatment and the **physical forms** of treatment. Physical treatments are described in the next chapter; at this point we are concerned only with those varieties of treatment which aim at influencing the patient's feelings and behaviour through some type of interpersonal relationship. All treatment of this type is known as **psychotherapy**.

It must however be understood that these two forms of therapy are not mutually exclusive; many patients, for example, will be receiving psychotherapeutic interviews from the psychiatrist at the same time as they are taking drugs which have been prescribed by him. Also, as will be seen more fully in the following chapter, physical treatments may in themselves have a profound psychological effect on the patient; many patients lose their symptoms, at least for a time, if they believe themselves to be receiving some powerful drug, even though they are being given a tablet which does not contain any active constituent. This important aspect of treatment, known as the **placebo effect,** is discussed further on page 353. Even psychotherapy may produce some of its beneficial result in this way—the mere fact that the patient is being taken seriously and interviewed regularly may be helpful to him to some extent, whatever takes place during the interviews themselves.

PSYCHOTHERAPY AND PSYCHOANALYSIS

The word **psychoanalysis** is used in two ways—firstly, to describe the theories formulated by Freud to explain the origins of normal and abnormal human behaviour (p. 10); secondly, to describe a specific method of treatment, also introduced by Freud, the principles of which underlie a good deal of modern psychiatric therapy. Psychoanalysis in its strict form is only carried out by a qualified psychoanalyst (p. 505) and is the most radical and ambitious weapon which can be employed in the treatment of psychiatric illness. It aims to trace the origins of the patient's conflicts back to his infancy and early childhood, because it is known that unhealthy patterns of behaviour established at that time will have persisted into later life; it is believed that, if these are uncovered and brought up to the surface, the patient can then start to deal with his problems in a healthy and mature way. Contrary to much popular opinion, it is not suggested that treatment of this kind will uncover one single crucial incident in the patient's early life; it has already been seen in other parts of this book that psychiatric illness is never caused by one all-important factor acting in isolation. Nor is it suggested that, as soon as important memories from earlier times escape from repression and become part of the patient's conscious awareness, the symptoms will then immediately disappear. On the contrary, the process of psychoanalytic treatment involves the realisation by the patient of the importance of a whole series of situations in his childhood development, as well as an understanding of the significance of his present patterns of behaviour, in the hope that he will reach a much greater degree of self-knowledge, not only in one special area but involving many aspects of his character and personality. This process of self-understanding is known as **insight** and many people believe it to be of crucial importance if really significant and lasting changes are to be brought about in the patient's feelings and behaviour.

An equally important component of psychoanalytic treatment is the relationship which develops between the patient and the psychoanalyst. Popular opinion has it that patients in prolonged psychiatric treatment invariably fall in love with

TREATMENT: PSYCHOLOGICAL METHODS

the person who is treating them; certainly in a successful treatment situation the patient will at times have highly important loving, even sexual, feelings about her therapist but it is equally true to say that at other times, perhaps even at one and the same time, she will experience very powerful aggressive and destructive impulses towards him. To explain these feelings Freud introduced the extremely important concept of **transference;** this describes the patient's unconscious readiness to transfer on to the therapist powerful emotions which were first aroused during her contact with her parents, which have no connection with the therapist's actual personality or behaviour but which are experienced towards him because

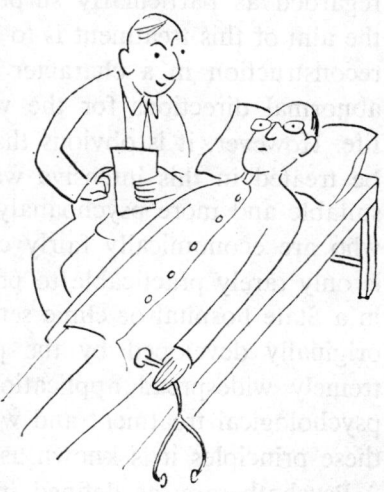

FIG. 23
The relationship which develops between the patient and the psychoanalyst.

he is for the time being a father-substitute or mother-substitute in her life. Transference is in fact a much more general phenomenon than this; very commonly a boy who has been frightened of a difficult, aggressive father will have similar feelings of fear when in contact with other powerful people in his environment, even though these new power figures are not difficult or aggressive people; he may become the office-boy described in Chapter 3 (p. 33) who quivers inside when ever he enters his boss's office, or the innocent pedestrian who nevertheless hurries guiltily by any passing policeman. Although transference assumes its most intense form during relatively long-continued psychiatric treatment procedures it is also of great importance to the nurse, as will be seen later in this chapter.

Psychoanalysis in the strict sense of the term requires the patient to attend for interviews of an hour's duration four or five times a week for at least two or three years and sometimes for a good deal longer. The length of this period will not be regarded as particularly surprising when one considers that the aim of this treatment is to produce a substantial degree of reconstruction in a character which has been developing in abnormal directions for the whole of the patient's previous life. However, it is obvious that only a very few patients can be treated in this intensive way; even if more patients were suitable and more psychoanalysts were available, only people who are economically fairly comfortable can afford it, as it is only rarely practicable to provide psychoanalytic treatment in a State hospital or clinic setting. Nevertheless the concepts originally developed by the psychoanalysts have found extremely widespread application in more modified forms of psychological treatment and when such treatment is based on these principles it is known as **psychoanalytic psychotherapy.**

Psychotherapy as defined in this way describes any treatment situation in which a trained person, usually but not necessarily a psychiatrist, sees the patient in a series of interviews which aim to bring about a favourable effect on those feelings and conflicts within him which are creating his abnormal behaviour. Because of our recognition of the significance of unconscious motives in determining human conduct, attention is paid in this form of psychotherapy to the **uncovering** of important problems which lie outside the patient's awareness. Such a treatment may be suitable for both inpatients and outpatients and may take place once, twice or even more times weekly, for a period ranging in duration from a few months up to several years. If treatment proceeds favourably, then it is hoped that there not only will be relief of the patient's symptoms but that certain changes will be brought about in his underlying personality which will make it less likely that he should develop symptoms again and also make his participation in life more satisfying and more rewarding.

TREATMENT: PSYCHOLOGICAL METHODS

Not all patients are suitable for this type of psychotherapy. Patients with neurotic reactions are generally considered to be most likely to benefit and for many or most of these some variety of psychotherapy is the treatment of choice. An increasing number of people believe that psychotherapy can bring about far-reaching changes in psychotic patients, particularly in those with schizophrenic reactions, but success here with psychotherapy alone always involves a very intensive form of treatment such as can only be provided in unusually fortunate psychiatric clinics. Even in a patient with a minor degree of organic brain damage psychotherapy is at times employed and can lead to his more efficient adaptation, if he is able through this treatment to deal more effectively with some of his conflicts. Psychotherapy also has a significant role in the management of some psychosomatic illnesses. Its place in the treatment of childhood behaviour disorders has already been considered in Chapter 13 (p. 295).

In general terms the patient who is likely to benefit from psychotherapy is the sort of person who has some degree of realisation that his past and present life experiences are tied up with his illness and who is able to talk about the various emotional components of his personality. The patient who wants to talk exclusively about his symptoms and who is not prepared or not able to look at the loves and hates and guilt feelings which are inside him is usually a difficult and often an impossible subject for this form of therapy. Even when circumstances seem to be favourable in the beginning, however, many patients break off their treatment in the fairly early stages and it is for this reason that psychotherapy is commenced for some extremely disturbed patients during hospitalisation, when it is not nearly so easy for them to avoid their regular treatment sessions. Patients who break off treatment usually do so because they find themselves becoming vaguely aware of frightening feelings which they had not suspected were part of themselves; these are often feelings stirred up in the transference relationship with their psychotherapist.

FACTORS INVOLVED IN SUCCESSFUL PSYCHOTHERAPY

It has been said above that, in the type of psychotherapy considered here, it is hoped that the patient will come to a clearer understanding of what he is really like as a person, the acquisition of this self-knowledge being called **insight**. Some of these truths about himself the patient will come to see spontaneously as he talks over his life situation with his psychotherapist; others are suggested to him by the psychiatrist in the light of the material which the patient discusses, these suggestions by the psychiatrist being known as **interpretations**. For example, the therapist may point out that while the patient has been talking about his mother he has been tearing viciously at a handkerchief and that this behaviour probably indicates a good deal of underlying destructiveness towards her. As treatment proceeds interpretations become deeper and more complicated—a young man may come to see that various aspects of his behaviour all represent a flight from facing up to an unconscious feminine component in his personality. Many of the psychiatrist's interpretations will be directed towards helping the patient see how he feels about the therapist himself; it is often more useful for him to understand his feelings in his present life situation than to talk in a theoretical way about remote events in his past. If a young woman has to learn, as many neurotic females have to learn, that she has a mixture of loving and aggressive feelings towards males with whom she is thrown into close contact, then it will be more convincing for her to see this in the first instance in connection with her feelings about the therapist, later coming to the realisation that feelings of this type are also experienced by her in her ordinary life. At times the therapist may also offer interpretations about the meaning of the patient's dreams.

It is very likely that other factors play an important part in the process of psychotherapy. Some patients lose their symptoms fairly rapidly without acquiring any increased degree of self-understanding and it is probable that for them the **support** which they derive from psychotherapy is of great value. For possibly the first time in his life the patient has found in his psychiatrist a professional person who is interested in him as an individual, who takes his complaints seriously and regards them as proper and important topics of conversation. He finds in psychotherapy that he can reveal numerous private doubts which he has had about himself for years and can discuss what he believes to have been his past failings. He is able to bring to the surface some aspects of his life which until this time had been surrounded by a wall of guilt and shame and finds that, even then, his psychotherapist remains a willing and sympathetic listener who attempts to understand him without making critical moral judgements about his present or past behaviour. Some psychotherapy relies almost exclusively on effects of this type, avoiding the uncovering type of approach which characterises the psychoanalytically based form of treatment, and is known as **supportive psychotherapy.**

Another important aspect of psychotherapy is known as **ventilation.** Many psychiatric illnesses have important origins in bottled up feelings of various kinds, particularly angry and destructive ones; some of these may be genuinely repressed, some are simply suppressed—that is, the patient is consciously aware of feeling this way but has not had the courage or chance to express himself. Release of these over-controlled emotions may bring a great deal of relief; a young man who has for some years harboured feelings of anger towards his father, whom he saw as cruel and disinterested, will tend to feel much better in himself if he can forcibly express these feelings to a psychiatrist, particularly when he finds that the latter accepts these without criticism and also gives him to understand that it is far from uncommon for people to have a good deal of anger towards their fathers.

Contrary to popular opinion, **suggestion** and **persuasion** play little part in psychotherapy, at least in any direct way. It is a common error to suppose that psychiatrists spend a good part of their time in arguing with their patients about their symptoms or in trying to convert them to the psychiatrist's own view of life. Persuasion in the usual sense of the term cannot possibly alter an individual's unhealthy attitudes nor cause his symptoms to disappear, for these attitudes and symptoms result from conflicts which as we know are quite deeply buried in the patient's mind.

SPECIAL VARIETIES OF PSYCHOTHERAPY

Hypnosis. Nurses are often surprised that treatment by hypnosis is not more frequently employed in psychiatry. Its " magical " flavour gives it a special fascination for many people and it has a particular attraction for some highly dependent individuals who hope that, by having hypnotic treatment, they can completely abandon any responsibility for getting themselves well and can shift the burden entirely on to someone else. Actually there is nothing magical about hypnosis, even though certain aspects of it are not completely understood; the practice of hypnosis requires no special gift and the hypnotic state can usually be fairly readily induced in another person who desires to be hypnotised and who has faith in the powers of the hypnotist. It is worth emphasising, however, that hypnosis should only ever be carried out by someone who has had substantial psychological or psychiatric training; amateur and untrained hypnotists, although they may be able to provide an entertaining spectacle on the stage, can in some instances cause serious harm to their subjects.

There are three possible therapeutic uses to which the state of hypnosis may be put. Firstly, hypnosis can be used to remove by direct suggestion neurotic symptoms which result from psychological conflict. This is an extremely dangerous proceeding, as might be expected from consideration of Chapter 9, in which it was learnt that neurotic symptoms arise as a defence against unconscious mental conflict. Sudden removal of such symptoms, therefore, without any attempt to deal with the underlying conflict, may frequently lead to the patient being in a much worse state than when he began treatment, even though the particular symptom for which he sought help has been removed; he may for instance become seriously depressed or panicky and some successful suicidal attempts have been reported immediately following treatment of this kind. A second and much more legitimate use is where the hypnotic state is employed to enable the patient to talk about problems which have been repressed from his awareness, or about which he would have had great difficulty in talking in the fully conscious state. This procedure is sometimes known as **hypnoanalysis.** The third and perhaps the most legitimate use of hypnosis is in the field of general medicine, not in psychiatry at all. It has great value in abolishing or diminishing pain of physical origin and has been successfully employed in obstetrics, in dentistry and as an aid to various forms of anaesthesia. It may be very effective in the alleviation of chronic pain due to organic disease, such as in terminal cancer, when its use may substantially reduce the amount of narcotic drugs required by the patient.

Narcoanalysis. The process of psychotherapy is sometimes hastened by the use of drugs, usually but not always given intravenously. Although these drugs are popularly known as "truth drugs", it is very doubtful whether they do in fact uncover material which had been genuinely repressed; more commonly they assist the patient to produce information about himself, communication of which has previously been blocked by excessive anxiety or guilt. Moreover there is no guarantee of the truth of the material produced in this way; on the contrary, in some instances elaborate fantasies are described which are deceptive and confusing. Occasionally these drugs are used by the psychiatrist for diagnostic rather than therapeutic purposes; for example, a patient whose diagnosis has been doubtful during ordinary conscious interviewing may under the influence of drugs reveal evidence of disordered thinking or of delusional beliefs which confirms the presence of a schizophrenic reaction.

The drugs most frequently employed are "Pentothal Sodium", "Amytal Sodium" and "Methedrine", either singly or in combination, all of which tend to diminish the patient's control over his thoughts and feelings. At times quite violent emotional reactions may occur after the drug is given and the nurse may be asked to stand by on such occasions; in any event she will be required to prepare the usual equipment necessary for intravenous injections.

Another type of drug altogether is lysergic acid diethylamide (LSD), usually given orally, which produces a severe though temporary disorganisation of the patient's personality and may give rise to hallucinations and feelings of depersonalisation and lead to a state which is similar in some respects to a schizophrenic reaction. In such a condition patients may acquire extraordinarily rapid and important insights into certain aspects of their personality; previously repressed events of childhood may come flooding into consciousness with great vividness and a profound emotional crisis may be experienced. This state is sometimes allowed to continue for two hours or more and, as the psychiatrist may not be able to be in attendance for the whole of this period, the nurse may be asked to stand by and maintain a supportive relationship with the patient during this time. It is important in these circumstances to keep a careful record of the patient's attitudes and statements for the guidance of the psychiatrist, who will probably discuss the material in later psychotherapy sessions with him.

Group Psychotherapy. Since World War II a great deal of interest has developed in the treatment of psychiatric illness by the use of group techniques. In its classical and best understood form (hereafter called **small group therapy**) this involves the treatment of a small number of patients, usually ranging from 6 to 10, by regular (usually weekly) sessions in which the aims are very similar to those of individual psychotherapy. The patients are usually those with symptom neuroses or borderline psychotic illnesses, though very similar techniques have also been applied to the treatment of chronic alcoholism, drug dependence, a variety of psychosomatic problems and have also been utilised in delinquent and prison populations. Usually the group is a **closed** one, *i.e.,* a fixed number of members begin treatment at the same time and remain together throughout their course of therapy. Group therapy of this type is regarded by its practitioners as having certain definite advantages over individual therapy, even though there may be less detailed analysis of the patient's earliest relationships which laid the foundation of his illness; in particular, patients learn a great deal about their current interactions with other people through experiencing and analysing these under the supervision of a skilled leader. Clinical experience repeatedly shows that group therapy can produce a degree of self-understanding and symptom reduction sufficient to permit the patient to function thereafter in a more mature and less troubled way. Patients are selected for group psychotherapy in much the same way as for psychotherapy in general (p. 331), but it is still far from clear which patients do better in individual treatment and which may make more progress in a group. Sometimes these two forms of treatment are combined, using the same therapist or different therapists.

With the growth of the therapeutic community idea, however, many other types of group have become commonplace within the psychiatric hospital (p. 409). Many units now commence each day with a group meeting attended by all the patients and most or all staff members. The primary purpose of this meeting is usually seen as providing a forum in which anyone may bring up personal or group problems, with the aim of promoting free communication and resolving where possible the difficulties that arise out of living together at close quarters over an extended period of time. Patients are encouraged to reach their own decisions about various administrative matters that affect their daily life in hospital, though the amount of decision-making that is entrusted to patients will vary according to the psychiatrist's own training and beliefs. Some psychiatrists, but by no means all, go even further and encourage intimate personal revelations and interpretations, by staff or by other patients, in such groups; such psychiatrists are those who tend to see the community meeting as the single most important factor in hospital treatment (p. 410). Nurses will be expected to play an active part in these meetings, which are usually followed by meetings of staff members only at which the events of the group session just completed are discussed and evaluated. These inpatient groups are of course *open* groups, members leaving the group at the termination of their hospitalisation and new members joining as soon as they are admitted. There is a wide difference of opinion as to whether *all* psychiatric inpatients are suitable for such treatment, or whether some selection should be employed.

Other group meetings, concerned with social and recreational activities, are also regular features of a modern psychiatric hospital. Nurses may be invited to lead such groups, and when sufficiently trained and experienced may also act as group leaders for smaller groups of patients (*e.g.*, a group of adolescents) who are discussing rather more personal material including their own deeper psychological conflicts. None of these group activities, however, should be confused with classical small group therapy as previously defined, which has much more radical aims and which attempts to bring about a very substantial change in the patient's psychological problems and the way in which he handles and expresses them.

It is perhaps impossible for the nurse to understand very much about small group therapy without participating in a group or observing a group in action. It is however helpful for her to have some general knowledge of what is involved for a patient undergoing this treatment. Though there are some exceptions, the majority of group therapists tend to be relatively non-directive in their approach, that is to say, they expect the group to talk about their problems and difficulties with little or no guidance from the leader. Each patient is encouraged to take a critical interest in the statements of the other members and to help them to understand the real significance of what they are saying. As in individual treatment, special notice is taken of the feelings stirred up in the members during the session and in particular the feelings which they experience towards each other and towards the group leader. No aspect of behaviour is too small to be scrutinised by the group should it appear to have some relevance and a substantial part of a meeting, for example, may be spent in looking at the particular seating arrangement taken up by the patients, or in trying to understand why a particular member is silent at some stage of the group proceedings. Free expression of feeling is permitted, patients being encouraged to be themselves and to act in a less defensive and controlled manner than they would do in ordinary social life. Patients can see in the group the effect on others of their own immature behaviour; moreover, their own reaction to the statements of other patients may make certain previously mysterious aspects of their own life more understandable to them.

Certain false beliefs about small group therapy are worth mentioning because they are commonly held by nurses. Firstly, as in individual therapy, the group does *not* consist of an attempt by the group leader to make everyone think and feel as he does; individual differences between people are tolerated and in fact encouraged and one substantial gain in patients undergoing group therapy is an increased respect for the attitudes and beliefs of others. Secondly, it is extremely rare for confidential material to leak outside the group room, the group quickly developing a morality and secrecy of its own. (One of the difficulties, however, of inpatient as opposed to outpatient groups lies in the fact that the group members in the former instance have to live for the rest of the day in a close and intimate contact with those people with whom a few hours before they were discussing highly personal problems.) It is also very uncommon for unhealthy relationships to develop between group members outside the group meeting hours. Finally, the danger that patients will to any extent copy other members' symptoms is not a significant one; perhaps for a brief period one patient may take over some of the undesirable attitudes and symptoms of another, but these tend to be quickly dropped unless they serve a special unconscious purpose.

Behaviour Therapy. This is a general term used to describe a number of different treatment procedures derived from a school of psychological thought known as learning theory. These techniques originated in psychological laboratories, and thus under somewhat artificial conditions; only fairly recently has there been any translation of findings from the laboratory situation into an attempt to solve " real life " problems. In brief, these treatments aim to help the patient " unlearn " various symptom patterns and forms of unhealthy behaviour, these being regarded as " learned bad habits " which have been acquired as conditioned reflexes; symptoms according to this view have arisen initially as responses to anxiety and mental conflict, but still persist even though the original anxiety-arousing situation has long since disappeared. The notion of the " symptom as a defence " (p. 131) is thus specifically denied by most learning theorists and behaviour therapists. Such a point of view is of course in strong opposition to the general theoretical scheme on which this book is based, but it should be noted that certain aspects of conditioning are not necessarily incompatible with the theory of personality development outlined in earlier chapters.

Treatments based on learning theory include aversion therapy (p. 374), reciprocal inhibition, positive conditioning and operant conditioning. In treatment by **reciprocal inhibition** the patient is repeatedly exposed in a setting of relaxed calm to situations, or to mental images of situations, which have previously provoked anxiety; the aim is to weaken the link between the specific situation and the anxiety response. This technique is often used with phobic patients, *e.g.*, those who have irrational fears of riding in public transport, of lifts, of injections, or of sexual intercourse. In **positive conditioning** the goal is somewhat different: the development of a normal

TREATMENT: PSYCHOLOGICAL METHODS

reflex which the patient has failed to acquire; enuresis (p. 286), for example, may be treated by the use of a machine which causes an alarm bell to ring when a pad on the bed becomes wet with urine.

Still more recently techniques of **operant conditioning** (sometimes called trial and error learning or reinforcement therapy) have been used with groups of hospitalised patients, or with entire wards, and have been reported to be successful in the removal of incontinence, hoarding habits, food refusal and bizarre styles of dress and in the improvement of personal hygiene and socially orientated behaviour. Operant conditioning consists of the selection, through experiment, of behavioural responses which are found to bring rewards in a given situation. (Basically this is how all of us acquire complex skills and habits, such as learning to talk.) The aim of the therapist is thus to reward behaviour regarded as desirable, in the belief that this rewarded behaviour will then tend to occur more frequently. For reinforcement to occur, the reward must be given immediately after the behaviour takes place, and must be seen by the patient as dependent on this behaviour; it can be either a privilege or some form of token which the patient can later exchange for a privilege.

Good results in terms of symptom removal and behaviour modification have been reported for many of these procedures, though the duration of the improvement is as yet uncertain; nor do we know much about the long-term effects on the personality dynamics of the patients so treated. As is so often the case with new treatments, their value has been asserted with considerable fervour and some of the sweeping claims made by some behaviour therapists do not stand up to critical examination. Certainly any talk of a complex and many-sided disorder such as homosexuality being cured by aversion therapy, as has been alleged, is completely nonsensical in anybody's terms. Moreover, the role of transference (p. 329) in these procedures has not as yet received adequate attention. Some of the successes reported from the use of operant conditioning in chronic wards may be explainable in terms of the identity and decision-making power which is given to the patients, in strong contrast with their previous lack of individuality and initiative; behavioural change might not be too surprising in these circumstances. In general, then, much more work remains to be done before we have an accurate appraisal of the size of the contribution that we can expect from these treatments in the future.

THE ROLE OF THE NURSE IN PSYCHOLOGICAL TREATMENT

Any patient receiving planned psychotherapy will at times find that this is a highly disturbing procedure. Powerful, hitherto unsuspected feelings may be stirred up towards the psychotherapist himself, towards parents or towards other significant people in his environment and patients almost invariably find at some stage, because their defences have to some extent been undermined, that they demand more warmth, love and support from the psychotherapist than he is able to give. It has already been said that, because of problems in the past with parents or parent-substitutes, the psychotherapist is commonly seen at times as cruel and rejecting and becomes the recipient of all the aggressive feelings previously experienced in the patient's life towards the "bad" parent but since repressed. All these strong emotions do not subside at the end of treatment sessions but inevitably flow over into the patient's everyday life to some extent and have a significant impact on his attitudes and expressed feelings towards the nursing staff.

Consciously or unconsciously, usually the latter, patients on the ward commonly act out tensions which have been stirred up in psychotherapy. Hostility towards the psychotherapist will frequently be displaced on to the nursing staff; the patient may act in irritating and annoying ways, he may be openly destructive, he may leave the ward without permission, be late for meals or leave the pantry in chaos. Sometimes it appears

TREATMENT: PSYCHOLOGICAL METHODS

that he is attempting to drive the staff into some act of retaliation and punishment which he unconsciously needs to allay his sense of guilt. Often he tries to " play one person against another ". In devious and subtle ways he may try to stir up resentment in the staff towards the doctor or may try to discover the nurses' feelings about him, seizing eagerly on any statement which he can interpret as being critical.

When his feelings about the psychiatrist are strongly positive then these too may be carried over on to other staff members, although there may at the same time be some resentment of nurses because they are able to achieve a closer and more personal type of relationship with the psychotherapist than the patient is able to do. At this stage he often tries to find out as much as he can about the doctor's private life, carrying this back into the treatment situation in an unwitting attempt to complicate and obscure certain basic issues. It is almost always important that the patient in psychotherapy should not in fact have too much intimate knowledge of this kind, which without doubt makes the treatment situation harder for him rather than easier. The nurse must therefore guard against letting him have other than general, non-committal information about the doctor as a person.

Another type of complication arises when the patient returns from his psychotherapy session in a tense and emotionally unsatisfied state and wishes in effect to carry on the treatment relationship with a nurse. If he finds her sympathetic, as indeed she should be, he may wish to continue discussion at quite a deep level and may try to coax her beyond her proper functions of gentle support, listening and encouragement. By flattery, by stressing the importance of her opinion to him, by direct and demanding questions, he may attempt to manipulate her into making her own interpretations on the material which he has produced and in particular he may try to get her to say something which differs from the doctor's view. Clearly he will only do this if the psychotherapist has said something painful or threatening to him, and it is a fairly safe assumption that a comment which disturbs him in this way will be the sort of home truth which hurts and which he is attempting to avoid facing. Under many guises he is really attempting to manipulate the nurse into propping up his own unhealthy defences and into protecting him from real understanding of himself. The nurse must also remember that, for similarly defensive purposes, the patient may deliberately or unconsciously misinterpret the doctor's remarks, trying to convince her how little he is understood by his psychotherapist and how wide of the mark the latter's comments really are.

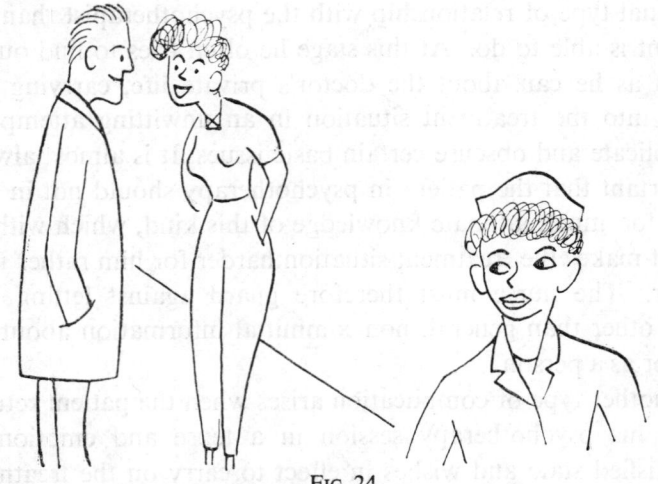

Fig. 24
A favourite patient of a doctor she admires.

The nurse's own feelings about the doctor introduce a further complication. It is only in fairly recent years that psychotherapy has been an accepted treatment in other than a very few hospitals and there is still a regrettable tendency amongst some nurses to see the term " treatment " as comprising only physical methods of care. Partly this is because the highly permissive role which the psychotherapist plays in his patient's life can lead him to tolerate, perhaps even encourage, behaviour on the patient's part which makes more difficult the

TREATMENT: PSYCHOLOGICAL METHODS

nurse's task of ward management and control; nurses at times resent what they feel to be the lack of enthusiasm which the psychotherapist shows for measures which they themselves regard as essential for proper ward discipline. Even if the nurse through her experience and training accepts psychotherapy as being a legitimate approach to a patient's problems, her attitudes in particular instances may yet be coloured by her own relationship with the psychotherapist concerned. If she has positive feelings towards the doctor this is likely to be of benefit to his patients, provided that they do not see her as being in competition with them for his interest and provided also that her admiration for his personality and methods do not completely blind her judgement and permit her to become unduly influenced by him and thus stop thinking for herself. (It is not unknown for a nurse to have conscious or unconscious feelings of antagonism towards a patient whom she senses is a particular favourite of a doctor she herself admires.) More importantly, her attitude towards the psychotherapist can be affected by hostile negative feelings; again she may or may not be aware of these. In these circumstances it is easy for her, often without realising what she is doing, to make remarks or even gestures which will be correctly interpreted as indicating her antagonism and which therefore make it doubly difficult for the patient to develop a helpful relationship with his therapist. These negative attitudes may be based on real difficulties she has with the doctor because of his own personality or because of temperamental or administrative differences between them; equally importantly, they may be derived from transference attitudes of the nurse herself who, like any other human being, can transfer on to the authority figures in her environment the sort of feelings she has had about an unsatisfactory parent in the past. Again we see that it is necessary for the nurse to be aware of herself and her own feelings, to recognise her hostility if it exists and to deal with it as best she can and, whatever her private prejudices, to refrain from saying anything in the hearing of patients which could be interpreted as a criticism of the importance of the relationship between patient and doctor.

Patients will sometimes reveal to nurses confidential information which they do not wish the doctor to know, partly because they find her in fact more sympathetic, perhaps partly because they are at the time feeling hostile towards him. The temptation to convey this information directly to the psychiatrist should be resisted (unless it should involve some real danger to the patient himself or to others), for relationships in the hospital must at all levels be based on trust; the nurse's correct procedure in this situation is to attempt to persuade the patient to discuss the particular incident or problem with the doctor or, in some circumstances, to obtain the patient's permission for the nurse herself to discuss the situation with him. It is nevertheless perfectly valid, indeed obligatory, for the nurse to report to the psychiatrist the patient's reactions before and after his treatment sessions and in particular to mention any pieces of behaviour which appear to have some connection with the patient's feelings about his therapist.

PSYCHOLOGICAL TREATMENT ON THE WARD

The most controversial topic in present day psychiatric nursing is the extent to which the nurse should herself become involved in the psychological problems of her patients. In some hospitals special training is given to selected nurses to provide them with a high degree of understanding of abnormal psychology and the dynamics of personality, some of these nurses being specifically called " nurse-therapists ". Such ideas are actively discouraged in other centres, where it is said or implied that the nurse is a totally unsuitable person to become involved with the patients' anxieties and complexes except at the most superficial level. It is the contention of this book that nurses do in fact become the recipients of the patients' strong and complicated feelings, whether they like it or not and regardless of whether this is approved of by their superiors. This problem will arise in any psychiatric hospital, but most

TREATMENT: PSYCHOLOGICAL METHODS

particularly in the all too common situation where there are relatively very few psychiatrists who are therefore unable to meet the personal needs of other than a small proportion of the large number of disturbed patients.

Some of the feelings which patients develop towards nurses will be on a basis of reality, that is to say, Mr. Smith likes Nurse Jones and finds her friendly and helpful because Nurse Jones is in fact like that; he dislikes Nurse Brown and is rather frightened of her because Nurse Brown's attitudes are in reality rather hostile and critical towards him. Many other feelings that patients have for nurses will be however on a transference basis; we have already seen that a relationship of any degree of closeness leads to the transferring of feelings which arose during an earlier experience in the patient's life. Mr. Smith may then feel that Nurse White is indifferent and unsympathetic towards him, even though Nurse White does not in fact feel this way at all, but because certain aspects of his dealings with her have stirred up, outside of his own awareness, old anxieties and resentments about his mother's indifference and lack of concern. Transference does not completely depend upon the actual age of the individuals involved; a nurse may be the recipient of feelings from a much older patient which were originally derived from that patient's relationship with his mother. Nor are transference feelings rigidly determined by sex, especially in a long-continued relationship; the ward sister, particularly if she is somewhat authoritarian in her approach, may well be the recipient in some instances of feelings which were originally stirred up by a powerful father. There are no general rules in this area; because every patient's past experience has been different there is no end to the possible variations in their transference feelings. A somewhat plain middle-aged woman may, for example, have feelings about a young good-looking nurse which are the same, without her realising it, as she experienced towards her younger and prettier sister.

Without a due recognition of the importance of transference the nurse may fall into one or both of two traps. Firstly, she may come to believe that patients who consistently show positive, loving feelings towards her are doing so entirely because of her own personality and charm; to keep herself on an even keel she needs to remind herself fairly constantly that many people tend to idealise nurses, to make them in their own minds the personification of goodness and kindness, because they are still unconsciously searching for the image of a good and perfect mother and would feel threatened if they found anything else in the nurse. The transference feelings of such patients may lead them to a quite uncritical and unreal view of the nurse, which in the long run will be good neither for nurse nor patient. The second problem arises if the nurse fails to realise that some hostile feelings directed towards herself have a similar transference basis. It is not easy for any human being to accept continuous hostility in a relationship with another person, whether this hostility be shown openly or in the more subtle form of passive aggression (p. 124). One of the most difficult tasks of the psychiatric nurse is to make it clear to her patients that she does accept their aggressive as well as their loving feelings, that they can express anger towards her without driving away her interest in them; she will be aided in this acceptance if she realises that this sustained hostility is not really directed at her, Nurse Jones the person, but against Nurse Jones simply because of her current place in the patient's transference feelings. A thorough grasp of this fundamental principle of human behaviour will make understandable to her a lot of the seemingly mysterious aspects of patients' reactions to her attempts to help them and she should be able to avoid being personally affronted by those patients who withdraw from her, who swear or who show open violence when she is trying so hard to be of assistance.

There is nevertheless one very real danger in this use of the concept of transference—that is, that the nurse will glibly explain away all the patient's attitudes towards her on this basis and will stop looking at herself to see whether in her own words or actions there might be some real justification for his feeling angry and hurt. One does at times observe instances in which the resentment which a patient shows to a nurse arises not from transference at all, but because the nurse is behaving in such a way as to warrant the patient's hostile feelings. Even the best-intentioned nurse will find that certain aspects of some of her patients do in fact make her angry, though this anger may itself have an irrational basis derived from her own childhood experiences; the patient's reaction to her may therefore be determined at least in part by her own conscious or unconscious feelings.

Though all this may make some intellectual sense to the trainee nurse, probably a vital realisation of the importance of transference will only come to her from some awareness of what this means in her own life. In the process of expanding her self-awareness she will probably come to see that some of her feelings about patients, about senior nurses, about psychiatrists or about significant people in her private life, are not only determined by purely rational considerations but that these too may have a transference component to them. If she is feeling angry with her ward psychiatrist, for example, she will do well to ponder whether his actual conduct is the whole reason for her resentment (which of course may well be the case), or whether in fact certain aspects of him as a person or certain characteristics of his behaviour have triggered off feelings derived from an earlier period of her own life. Though she will not necessarily need to understand the origins of such components of her own personality, she will certainly be a more effective nurse if she can really feel that, in herself as well as in her patients though to a different extent, past and hitherto forgotten feelings keep cropping up and to some extent distorting current relationships.

In the light of the above considerations we can now examine the role and responsibility of the nurse when confronted with those patients who are *not* receiving any organised psychotherapy from another staff member and who select her as the person with whom they wish to discuss their illness and problems. The nurse at the very least must be capable of sympathetic listening and should be prepared to fill such a role on any occasion when her attention is not otherwise completely distracted by important tasks; a patient may choose to talk about himself when walking in the grounds with her, when helping her make a bed or when "sitting out" with her at a social function. As has been indicated earlier in this chapter, and as some religious groups have known for many centuries, a great deal of relief can be provided for a tense, disturbed person by simply giving him the opportunity to talk himself out, with occasional nods and reassuring noises to indicate continuing interest. In Chapter 20 it is stressed how much may be learnt about the patient and his background through apparently random conversation and it may also be that his account of what appear to the nurse to be trivial issues does in fact afford him a good deal of satisfaction and comfort. Sympathetic listening is a more difficult task than it appears; there may be for some nurses an almost irresistible temptation to take the lead, to direct the conversation into "loaded" areas and in some way to show off their superior knowledge and training. All that has been said earlier about the value of support and ventilation in formal psychotherapy is equally applicable when the patient is talking in a quite informal way to a nurse; it may well be that she is the most suitable person to provide him with an outlet for pent-up feelings and that her toleration of these is a positive therapeutic experience for him. Unlike the usual conventions of social conversation, free communication in the nurse-patient relationship is to be encouraged, rather than discouraged, and the verbal expression of antisocial impulses should be tolerated without moralistic comment, even when these are directed against the staff or against herself personally.

The situation is more difficult with those patients who attempt to manipulate the nurse into a frankly psychotherapeutic position. Earlier in this book (p. 19) it was stressed that the nurse's role is never in any circumstances an interpretative one and that she is required to resist any temptation to discuss with a patient the inner meaning of his behaviour, to attempt to analyse his dreams or point out the significance of his childhood experiences. (This inclination to analyse the patient's attitude may be particularly strong when he is behaving towards her in a critical and destructive way.) It is repeated that it is only the psychiatrist, or in some circumstances the psychologist or psychiatric social worker engaged in long-term therapy, who is in a position to gauge the correct time for interpretation which, if premature, will only increase the patient's anxiety and cause him to retreat further into his defensive shell.

It is difficult also for the nurse to get out of the habit of reasoning in a purely intellectual fashion with psychiatric patients; one sees this sort of technique paying dividends with one's family and friends and tends to forget that the emotionally disturbed person is so powerfully motivated by deep unconscious drives that he is little if at all accessible to the sort of argument which would impress other people as being rational. For a certain sort of nurse there is always the temptation to give advice; on odd occasions it will work, much more frequently it will not, with the result that she either feels personally upset or tends to blame the patient for failing to respond to such wise counsel.

The achievement of the psychiatric nurse in this sphere of her work is intimately connected with the attitudes which she expresses towards her patients and with the feeling of acceptance which they sense to be coming from her, even though they may not be able to put this into words. Some experienced nurses can use kind and supportive phrases, yet without genuine warmth behind them or even with an underlying resentment, both of which attitudes will invariably be detected and responded to by her patients. It may then well be that in many situations it is as important to consider how the nurse feels as it is to look at what she actually does and says; once again we are brought back to the significance of the nurse-patient relationship.

17

PSYCHIATRIC TREATMENT.
B: PHYSICAL METHODS

AT the beginning of the previous chapter it was pointed out that there is no watertight division between those methods of treatment described as psychological and those which are of a physical kind.

This is particularly obvious in the case of treatment using various drugs. Cynics have said for a long time, and not without reason, that doctors get the best results from a drug when it is new, at a time when both the patient and the doctor himself have great enthusiasm for the preparation and great faith in its possibilities. Medical journals are regularly full of excited accounts of some new tablet which is said to bring about dramatic results in a particular form of psychiatric illness; in the same journal 12 months or so later one is very likely to find a much more cautious report of its value now that its newness has worn off. It is now known that those psychiatrists who are enthusiastic about the value of drug treatment do in fact achieve better results with drugs than those who are sceptical about them; this does not only mean that the enthusiastic ones may rate the patient's improvement more highly, but that some patients do in fact feel better when treated by such a person. The same sort of problem arises with many individual patients to whom a drug, new or old, is being given. The psychiatrist prescribes the drug in the outpatient department and at the patient's next visit a fortnight later she reports very great improvement; at first sight this looks like a clear-cut success for drug therapy, until on closer interrogation the psychiatrist hears that her improvement set in only an hour after taking the first dose, long before this particular drug could possibly have had any physical effect on her.

Moreover, some studies suggest that the attitude of the person who actually administers the drug is also of significance; in hospital practice, of course, this is almost invariably the psychiatric nurse. In one hospital it was found that when the nurses believed that the pills they were administering were powerful tranquillisers the patients' behaviour moved in the direction of greater tranquillity; the pill in fact contained no active drug at all and, when the nurses were given this information, the patients' behaviour rapidly returned to its previous state!

The patient's expectations concerning his treatment play a very great role in determining his response. Numerous studies have shown that roughly 30 *per cent* of people are **placebo reactors**—that is to say, they will show some degree of response to any preparation given to them, whatever its content. In certain drug trials, in which some patients are receiving the drug to be tested and another group of patients having pills which look exactly similar but which do not in fact contain any active drug, many of the latter group respond in the same way as those receiving the drug and, in addition, in some cases develop some of the side-effects shown by the drug group. The advertisement columns of the daily papers are full of the stories of placebo reactors: Mr. J. G. of North Y. writes enthusiastically that " since taking your famous remedy I have not had a single cold ", even though there may be no ingredient in the preparation which could possibly account for this stupendous result. The role of faith in medical treatment is very significant, and from all sorts of sources one obtains evidence of the way in which such faith may in fact bring about real bodily changes, often of a quite dramatic kind which in some instances may be labelled as miraculous.

Another important issue related to the psychological effect of drug treatment is concerned with the gratification of oral needs which may be provided in this way. From repeated observations of patients receiving psychotherapeutic interviews at the same time as drug treatment is being given, there can be no doubt that for at least some of these persons the fact that they are being given something to chew or suck or bite or swallow does, at a partly or wholly unconscious level, fulfil some of their oral dependent needs (p. 38). Because the doctor or nurse is giving him *something*, whatever this something may be, the patient feels that he is being kindly treated and it is for this reason that the type of person previously described develops a quick though temporary relief of symptoms within a few hours of receiving some medicine. Some patients will become furious if they are refused drugs though in some instances the more insightful amongst them can realise after a little introspection that in fact the tablets they were receiving were doing them little or no good.

For all these reasons the nurse should retain a healthy scepticism about the value of the physical treatments, and particularly the drug treatments, which she is giving on her wards, just as she should avoid being carried away by the claims of those enthusiasts who maintain that psychotherapy is the answer to all the troubles of humanity. Many psychiatric illnesses, particularly some of the neurotic reactions and not a few depressions, tend to have periods of seemingly spontaneous improvement which may be quite long-lasting (p. 211), so that it is always difficult to be certain in a particular instance whether the beneficial effect noted in the patient is due to the drug or due to this unpredictable remission. The admission of a patient to a good psychiatric hospital may in itself substantially relieve his distress in some cases. Because of these factors and the placebo effect previously mentioned, it is now recognised that no definite conclusion can be reached about the value of any particular drug until it has been subjected to what is known as a **double-blind trial**—that is, a trial in which some patients have received the active drug and an equal number of patients have received a pill of exactly the same appearance but containing no active constituent, with

TREATMENT: PHYSICAL METHODS

neither doctor nor patient knowing which pill is given to each individual. From what has been said above, it might be regarded as justifiable to insist that the nurse should also be unaware of the type of pill she is administering, if her observations of the patient's behaviour are to have any scientific value.

Though the foregoing remarks have largely centred on the psychological problems associated with the administration of drugs, there is little doubt that some of the same principles apply to the use of other physical treatments; some of these will become apparent later in this chapter.

ELECTROTHERAPY

The term electrotherapy embraces all those forms of treatment used in psychiatry wherein some type of electrical stimulation is applied to the brain. There are many isolated reports of electricity being used in psychiatric illness during the nineteenth century, but the systematic development of this form of treatment dates only from 1937. (For a few years prior to this convulsions were being produced by the intravenous injection of "**Cardiazol**" (pentamethylenetetrazol) and this form of treatment has its occasional advocates at the present time.) Electrotherapy is still commonly referred to as **electroconvulsive therapy** and is abbreviated as **ECT,** but it is now regarded as very doubtful whether the production of a convulsion is an essential part of the treatment.

If a therapeutic dose of electricity is applied to the head then the normal result is a convulsion which resembles in all important respects the *grand mal* seizure of the epileptic patient (p. 272). Present day practice however almost invariably involves the use of a **relaxant drug** together with a barbiturate, both of which are given by intravenous injection immediately prior to the treatment. The purpose of the relaxant drug is to bring about such a degree of muscular relaxation that the convulsive movements are very substantially modified or virtually abolished, the net result being that the possibility of damage to the muscles, bones and joints is very greatly reduced. The barbiturate is given at the same time merely because the experience of being fully paralysed by a relaxant drug is a most unpleasant one for the patient if he is not simultaneously put into a light sleep. The principles of management are essentially the same whether relaxants are used or not.

Electrotherapy is sometimes popularly known as "shock treatment"; this is an extremely unfortunate term and one which the nurse should avoid using, most particularly in the patient's hearing, because it is a phrase likely to produce a great deal of unnecessary apprehension and create in his mind the completely false idea that the treatment is highly dangerous. This is far from being the case; despite the number of possible complications listed below, the nurse is in a position to reassure any fearful patient that the risk in the treatment is exceedingly small and that, moreover, it is painless and has few or no unpleasant sequelae.

Indications. Electrotherapy is still of great value in depressive illnesses, particularly those of psychotic type, and most especially in that group of depressions known as involutional melancholia (p. 248). It is usually helpful in those schizophrenic reactions where catatonic features are prominent and also when there is a marked and relatively recent paranoid component; unfortunately some schizophrenic patients may not be improved and may even be made worse by electrotherapy and it is not always easy to identify these individuals in advance. In those neurotic illnesses where depression is a conspicuous feature electrotherapy may be of some value, though the results are not likely to be as spectacular as one commonly sees in the previously mentioned types of depression. Some psychiatrists will employ intensive electrotherapy in the treatment of manic reactions, though there is an increasing tendency to use lithium salts or large doses of tranquillising drugs in this illness. Occasionally the psychiatrist prescribes a very short course of electrotherapy for an epileptic patient, usually one who is known to show a progressively mounting disturbance of his mental function prior to a seizure; the electrical current in this instance produces an epileptic fit prematurely and usually cuts short the psychiatric symptoms.

Contraindications. Electrotherapy is not used in those psychiatric patients who are known to have any significant degree of organic brain damage—for example, in psychotic reactions due to senile brain changes or to arteriosclerosis. In such cases the already existing confusion is likely to be much exaggerated by the use of this treatment. It is also uncommon for it to be employed in neurotic illnesses characterised by great anxiety, for in the majority of these the patient's apprehension and distress are likely to be increased.

The physical contraindications are much less important now that relaxant drugs are so widely used and it is uncommon to find a patient denied electrotherapy if his mental condition is such as to warrant it. Nevertheless special care is taken in patients with a history of serious cardiovascular disease, particularly if there is incipient or actual heart failure or a history of recent myocardial infarction (coronary occlusion). Asthmatic patients may be treated, but not during an acute attack. Active bone disease is generally regarded as a contra-indication, due to the heightened risk of fracture, but profound paralysis brought about by a large dose of muscle relaxant may allow even these patients to receive treatment. Its use in pregnancy poses no particular danger to the mother or to the foetus.

Here is as good a place as any to stress the unfortunate uses to which electrotherapy can possibly be put in a large and understaffed psychiatric hospital. It is not rare to find in these circumstances that the treatment is used by the staff, occasionally consciously but more commonly unconsciously, as a form of punishment for unruly and refractory patients. When the psychiatrist is looking after several wards containing long-stay patients, so that he has little time to investigate the detailed behaviour of each individual, he has to be guided to some extent by the reports and recommendations of senior nursing staff and in these circumstances a particular responsibility falls on the nurses to ensure that the unjustified use of electrotherapy is vigorously avoided. There are some schizophrenic patients, it must be admitted, who do pose less trouble for themselves and for the staff and other patients if they receive occasional electrical treatments, but they are few in number since the tranquillisers have been introduced. In any event, whether electrotherapy or tranquillising drugs are used, there is never any justification for employing such treatments purely to subdue an otherwise difficult patient, unless all other possible avenues of doing so have been explored. It is poor nursing to recommend the suppression of a troublesome symptom by a non-specific physical treatment without attempting to find out what is behind it and what factors in ward life or in the patient's contact with others are causing the behaviour to appear.

The Technique of Treatment. This is divided into four phases:
1. Preparation of the patient.
2. Preparation of the equipment.
3. Management of the convulsion.
4. After-care.

1. PREPARATION OF THE PATIENT

(a) The patient is usually informed on the preceding night that treatment is to be administered on the following day; it is important that the nurse should firmly reassure him that the procedure will be harmless and painless. Nocturnal sedation is frequently prescribed. Consent must be obtained from voluntary patients and from the parents of minors.

(b) Fasting for at least five hours before the treatment is essential, as in any other procedure involving loss of consciousness. Temperature, pulse and respiration should be checked prior to treatment.

(c) Diversion and occupation should be available for the patient while he is awaiting treatment. There can never be any justification for placing him in a situation where he can see

Plate I

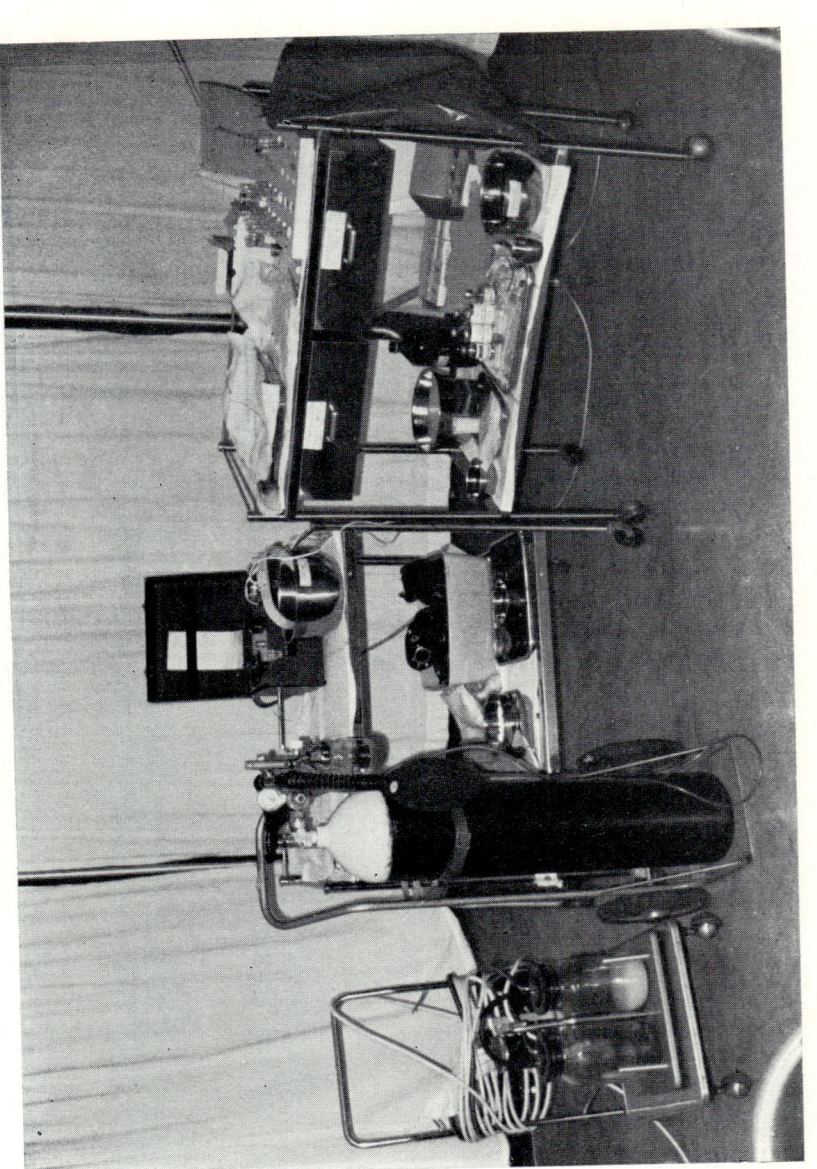

Typical arrangement of equipment for ECT, including (from left to right): electric sucker; oxygen cylinder with attached inflating apparatus; trolley with electrotherapy machine and headpiece, with electrodes in bowl of saline; second trolley with drugs, chart, emergency gear and drawers containing sterile syringes and needles.

Facing page 358

TREATMENT: PHYSICAL METHODS

any of his fellow-patients receiving their own treatment or hear any of the incidental noises which may accompany this.

(d) Hair-clips, pins, jewellery and false teeth must be removed; any tight clothing is loosened, and the patient should be encouraged to empty his bladder just before entering the treatment room.

(e) Premedication with intramuscular atropine sulphate (0·6-1 mgm.) is sometimes ordered. This must be given 30 minutes before treatment, this timing being critical if the effect of the drug is to be at its peak. Since this may be difficult to achieve with precision, one frequently finds that atropine is given intravenously at the same time as the anaesthetic is administered.

2. PREPARATION OF THE EQUIPMENT

The following equipment will be required in the treatment room and it is the nurse's responsibility to see, not only that it is there, but that it is in satisfactory working order.

(a) Electrotherapy machine, of the type employed in the hospital.

(b) Electrodes, usually mounted in a headpiece, but sometimes separate.

(c) A bowl of saline solution, with which the electrode pads must be moistened before use to ensure good electrical conductivity.

(d) Oxygen cylinder, checked for contents, with the apparatus for inflating the lungs (see illustration).

(e) Syringes and needles for drawing up and injecting the appropriate drugs.

(f) Tourniquets, swabs, solutions and bowls; elastoplast for applying pressure dressings to the site of venepuncture.

(g) Pharyngeal (Guedel) airways, laryngoscope, endotracheal (Magill) tubes and the appropriate connections.

(h) Mouth gags, which may be rubber, covered with cloth. It is important that, whatever material is used, the gag should be broad, so as to spread the load over the maximum number of teeth. Airways are NOT suitable for use as mouth gags, as they are too narrow, and serious damage to the teeth and/or jaws may result.

(*i*) Sucker, with a number of metal handpieces which can be replaced as used (otherwise each time the machine is employed, the handpiece must be sterilised before it can be used on another patient).

(*j*) The intravenous anaesthetic agent currently used in the hospital. This may be " Pentothal " (thiopentone), which is perhaps the commonest, " Brietal " (methohexitone) or " Epontol " (propanidid).

(*k*) The muscle relaxant drug or drugs: " Brevidil " (suxethonium), which must be mixed immediately prior to use, and is supplied in ampoules as a dry white powder, or " Scoline " (suxamethonium, "Anectine "), which is already in solution but which must be kept in a refrigerator, otherwise it will rapidly lose its potency.

(*l*) Atropine, in ampoules of 0·6 mgm. (where the drug is given at the time of induction it is usually mixed with the dose of " Pentothal ").

(*m*) The beds or trolleys on which the treatment is given must be firm, and of a convenient height to enable the anaesthetist to attend to the patient without too much stooping. Pillows and mattress should be covered with a mackintosh. An appropriate covering for the patient after treatment has been given should be provided.

(*n*) The patient's chart should accompany him to the treatment room, so that all relevant details can be recorded thereon, and to enable the medical officer to check any information concerning the patient's condition before giving the treatment.

3. MANAGEMENT OF THE CONVULSION

(*a*) *Posture.* The patient is allowed to lie comfortably on his back with a small pillow under his head. The legs should be uncrossed and the feet and hands exposed, since it is here that the signs of the clonic phase (p. 272) can best be seen.

TREATMENT: PHYSICAL METHODS

(b) The intravenous anaesthetic agent, with or without atropine, is administered first, followed by the muscle relaxant. As the patient loses consciousness, and subsequently becomes paralysed, oxygen is administered by the medical officer and the lungs are inflated with this gas for about 30-45 seconds, until the action of the muscle relaxant has reached its maximum and the patient is fully paralysed. Some doctors remove the pillow while inflating the patient, others do not.

(c) The shock is then administered; there will be a violent clenching of the jaw, though other muscles of the body will contract only slightly. The reason for this difference is that muscle relaxants cannot prevent contraction due to *direct* electrical stimulation, the placement of the electrodes allowing current to flow through the muscles of the jaw as well as through the brain. Hence it is important to use a mouth gag; in addition, the lower jaw should be held firmly closed against the gag by the nurse before the shock is given. This is the only restraint required for the patient undergoing modified electrotherapy.

(d) Following the initial clenching of the jaw (usually accompanied by a slight stiffening of the rest of the muscles), there occurs a modified clonic stage of a *grand mal* convulsion. It can be seen in the muscles of the face (especially around the eyes) and in a tremor of the hands, with the feet assuming a characteristically contracted position. This lasts for a varying time, up to two minutes at the most, and during this period the patient is not breathing adequately. Hence the importance of the *prior* administration of oxygen, so as to prevent cyanosis occurring during the fit.

(e) When the fit subsides the medical officer once more ventilates the patient with oxygen until he is breathing adequately without assistance.

(f) At this stage the (still unconscious) patient is turned onto his side and *nursed in the semi-prone position until consciousness is regained*. Nursing supervision during this period is essential. Patients recovering from anaesthetic and/or ECT should never be left unattended.

4. AFTER-CARE

(a) During the period of unconsciousness the closest attention must be paid to the patient's airway and skin colour. Any suggestion of respiratory difficulty or cyanosis must be brought immediately to the medical officer's attention, and in the meantime the nurse should endeavour to clear any obstruction. If the patient's own respiration should appear to be inadequate, mouth to mouth artificial ventilation should be commenced.

(b) After waking for the first time the patient may return to dozing in the semi-prone position which has been maintained until this time. More often he will sit up and may attempt to get off the bed.

(c) At this stage tactful restraint is often necessary, as the patient's ability to stand or walk may still be so impaired that he might undergo serious injury if allowed to get up.

(d) Confusion for a varying period after treatment is the rule. Rarely a patient may become quite difficult to manage, but the disorientation and disturbance of behaviour are temporary and usually do not require treatment.

(e) Under no circumstances should patients who have received ECT be allowed to leave the room or building without an escort. If they are outpatients a friend or relative must collect them. The patient must make no attempt to drive a vehicle for at least 24 hours.

Complications. The following should be noted:

Injuries to the tongue, teeth or lips, due to misplacement of the gag, may occasionally occur, but are usually minor.

Headache is a common complaint during the recovery period, and should be treated with an adequate dose of aspirin, unless the patient suffers from a disorder which contraindicates its use (*e.g.* peptic ulcer).

Memory defects. Prior to the advent of unilateral ECT, some degree of confusion almost invariably followed the administration of the treatment, and in quite a few patients a series of treatments created a patchy amnesia which was often very distressing, although a permanent memory loss of any consequence was rare. Now that it is increasingly common for the current to be administered by applying the two electrodes to the non-dominant side of the scalp, rather than placing them one on each side, such consequences are even less likely to occur. If the patient has been properly selected, so that underlying organic brain disease has been satisfactorily excluded, then any slight disturbance of memory can be dealt with by reassuring him that it is most unlikely to last and that in any event important things will be retained.

Confusion. More serious is the development of confusion which outlasts the first few hours following treatment. This is commonest in elderly patients and must be immediately reported, as it may well cause the psychiatrist to discontinue treatment lest the confusion become worse or even permanent.

Fractures are virtually unknown since modified treatment has become almost universal. Occasionally, due to an error in the administration of the relaxant (*e.g.*, if it is not given into the vein), a patient may accidentally have an unmodified fit. Complaints of back, jaw or limb pain after such an event warrant investigation for the presence of fracture or dislocation, and should be reported to the doctor.

Death is exceptionally rare as a consequence of ECT or its accompanying anaesthesia. Adequate oxygenation before, during and after treatment is the best safeguard against such a disaster. It is probably true to say that the risks of ECT are less than those of the anti-depressant drugs, if it is admitted that very occasional patients use these as a successful means of suicide.

MODIFIED INSULIN THERAPY

The use of moderate doses of insulin, to produce a mild disturbance of consciousness short of coma, is still in favour in some psychiatric clinics, though much less so than a decade or two ago. It may be of benefit as an auxiliary treatment for some neurotic patients who are tense, anxious, anorexic and sleepless, or where there has been considerable reduction in their normal weight. It may have some value in the relief of anxiety symptoms remaining after a relatively satisfactory course of electrotherapy in a severely depressed patient. It is also at times employed in the management of states of restlessness and anxiety which may follow the withdrawal of drugs from drug-dependent people. The dosage of insulin ranges from ten units up to a usual maximum of 100 units, the resulting drowsy and slightly confused state being terminated by the oral administration of an appropriate amount of glucose. Probably here also, though to a lesser extent than with insulin coma therapy (p. 231), the quiet efficiency and personality of the nurse are of therapeutic value, and during the treatment some patients may have an increased accessibility to therapeutic interactions with her.

CONTINUOUS NARCOSIS

The aim of this treatment is to keep the patient in an almost continuous state of sleep by the use of large doses of sedatives and hypnotic drugs, it being generally regarded as desirable that he sleep for 20 out of each 24 hours for a period of three to four weeks.

Though it appears to be still valued by some Russian psychiatrists it has been almost entirely abandoned in the Western world, where by and large it is considered that its very real dangers outweigh any potential benefits it may confer.

SEDATIVES AND TRANQUILLISERS

All drugs of consequence will of course be ordered for the patient by the psychiatrist, but it is nevertheless necessary for the nurse to have a clear idea of the drugs that are being given and of what it is hoped to achieve by their use. It should be hardly necessary to stress that in psychiatry, as in any other branch of medicine, a heavy responsibility rests on the nurse to see that, in the giving of drugs and medicines, the doctor's orders are faithfully carried out, that the patient does in fact receive the specified drug in the specified amount and that the effects of the drug are carefully and accurately reported. When dealing with some unco-operative psychiatric patients there may be an additional problem in that one cannot be certain that the drug is actually taken by the patient simply because it has been handed to him, and in such circumstances special observation will be required. The nurse should also remember the points raised earlier in this chapter concerning the psychological aspects of drug administration; the enthusiasm or otherwise with which she dispenses her pills may well have a significant influence on the result achieved.

Sedative Drugs. These drugs produce a general calming effect on the patient together with some degree of drowsiness. **Barbiturates** were for many years the most commonly used drugs of this class, including both longer-acting substances such as **phenobarbitone** and short-acting ones such as amylobarbitone ("**Amytal**"). It is now generally acknowledged that these are poor drugs for psychiatric patients, as they may increase depression and particularly in elderly patients may lead to some degree of confusion. Moreover, they are undoubtedly drugs of dependence. The development of the class of drugs known as **minor tranquillisers** (p. 370) has greatly reduced the number of prescriptions written for barbiturates, though it should be noted that these new substances are in fact, pharmacologically speaking, only more elegant sedatives, and many of the same hazards are involved in their use.

Hypnotic drugs are those used to induce sleep and are an important part of the care of the psychiatric patient in some instances. It is however necessary to point out that a psychiatric ward in which many patients are receiving large doses of hypnotics, night after night, is probably a ward in which the level of nursing care is not as high as it should be; it is pointed out elsewhere (p. 465) that the need for nocturnal sedation can be greatly reduced if the nurse ensures that the patient receives adequate occupation, recreation and mental activity during the day. In other instances the quiet, confident attitude of the night-nurse herself will exercise a calming effect on the patients in her care and it will be noted that, even with the same group of patients, some nurses require to use far fewer hypnotic drugs than their colleagues. The number of these drugs is very large indeed and the particular preparation employed will always be specified by the psychiatrist; no attempt will be made to list them here.

Particularly in those patients whose stay in hospital seems likely to be lengthy, the routine use of hypnotic drugs should be avoided wherever possible, as it will not be helpful to the patient to bring him to a stage where he is quite unable to sleep without their aid. Moreover, although insomnia is a common, genuine and occasionally serious problem in psychiatric patients, the nurse will quickly note that in fact many patients sleep rather more than they realise and close observation of their sleeping patterns will suggest that their demands for drugs are not really warranted. Other patients sleep adequately and soundly, yet still feel that they are having less sleep than they should, although they function quite satisfactorily on the amount they do receive. In these and other instances the nurse must precisely report the patient's sleeping habits, in order that hypnotics may be dispensed with in those cases where this is possible.

Major Tranquillisers. The development since 1952 of tranquillising drugs, sometimes known as **ataractics,** has made a very great difference to the practice of psychiatry, particularly within the psychiatric hospital. These drugs differ from sedatives in that, as their popular name suggests, they quieten the patient's disturbed behaviour and calm his agitation without having any major sedative effect and therefore without the induction of sleepiness. Though each new drug has been tried out in the management of neurotic reactions, it does not appear that any of them have any particular place here, and without doubt their major effectiveness is with psychotic patients and in particular with those who are overactive, fearful, restless, impulsive or destructive. Above all they have been useful in the management of patients with advanced schizophrenic illnesses; many of these patients, because of these drugs, are able to live outside the psychiatric hospital whereas they had previously spent many years within its walls. Their value in acute forms of psychotic illness is also substantial, and in many instances they are the treatment of choice in acute schizophrenic disorders; in acute manic reactions they have an undoubted place, though without the specific action of lithium salts on manic symptoms. With chronic psychotic and particularly chronic schizophrenic patients treatment requires to be long-continued; patients are usually discharged from hospital while still taking the drug and in many instances continue to take it for months or years after their discharge while being supervised at an outpatient level. The same is true for most patients who have been treated for an acute illness. It is obvious therefore, despite the optimism of a few years ago, that the presently available drugs do not in any sense cure schizophrenic or any other forms of psychiatric illness but merely provide in many instances an effective method of modifying distressing symptoms and of bringing disturbed behaviour under more efficient control.

The first tranquillising drug to be developed was " **Largactil** " (chlorpromazine, " Thorazine "), which came on the market in 1952. Since then an extremely large number of major tranquillisers have been produced, some of which have had little apparent additional merit, but others have won a secure place, either by a somewhat lesser liability to produce toxic or side-effects, or because they appear to be valuable for some patients who show a less than adequate response to " Largactil ". " **Melleril** " (thioridazine) in particular is favoured by some psychiatrists because of its lesser toxicity, and " **Stelazine** " (trifluoperazine) is usually considered to have special value by reason of its capacity to activate the chronic, rather apathetic schizophrenic patient and create in him an increased interest in his surroundings. Other drugs which are relatively commonly employed by particular psychiatrists for particular purposes include **"Anatensol"** (fluphenazine, "Moditen"), **"Serenace"** (haloperidol) and **"Trilafon"** (perphenazine, "Fentazine"). Fluphenazine has found a special place because it is available in two long-acting injectable forms, which may exert effective control over psychotic symptoms when depot injections are given at two to four-weekly intervals; such medication schedules have the additional value of providing an acceptable rationale for a regular contact between discharged patient and community nurse, which will probably form an essential part of his after-care programme.

These drugs all have their own particular dosage schedules, details which the nurse will quickly learn in her own clinical work. It should be noted, however, that for any particular drug the required dosage may vary over a wide range. " Largactil ", for example, may produce a beneficial response in some mildly disturbed patients in a dose as low as 25 or 50 mgms. t.d.s., but in the acute psychotic reactions it is unusual to see much response under 300 mgms. per day and at times dosages up to 1,200 or even 2,000 mgms. per day have been employed. Once his disturbance has been brought substantially under control, the patient is usually maintained on a much reduced dose, in the case of " Largactil " this varying from 100 to 600 mgms. per day. Some of these drugs are also prepared for parenteral administration, for use when urgent action is required to bring particularly disturbed behaviour under rapid control.

In addition to their value in the acute and chronic functional psychotic illnesses, ataractics can also be very useful in modifying the restlessness and anxiety which are sometimes features of organic brain disease, for example, in the apprehensive, agitated senile patient. They may also be effective, in much larger doses, in the management of acute organic reactions which show a great deal of confusion and agitation. They are not generally used when depression is a marked feature of a psychiatric illness, as this symptom may be worsened by these drugs: in some such patients, however, a small dose of a tranquilliser may usefully be combined with an anti-depressant drug.

The drugs may have many possible side-effects, though it is rare for these to be of serious significance. The nurse, however, should be on the look-out and report them should they seem to be in any way distressing. Patients may complain of dryness of the mouth, marked constipation, mild fever, sensations of dizziness and faintness, blurring of vision and local skin irritations. " Largactil " may lead to a great increase in the sensitivity of the skin to light and when early signs of this occur the nurse should ensure that the patient's skin is not exposed to strong sunlight. More serious complications are not unknown; jaundice, produced by obstruction to the flow of bile within the liver, is a very occasional toxic effect of " Largactil ". A very few cases of agranulocytosis (that is, a great reduction in the number of white corpuscles) have been recorded and, rare though this complication may be, the occurrence of sore throats or mouth ulcers, particularly if associated with fever, should be immediately reported. Pigmentation of the skin and eye has been noted to occur with long-continued use of " Largactil ", while " Melleril " in very high dosage may cause retinal pigmentation.

Most commonly and importantly of all, these drugs are capable of producing symptoms and signs indicating interference with the function of the extrapyramidal portion of the nervous system. The resulting picture may resemble Parkinson's disease (p. 266), with its tremor and rigidity, but other important complaints are of akathisia, in which the patient has " restless legs " and finds it impossible to sit still or relax, and various tonic spasms of the muscles, commonly those of the head and neck, so that there may be violent contraction of the jaw muscles, or sudden and sustained twisting of the neck. Some of these acute symptoms are alarming, but the condition is not as serious as it may first appear and can be reversed by the administration, intravenously if necessary, of anti-Parkinsionian drugs such as "Artane" or "Cogentin" (p. 270). Commonly these drugs are continuously administered together with the tranquilliser from the beginning of treatment. Clinical experience suggests that "Stelazine" and "Serenace" are particularly likely to produce rather dramatic symptoms of this nature.

Lithium Compounds. In 1949 the Melbourne psychiatrist Cade noted that compounds containing lithium seemed to exert a strikingly beneficial effect on manic patients. This observation gradually led to a substantial volume of research, in Australia and elsewhere, which has demonstrated the validity of this finding and has established even more clearly that the regular administration of lithium to patients with classical manic-depressive illness will significantly reduce the liability to relapse in this notoriously relapsing syndrome. The compounds are potentially toxic, and are therefore administered with substantial care, a common practice being to discontinue the medication for one day in each week. Maintenance dosage usually involves the administration of 0·5-1·0 Gm. per day, but the really important issue is to achieve a blood level within a safe yet effective range, and blood samples will be regularly sent for biochemical analysis in order to keep a check on this.

Minor Tranquillisers. It has already been pointed out that the major tranquillisers are usually ineffective in the treatment of neurotic patients. More recently, however, there have been developed some substances of a different chemical composition which do seem to have the effect of reducing severe anxiety, at least to manageable proportions, when this seems a desirable goal. These drugs are sometimes known as the minor tranquillisers, and the two which have been used most extensively are "**Librium**" (chlordiazepoxide) and "**Valium**" (diazepam). They are relatively safe drugs, but in at least some neurotic patients there is the very real risk that a dependence on them may fairly quickly be established, which may leave the patient worse off than before.

ANTI-DEPRESSANT DRUGS

For many years various drugs have been used to stimulate and activate depressed patients, in the knowledge that in some instances there would be an accompanying elevation of mood. The chief members of this group are the amphetamines, particularly "**Dexedrine**" (dexamphetamine) and "**Methedrine**" (methamphetamine). They are, however, very unsatisfactory drugs, for this or any other purpose; patients may become overstimulated and overactive, appetite is reduced, and there may be a considerable increase in depression when the stimulant effect wears off. Moreover, drug dependence and even a psychotic reactions (p. 201) are real possibilities when they are given for any length of time. Probably the only remaining indication for their use is in some of the childhood behaviour disorders (p. 295).

In recent years there has been developed a completely new class of drugs which have specific anti-depressant properties, which produce much less general stimulation and which carry little or no risk of dependence. In major depressions, particularly those showing the features of psychotic depression (p. 247), "**Tofranil**" (imipramine) is undoubtedly effective, as is "**Tryptanol**" (amitriptyline, "Laroxyl", "Tryptizol", "Elavil"), the latter being perhaps specially valuable for older, agitated depressive patients. Both these drugs have relatively minor side-effects in the great majority of patients, but are prescribed with great care, if at all, in patients with prostatic enlargement or raised intraocular tension, due to the risk of precipitating urinary retention or glaucoma. They require continuous administration in adequate dosage for one to three weeks before the patient experiences maximum benefit, so that they are of little value for the very acutely depressed patient whose symptoms usually require the rapid relief which can be expected from electrotherapy. Some of the newer derivatives of these substances are claimed to have a more rapid effect, and/or to have less pronounced side-effects; drugs such as "**Allegron**" (nortriptyline, "Aventyl"), "**Pertofran**" (desipramine), "**Surmontil**" (trimipramine) and "**Concordin**" (protriptyline) all have their advocates.

Anti-depressant drugs of a different type, known as **monoamine oxidase inhibitors,** are claimed to be of particular value in depressions with marked neurotic features, though the evidence for their effectiveness is far from conclusive. The most widely used drugs of this class are "**Marplan**" (isocarboxazid), "**Nardil**" (phenelzine) and "**Parnate**" (tranylcypromine). With all of them there is some slight risk of liver damage, other drugs such as "**Marsilid**" (iproniazid) having been almost completely abandoned because of this possibility. In rare instances they may produce paroxysms of hypertension, extremely severe headache and even the occurrence of a subarachnoid haemorrhage; a few deaths have been reported. The nurse must therefore report immediately any complaint of headache in patients receiving these drugs. The risks from these drugs are enhanced if the patient eats, or is given, any of the following substances whilst under treatment: (i) adrenaline or any related compound; (ii) "Pethidine" (Demerol, meperidine); (iii) barbiturates; (iv) steroids; (v) hypotensive agents; (vi) alcohol; (vii) cheese. It is also customary to avoid the combination of any of these drugs with the anti-depressant drugs of the type mentioned in the previous paragraph; if a change is made from a drug of one class to a drug of the other class, it is usual to allow a week or 10 days to intervene between the two drugs.

The nurse must be clear that neither anti-depressant drugs nor tranquillisers lessen in any way her responsibility for good nursing care. The original hope that these drugs would "cure" psychiatric illness has not been realised and, in view of what has been previously said about the complexity of the causes of emotional disorder, this should hardly be a matter for surprise. On the contrary, the new drugs provide a special challenge to the nurse in that, through the control of disturbed behaviour and the relief of distressing symptoms in a more rapid way than was previously possible, the patient is brought more quickly and more comfortably into an effective contact with his environment; he is thus more accessible to the full range of social, occupational and recreational techniques which the nurse is able to use in order to facilitate the emergence of healthier patterns of living.

THE DRUG TREATMENT OF ALCOHOLISM

Except in those cases where alcohol addiction arises as a symptom of another major psychiatric disorder, it is believed to develop on the basis of a character neurosis (p. 197), yet for various reasons the alcoholic patient is often unlikely to benefit from psychotherapy alone. Probably the best results obtained at present with this group of patients are through the use of psychotherapy in conjunction with the drug "**Antabuse**" (disulfiram), a compound which in combination with alcohol produces a toxic substance which causes the patient considerable physical discomfort. The organisation known as **Alcoholics Anonymous** may also be of great value for certain patients.

The treatment is usually commenced in hospital, alcohol having first been completely withdrawn. The drug is given for a few days in order to develop a high concentration of "Antabuse" in the body, then the patient is given a test dose of alcohol so that he will experience for himself the effect of combining alcohol intake with this medication. In a typical case the result is most unpleasant; there is flushing of the face, vasodilatation with a sensation of great heat, raised pulse rate, dyspnoea, nausea and sometimes copious vomiting. If due care has not been taken with the dosage, these effects may even lead on to disturbance of the heart rhythm and cardiovascular collapse. After one or more of these tests the patient is usually discharged from hospital and is instructed to continue with his "Antabuse" medication in a specified dosage. The effect does not persist if he ceases to take the drug, so that naturally this regime is only of value when the patient is reasonably co-operative; at times his co-operation is made more likely by arranging for his wife to present him with his tablet each morning. The treatment however is not likely to be successful unless the patient keeps in regular contact with his medical adviser for support and psychotherapy.

Another form of treatment for well-motivated alcoholic patients is **aversion therapy.** One form of this treatment consists of the repeated administration of alcohol in combination with an emetic drug, usually apomorphine. A conditioned reflex is built up so that in a successful case, after a series of trials, even the sight and smell of alcohol are enough to make the patient vomit even though no emetic drug is now being given. More commonly today the administration of alcohol is accompanied by painful electric shocks delivered to the body. Here too a conditioned reflex is built up and the smell or even the thought of alcohol will thereafter evoke strong feelings of discomfort associated with the earlier painful experiences.

The Nurse's Role in Drug Treatment

It has already been pointed out (p. 365) that the nurse plays a very responsible role with any patient who is receiving drug treatment. She should report the effects that she observes, whether these be the expected ones or unwanted side-effects; details are extremely important to the doctor, who may well decide to reduce or to increase the dose on the basis of what he is told by the nurse. Instructions concerning the timing of drug dosages must be carefully followed—too commonly one finds a four-hourly schedule, for example, " adjusted " by the nursing staff to suit administrative convenience, so that the drug in fact is being given at quite irregular intervals, with consequent difficulty in gauging its effect. The timing of premedication prior to electrotherapy also needs to be strictly observed.

The nurse is responsible for seeing that the patient on leave from the hospital, and his relatives, clearly understand the doctor's instructions concerning drug administration and the dietary restrictions which may need to be followed with certain drugs.

TREATMENT: PHYSICAL METHODS

The legal aspects of the storing, recording and administration of drugs are important parts of the nurse's responsibility. Certain drugs listed in Government acts and ordinances must be checked regularly and the amount on hand recorded in a special register. It is necessary for such drugs to be kept in a locked cupboard, the key of which is retained by a registered nurse; when any such drug is given to a patient both the preparation and its administration require to be checked by a second nurse.

CEREBRAL SURGERY

Surgical operations on the brain are of course widely used in many forms of nervous system disease, but the subject is confined here to those procedures which are occasionally

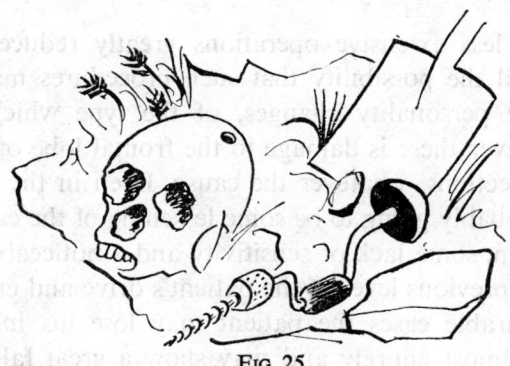

FIG. 25
Cerebral surgery in primitive times.

employed in the treatment of severe and intractable functional mental disorders. It has already been noted in Chapter 1 that in primitive times holes were sometimes bored in the skull of mentally ill patients, but it was not until 1937 that a scientific approach was made to the use of brain surgery in psychiatric illness and the modern era of **psychosurgery** began. These procedures, like the tranquillising drugs a decade or so later, were at one time thought likely to "cure" a large number of psychiatric illnesses, but these hopes soon proved to be unfounded and it is now recognised that operations of this type are only indicated in an extremely small number of psychiatric patients, and then only when there has been an extended trial of other forms of therapy appropriate for the particular case. The most suitable patients are those with a chronic, agitated form of depression which has totally failed to respond to electrotherapy or to drug treatment, or where the response to these treatments has been of extremely short duration; the relief from anxious misery is sometimes very striking in these cases, even in patients over the age of 60. In the 1950's a large number of these operations were done on chronically overactive schizophrenic patients, and in cases of intractable neurosis where there was disabling anxiety and tension, but it is now considered, except by a handful of enthusiasts, that the operation has little or no place in the management of these illnesses.

Though less extensive operations greatly reduce the risk, there is still the possibility that such procedures may lead to undesirable personality changes, of the type which may be seen whenever there is damage to the frontal lobe of the brain or its connections, whatever the cause. Even in the best cases there is probably going to be some lessening of the capacity for self-criticism, some lack of sensitivity and a noticeable diminution in the previous level of the patient's drive and enthusiasm. In unfavourable cases the patient may lose his interest and ambition almost entirely and may show a great falling off in the level of his social consciousness, so that he makes inappropriate, embarrassing remarks to others and, in the worst instances, performs antisocial acts, sometimes of a sexual kind, completely out of keeping with his previous behaviour. There is sometimes a persistently silly and fatuous mood and a great deterioration in personal habits. An intensive rehabilitation programme may help to minimise these effects when they occur.

A large number of operations of this general class have been devised, the details of which can be located in a textbook of surgical or neurosurgical nursing should the need arise. There also the nurse will find details of the pre-operative preparation of such a patient and information about his post-operative nursing care. There are many other diagnostic procedures which may be carried out in a psychiatric hospital which contains a neurosurgical unit, but the details of these, and the nurse's task in relation to them, are beyond the scope of this book.

CONCLUSION

The development of physical forms of treatment during the past 30 years has revolutionised the psychiatric hospital and considerably modified the work of the nurse. Real psychiatric nursing has been made in many respects much easier and more interesting now that many effective symptomatic treatments are available; schizophrenics long out of contact with their environment, depressives previously destined to many months of gloom and isolation, these and many other patients have been rendered much more accessible to social influence and the nurse's task has therefore been made much more rewarding. Though physical treatments are not by any means the only important factors, they have certainly been very significant in leading to the development of more open types of hospital environment and in giving to the general public tangible proof of the value of psychiatric treatment. But the use of these treatments increases rather than decreases the need for skilled psychiatric nursing based on a sound knowledge of interpersonal relationships; enough has been said during this chapter for the nurse to realise that they are largely of symptomatic value and that her own special skills are still required in every case of psychiatric illness. It was said in Chapter 1, and is repeated here, that the nurse must never allow her participation in physical treatment, dramatic as this at times may be, to reduce her to the status of a mere technical assistant to the psychiatrist.

18
REACTIONS TO ILLNESS AND HOSPITALISATION

When a person develops an illness, and especially if he requires admission to hospital, his previous personality and past experiences will have a profound effect on his own attitude towards his sickness and towards the hospital and its staff. All the various patterns of defence which he has previously acquired in order to deal with stressful situations will again be brought into play and it can be expected that he will attempt to cope with this new problem situation in much the same way as he has coped with problems in the past.

Different societies have many different ideas about the proper handling of sick people, and may in fact have varying views on the nature of illness itself. In some primitive cultures the sick person is treated as a God (Fig. 26) whereas in others he is punished and rejected. In highly industrialised Western communities there is a demand for a hospital system to look after the sick person until he is healthy again, this demand being clearly shown by the presence of national health schemes, government budgets and legislation. This is in one sense a logical development, for the hospital is the hub of scientific and technical advances concerning the diagnosis, treatment and prevention of illness. On the other hand this great dependence upon the hospital can in part be viewed as a reflection of society's anxieties, fears and guilts about disease. This becomes particularly apparent when one is talking about psychiatric illness for here, even more than with physical sickness, society's way of coping has been almost completely by means of isolation and hospitalisation.

Being admitted to hospital means different things to different people; the very act of admission marks the beginning

REACTIONS TO ILLNESS

of a special relationship between hospital and patient. This relationship is most commonly voluntarily requested by the patient in order to satisfy his needs but, in certain psychiatric illnesses, it may at times be imposed on him as a result of a legal decision. The meaning of hospitalisation to any individual will therefore depend, not only on his personality and

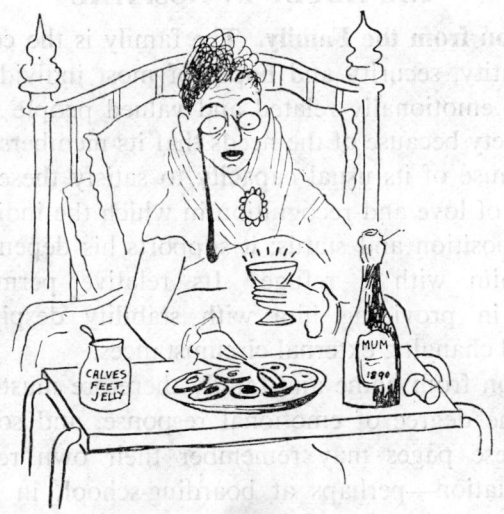

Fig. 26
In some primitive cultures the sick person is treated like a God.

past experience, but also on the way in which he perceives his current situation. Hospital may represent a service benevolently designed to allow recovery from illness, it may be seen as a haven which will protect him from his impulses and fears, to some it may be perceived as a final retreat or exclusion from society while to others the imposition of hospitalisation is felt as a hostile attack, an unwarranted imprisonment confirming their beliefs of persecution. Depending upon the way in which hospitalisation is perceived the patient's reaction may range from trust to distrust, from dependence to scornful rejection—needless to say, these emotions will colour his attitudes towards the hospital staff and its treatment procedures.

Hospitalisation also requires the separation of the patient, often abruptly, from much that is familiar to him—from his family, his occupation and his community contacts. Deprived of these supports he will feel some degree of anxiety, the extent of this also being largely determined by his previous personality.

THE ADULT IN HOSPITAL

Separation from the Family. The family is the central core of the identity, security and hopes of most individuals. It is a group of emotionally related and valued people which persists in society because of the needs that its members seek from it and because of its usual capacity to satisfy these needs. It is a source of love and recognition in which the individual has a definite position and status; it supports his dependency and provides him with a refuge. Its relative permanence is important in providing him with stability despite shifting stresses and changing external circumstances.

Separation from home and family therefore must inevitably arouse some degree of emotional response, and some nurses reading these pages may remember their own reactions to such a situation—perhaps at boarding-school, in the armed forces or upon entering nursing training school for the first time. It is no accidental combination of words that leads to the term " homesickness " being part of our language. This can be a real mood of sadness in which there is a yearning for a familiar face, voice or experience characteristic of home life.

The patient in hospital, in many instances already perplexed and confused by his illness, may suffer further anxiety from this separation, both from his own sense of loss and because of fears and guilts concerning his family arising out of his sickness. He may react with despair because he sees hospitalisation as the ultimate proof to his family of his hopelessness and incurability. On the other hand, this separation may produce hostility because it is seen by him as a result of rejection by the family, indicating its failure to stand by him when he needs it most. These reactions, real enough to many individuals in the light of current circumstances, may be much exaggerated if they also represent, consciously or unconsciously, a repetition of an earlier experience which involved separation from parents, together with the anxiety, fear and anger which went with this—these emotions of childhood may have been deeply repressed, only to be reawakened in this new situation. Another patient may unconsciously equate the hospitalisation experience with earlier punishments which he feared or perhaps expected because of rivalry with other members of the family.

Separation from Work. The importance of work to the adult has already been mentioned in Chapter 4 (p. 66). It provides the basis of his financial security, it forms a significant element in the maintenance of his identity and is essential to him if he has hopes of achieving various future goals. Hospitalisation is usually accompanied by financial problems and frequently by economic hardship. The patient may well have real concern about his ability to hold down a job in the future; there may be a lurking suspicion that his wage-earning capacity has ceased or at least been greatly modified and this intensifies his fears both for his own and his family's subsequent well-being.

In addition, the work situation provides the person with real gratification arising from his status and acceptance therein and from his ability to contribute; cessation of work is usually accompanied by an awareness of loss (p. 74). Money itself may also have been unduly important to the individual, symbolising power and security to a pathological degree; for some people money has been used in much the same way as a defence mechanism and as a means of ensuring self-protection. The adult who has used money to buy emotional satisfactions or status will have grave anxiety if the source of his income is interrupted.

Separation from the Community. Social interests may have considerable importance in stabilising the individual's adjustment to himself and to the world around him (p. 66). Hospitalisation will lead to some extent to a loss of these social experiences and their resulting satisfactions; if these were particularly significant, this factor may create further anxiety.

Problems in Hospital

The patient entering hospital steps from his familiar environment into a new and strange one. Whereas he was formerly fully responsible for himself and perhaps for others, as a patient he enters into a new type of relationship with unfamiliar authorities on whom, at least to some extent, he is required to depend. The hospital community, like any other community,

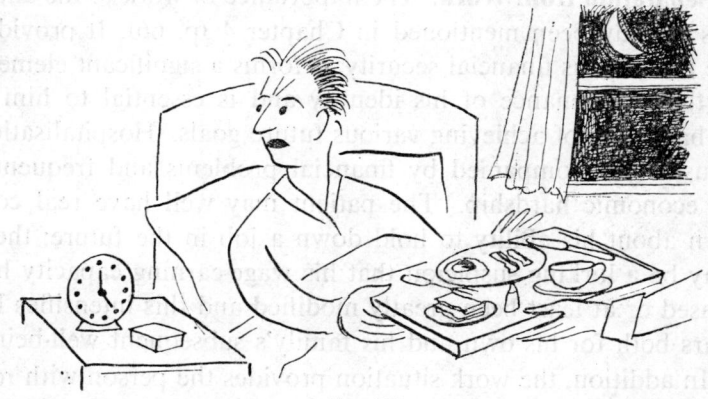

Fig. 27
Changes in food and eating patterns.

runs with the aid of a certain code of behaviour which has been designed for its efficient function; rules and regulations are always necessary although, as will be seen in the following chapter, some of these may in the case of psychiatric illness defeat the primary aims of treatment.

Hospitalisation must interfere to some extent with the patient's usual pattern of life. His various routines, tastes and preferences, built up over the years, are now largely disregarded and he is required to accept new habits, basically directed towards his well-being though perhaps not initially accepted as such by him. Changes in food and eating patterns, in bathing and toilet functions, in daily activities and sleeping rituals are all required for ward convenience but provide personal upset for many patients. With the best of intentions the hospital might take away the patient's spectacles or even her wedding ring; the former act may leave her in a world of vague forms, perhaps unable to locate the few possessions she has—the latter practice (now fortunately almost completely outmoded) frequently created in psychotic patients further anxiety and confusion due to new uncertainty about their identity.

There are also the numerous difficulties which arise from the unknown situations in the hospital and from fear of what is going to happen next. The unfamiliar almost always creates anxiety, even in the best-adjusted person. Often the patient's fears are unjustified, especially when they arise from serious misconceptions about certain aspects of hospital procedure and his treatment; many adjustment problems can be avoided if the patient and his relatives are provided with simple factual information about hospital routine.

The patient is also surrounded by a wide variety of people; he is required to meet and to trust many unknown persons and to establish new relationships with various staff members and with his fellow-patients. Because hospitalisation must inevitably involve some degree of dependence, some awareness of a need for help and a sense of being in the hands of others, it is hardly surprising that the hospital staff tend to be seen in the same sort of way as parents were seen when the patient was a child and looked to them for protection. Some patients will for these reasons see hospital staff members as trustworthy, friendly and supportive, whereas others will see them as rejecting, hostile and disinterested. (Have you by now observed the patient who is reduced to abject fear by the presence of the superintendent, the matron, or even the ward doctor and sister?) Naturally these attitudes, arising on a basis of **transference** (p. 329), will make themselves apparent in the patient's behaviour and will influence to some extent

PSYCHIATRIC NURSING

the course of his illness and the speed of his recovery. Likewise his response to other patients will be partly determined by his successes and failures in relation to other people throughout his life.

With psychiatric patients, adjustment to these new surroundings is an essential first step towards the restoration of emotional well-being. The role of "patient" is difficult for

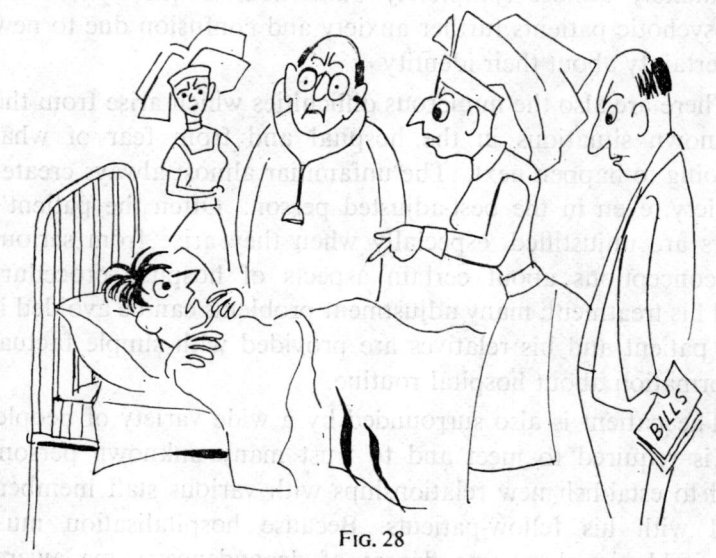

FIG. 28
Patient reduced to abject fear.

some individuals to accept; for weeks or months they retain conflicting and hostile attitudes towards themselves and their surroundings. Because of these attitudes illness and treatment may not be accepted rationally; sickness may be completely denied, it may be exaggerated and prolonged or, on the other hand, the help which the hospital might give is summarily rejected. All these adjustment problems will be made substantially easier if from the beginning the patient is met with trust, understanding and consistency, for these are the attitudes which will encourage a sensible acceptance of the hospital and its staff.

Of course the danger is always present that the patient may come to adjust to hospitalisation almost too well, so that he sees the hospital as a refuge wherein he can escape forever from the difficulty of coping with real life situations. Recovery may then be seriously threatened, because the patient gives up responsibility for his own life and leaves it to the hospital to take care of his needs. Sometimes patients recently discharged from a psychiatric hospital will return imploring to be readmitted and this must be counted as a failure on the hospital's part, even though it may not always have been preventable. A parallel can be drawn with the social situation at the end of World War II when many servicemen, suddenly deprived of the administrative machine which had planned their lives for them, were " lost " and unable to adjust to the demands of civilian life.

THE CHILD IN HOSPITAL

During the last 20 years great interest has been shown in the effects on the child of separation from the home and family, particularly in relation to hospitalisation. The possible effects of this separation, particularly a break in the continuity of the relationship between mother and child, vary with the child's age. It is not until the latter half of the first year of life that the child is capable of forming meaningful relationships with the objects in his surroundings. After this time it is always possible that separation will produce a substantial emotional reaction in the child, sometimes even a major infantile depression (p. 40).

When considering children in hospital we must always remind ourselves that the child's thinking is not governed by normal adult logic but has many elements of a primitive and magical kind (p. 50). Unpleasant feelings arising out of illness will tend to produce insecurity, and he may interpret these feelings in what are to us quite peculiar ways. They may, for instance, be seen as punishment for his badness or as the result of somebody's anger being directed towards him;

in these circumstances he will obviously have an even greater need for the parents whose presence and love provide reassurance. To be hospitalised at this stage may be seen as a rejection and as evidence that he cannot trust his family to look after him when he most needs them. He may react with despair or anger and be further frightened by his own destructive wishes.

For this and other reasons hospitalisation may result in regressed behaviour, evidenced by a return to earlier levels of eating, sleeping, toilet and even speech activities. Such a child can hardly be overlooked, but another equally disturbed youngster who feels depressed and hopeless may not be recognised as distressed by the nursing staff because " he is no trouble in the ward ". Sometimes there is no apparent disturbance whilst in the hospital environment, but on returning home the child's anxiety is expressed in a fear of being left alone, in nightmares, bed-wetting, destructive behaviour, nail-biting or temper tantrums. Not infrequently the results of separation may be more serious and longer-lasting than the effects of the illness itself.

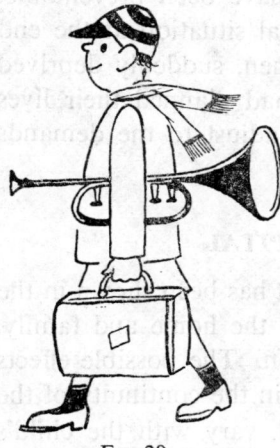

FIG. 29
He may be allowed to take something from home.

To help overcome the difficulties arising from separation frequent and regular visiting should be encouraged in order to permit the child to retain some contact with the security of his previous existence. In some modern centres the mother is encouraged to live in the hospital with her sick child and to take a large share of the responsibility for his care. The strangeness of new experiences may be partly offset by allowing him to take something from home, such as his favourite teddy-bear or the battered suitcase in which his valuable personal possessions are stored. Consistent tolerance expressed by the nursing staff will help support him through his indecisions and fears. However, despite all these precautions, hospitalisation must inevitably create some stress for every child, and the parents should be advised of the difficulties which might possibly emerge and should be supported by the nurses in coping with them.

PATTERNS OF ADJUSTMENT

Throughout the history of man it is strikingly evident that psychiatric illness has been taken to mean that the affected person is in some way basically different from the other people in his surroundings (p. 5). These attitudes still tend to persist in our so-called rational, civilised society. It is not unusual to note the amazement of some students or visitors to psychiatric hospitals as they exclaim " but they look just like you and me ". Sometimes the impression is gained that those people who have had no contact with psychiatric illness expect psychiatric patients to have horns and a forked tail. Even in some people with clinical training and experience it is not unknown to hear the allegation that psychotic behaviour is occurring " because he is mad, he is mental, unlike us, there is something wrong with his brain, he was born that way "— even though the patient for the first 30 or 40 years of his life has behaved in a manner which is to all intents and purposes rational. Such views are partly due to ignorance, but they are also born of fear. As children many of us heard talk of " looney bins " and " mad people " being whisked away in " green carts ". This was the point of no return; the whole business was inexplicable and frightening. The implications of psychiatric illness are so complex and threatening that many people take refuge from their fears by noisily asserting " it can't happen to me ". There is abundant evidence that these attitudes are defences designed to protect and secretly reassure the individual against the awareness of a terrifying possibility.

Our understanding of illness as a stress situation is increased by recognition of the extent to which unconscious, as well as conscious, factors may direct human motivation. Even a mild bout of some trifling physical illness tends to produce personal discomfort and annoyance because it stops us doing something which we had planned; this inconvenience and frustration is often apparent in ordinary behaviour, directed at workmates, a family member or the cat. If it is a major physical illness, the patient's reactions are correspondingly more intense. We have already seen that there will be concern about his future, his job, his finances, his family and whether he will recover; these anxieties will be added to in many instances by unconscious fantasies concerning the meaning of his disease. All this will be reflected in his behaviour; he may be tense, despondent, childish, clamouring for attention, demanding reassurance or aggressing at cruel fate. These responses can be commonly witnessed in any general hospital by anyone who takes the trouble to look for them.

If these are the reactions to illnesses which are physical in nature and therefore to some extent objective and understandable, it is hardly surprising that even grosser variations of behaviour may be noted in psychiatric patients who are experiencing fluctuating emotions, irrational fears, destructive wishes, inexplicable changes in bodily sensations and unpleasant alterations in the world around them. Such a patient also has to cope with the prejudice and even open hostility which may be aroused in society by the knowledge that he is mentally ill. To deal with the anxieties which arise from an awareness of psychiatric illness the patient will unwittingly seek to bring defence mechanisms into play; they will be essentially of the same nature as those described in Chapter 5, but with certain special features which warrant extended description in relation to this particular setting. Many of them will also be observable in some non-psychiatric patients in a general hospital.

Denial

Four types of denial reaction (p. 93) are quite commonly encountered at the beginning of illness and hospitalisation.

(*a*) The denial of any illness or problems. Here the patient asserts " nothing is wrong with me " because the implications behind illness are so frightening that he cannot accept them. This view will be maintained unless and until he can establish trust in the hospital and its staff.

(b) Denial of any emotional illness. This patient says, in effect, " my trouble is all physical ". Most people find it less disturbing to see themselves as physically, rather than psychologically sick. Moreover an allegedly physical illness will tend to evoke the support of relatives and friends, whereas a frank psychiatric illness may cause some of them to shun him.

(c) Denial of any physical illness. This patient says, in effect, " it is all emotional ". This defence is not uncommon amongst those suffering from progressive organic reactions. The patient at one level realises that his mental faculties are deteriorating and that his memory is failing, but rather than face this frightening knowledge he asserts that his difficulties are purely " due to worry ". Such a patient will try to protect himself from anxiety by avoiding those tasks or experiences which might highlight his deterioration.

(d) Denial in euphoria, elation and excitement. This is basically a defence against depression and tends to arise in some individuals in those circumstances where depression would be an appropriate response—for example, prior to extremely hazardous surgery. In its grossest form it is responsible for the appearance of frankly manic behaviour.

Suppression

This is a conscious attempt by the individual to forget or to rid himself of ideas and feelings which stir up anxiety and guilt (p. 90); for example, the woman who has impulses to harm a member of her family will commonly endeavour to suppress these by formal, deliberate control. This process is frequently accompanied by considerable tension. Such patients in hospital may attempt to deal with the situation by keeping themselves fully occupied throughout all the waking hours; without constant activity they may find that painful and distressing thoughts rise into consciousness.

Rationalisation

This mechanism is used by the individual to construct a plausible, socially acceptable reason for his behaviour rather than acknowledge the existence in him of unacceptable or anxiety-producing motives (p. 99). It is common for illness to be explained as " due to overwork " rather than admit to insecurity, guilt, feelings of incompetence, disharmony in the family and so on. This technique does not alter the basic conflict; it simply provides an excuse and an escape. Rationalisation is often used to attribute the blame for illness to another person or object; the patient unable to contemplate his own shortcomings may see the hospital staff as hostile and destructive, and at this point rationalisation is of course very close to projection (p. 100). The term rationalisation is also sometimes used to describe that process whereby a psychotic patient who has had peculiar delusional experiences erects complex and even more delusional explanations to justify the strange happenings which he feels to be occurring inside himself or in his environment.

Regression

This is one of the most frequent reactions to stress and is commonly encountered in illness (p. 99). Here the patient seeks to deal with anxiety by falling back on to earlier, immature forms of behaviour which achieved some degree of comfort for him in childhood. Rejection of personal responsibility, impatient and demanding behaviour, attempts to gain the nurse's complete attention at all times, querulousness, sulking and tears, demands to be fed, washed and dressed—these are some of the expressions of regressive defences. Incontinence may also be a manifestation of regression—as well as evidence in some instances of the patient's hostility towards the hospital or to some of its staff members. Sometimes regressive behaviour takes the form of attempts at **manipulation** of the staff. Through this technique the patient seeks to engineer situations in which he will gain the satisfaction he seeks. The expression of suicidal threats is one outstanding way in which a patient may draw more attention to himself (p. 150); others may set out to anger the nurses because of some complicated satisfaction which this brings derived from early childhood experience. To achieve these needs the patient may play other patients against the staff, or staff members against their colleagues. Some do this with considerable skill and there will be an increase in tension on the ward until this manoeuvre is recognised and dealt with as effectively as possible.

Overdependency is another instance of regression, a form of escape which involves a turning away from problems and their frustrations, a special kind of avoidance in which the individual simply quits and seeks to be rescued from his difficulties by complete dependence on others. The most obvious example of such a reaction is shown by the patient who says, " here I am, it's your problem, now fix me up "; many do not say this in so many words but express it quite clearly in their actions. Built in to this claim is a child-like plea to be returned to the breast and be fed, comforted and completely protected. Such a patient will stoutly resist contributing towards his own recovery; instead of looking constructively at his own behaviour he often clamours for hypnosis or the " truth drug " so that he will " wake up cured ".

Fantasy

Fantasies and day-dreams substitute imaginary satisfactions for unrewarding real experiences. Faced with sickness some patients retreat increasingly into a fantasy world of their own making, where grandiosity replaces feelings of inferiority and dreams of exceptional ability mask ideas of incompleteness and inadequacy. This behaviour may appear as the creation and exposition of a new philosophy, art, religion or mechanical invention in which the patient remains completely engrossed. He may fantasy his own death so that he can then visualise the family's guilt and remorse for their failure to understand and support him. This is very like the child who day-dreams that he dies or goes far away so that his parents will be sorry for what they have done to him.

Seclusiveness

The seclusive person moves away from his surroundings either because he finds there some threat to his existence or tranquillity or because he sees inside himself emotions which could threaten his future if they became apparent to others. If he perceives the other patients and staff as hostile and destructive he may then try to isolate himself; conversely, he may feel that his own thoughts and feelings would lead other people to punish him in retaliation. The nurse must recognise that any movement towards seclusiveness, either in a literal physical sense or by establishing a mental isolation from his surroundings, is evidence of considerable tension in the patient.

Apathy

A state of apathy may be precipitated by extreme frustrations which lead a person to feel that he has been abandoned; we have already seen that in some patients the process of hospitalisation may create feelings of being unloved and unwanted. Apathy quickly leads to a state of social atrophy, a condition which the nurse will still encounter in some patients in chronic wards. Current psychiatric literature is full of studies which emphasise the improvements which have followed the introduction into these wards of treatment programmes designed to allow the patient to see that he is wanted, valued and recognised as a person and not simply as a number, a diagnosis or a barely tolerated occupant of a hospital bed. Modern rehabilitation programmes are based on the realisation that apathy is the greatest single difficulty which must be overcome in the management of advanced psychiatric illness.

Depression

We have already discussed in detail the various depressive illnesses (Chapter 11), but depression is also a possible reaction to many stress situations, including illness and hospitalisation. In this sense it does not by its occurrence indicate the presence of any one illness but is a reaction commonly encountered in various psychiatric disorders as well as being seen with considerable frequency in physically ill patients in general hospitals. It may occur for a variety of reasons; it is often, for instance, a fairly simple and understandable reaction to loss and separation, as is commonly seen in the hospitalised child. The loss may be a bodily one; some surgical patients who have undergone an operative procedure resulting in the removal of a part of their body become mildly or even severely depressed during the convalescent period. Other forms of depression may be related to guilt arising from hostile wishes or from a feeling of having "let the family down". Turning of destructive wishes against the self (p. 102) is important in some cases. In some instances the depressed mood leads on to major feelings of hopelessness and worthlessness, sometimes coupled with self-destructive thoughts or impulses, and at this point one is dealing with a major depressive illness.

Aggression

Persons with a good deal of latent aggressive feeling may have this emotion greatly stimulated by illness and hospitalisation. The nurse must train herself to recognise that these aggressive feelings may not be directly expressed, but may be displaced on to a substitute object or person, or may come out in a variety of disguised ways.

Displaced Aggression. This is so much a part of daily life that the phrase " don't take it out on me " is familiar to all of us. Through this technique the individual eases his angry feelings by aggressing at an object or person who is not however the proper target of his hostility. It is a very common way of dealing with frustration and every day the hospital ward provides examples. Perhaps the patient feels neglected, or he has been denied a privilege he sought; he may be annoyed by his family's attitudes towards his illness, by the hospital's decisions and restrictions concerning him or by the behaviour of the staff and other patients. The complaints, however, may not be directed at any of these persons but in one very common example of displacement are focussed entirely on the quality or quantity of the food which is being served. This mechanism, as has been said, is not the exclusive property of psychiatric patients; the nurse herself who has been annoyed by a colleague or exasperated by a hectic day full of irritating frustrations may direct her own angry feelings towards the patients or other quite innocent staff members. Good psychiatric nursing involves looking past the patient's immediate reaction in an effort to detect the underlying cause of this behaviour and will be aided for each nurse by a recognition of processes of this type in herself.

Over-conforming. At first this may not be recognised as related to anger, because it is based on the mechanism of reaction formation (p. 95). Such a patient is angered by the demands and restrictions imposed on him, but instead of showing overt anger he behaves according to the letter of the law, a phenomenon which, when it occurs in industrial relations, is known as a " regulation strike ". For example, a nurse asked a patient to collect and burn all the loose papers in the patients' lounge room; he duly gathered up the newspapers, the sheet music from the piano and a dress pattern spread on a table and burnt the lot because " I was only doing what the nurse told me—she said *all* the papers ". A carelessly stated request by a member of the hospital staff may allow aggression to be expressed in this way.

Superiority. Many patients who are frightened by sickness and who are unable to face their own interpretation that sickness equals weakness react towards healthy people with claims of their own superiority. Many a nurse has been made to "feel small" by a patient who continually is emphasising that his educational, social, vocational or economic background is superior to her own. This is a form of aggression designed to hide latent insecurity and inferiority.

Negativism. Aggression here appears in pretty thin disguise. The negativistic patient may never talk about his aggressive feelings, but shows them very clearly by his persistent refusal to co-operate in ward routines. Often this lack of co-operation takes extremely subtle forms, so that the nurse may be tempted to believe that the patient is "just stupid", or even slightly deaf, or in some instances she may feel that he is too preoccupied with his own troubles to have attended to the request that she has made. This is one of the classical forms of **passive aggression** (p. 124), and may in some instances be carried on behind a pleasant facade of what looks like smiling agreement.

Criticism. Some patients discharge their aggression through an extremely critical examination of the staff and of the hospital's procedures. Often these complaints are voiced chiefly to other patients and only indirectly reach the ears of the staff. Claims of incompetence, prejudice, emotional bias or inconsistency may be made concerning a doctor or nurse, the intention being to reduce confidence in the particular person or to make the individual uncertain of himself. These attacks may be delivered with considerable skill and sometimes with an acute insight which makes them all the more difficult to handle; an example of this is the patient who, seeing her doctor wearing a white coat which was unusual for him, quietly remarked "he must feel more insecure than usual today". An important part of ward administration is to ensure, through group discussions or some similar technique, that this type of behaviour is brought into the open, because it is only possible to cope with it when it comes out from under cover.

Paranoid Projection. Aggressive feelings are commonly dealt with in the hospital situation by being projected—that is to say, other people are said to have those feelings or thoughts which are too disorganising and threatening for the patient to admit as parts of himself (p. 100). Many patients hospitalised for medical and surgical illness, quite apart from those in a psychiatric ward, show tendencies of this kind; a common manifestation of this is known as **scapegoating,** by means of which the patient attributes all his difficulties to the hospital's incompetence. If he does not respond rapidly to treatment, or if accidental circumstances prolong or complicate his stay in hospital, then this is all unwittingly seen as a product of the hospital's disinterest in him or active dislike of him. In even more serious cases the patient's projective mechanisms lead him to incorporate the hospital or its staff into his own frank delusional system, so that he comes to see them as agents of some conspiracy plotting to harm him.

CONCLUSION

In this chapter there have been indicated some of the stresses which are posed for adults and children by illness and hospitalisation and some of the more important methods by which patients seek to relieve the tensions created by these situations. The more that these forms of defence are comprehended, the more will the nurse develop an understanding of the patient's deeper and more significant anxieties. Knowledge of this kind is, in addition, a considerable help to the nurse, for she should then be able to understand that in many instances unpleasant aspects of the patient's attitude to herself are not a true indication of her own personality and competence but provide evidence of the pathological way in which he is attempting to deal with a stressful situation. Hospitalisation and illness must always be, in varying degrees, frightening and uprooting experiences; both in the patient and the family there will be liberated anxieties, fears, guilt and other emotions, both these and the defensive techniques employed reflecting in large measure their previous life experience. It is for the hospital staff to use its knowledge and resources to ease both the patient and his family through this period of turmoil.

19

THE PSYCHIATRIC HOSPITAL AS A THERAPEUTIC COMMUNITY

IN the previous chapter we examined briefly some of the difficulties which are posed for every patient confronted with a hospital environment (p. 382). Many of the comments made there were applicable to any form of hospitalisation, whether for a medical, surgical or psychiatric illness, and in this chapter we deal in more detail with some of the specific problems which arise in a psychiatric hospital, with particular reference to the unfortunate impact which these may have on the patients under care. Whilst it is true that in any form of illness the untoward effects of the hospital environment may work against the patient's recovery, this possibility is magnified a hundred times when one is dealing with illnesses which are largely or wholly psychological in their implications.

In Chapter 2 the objectives of hospital care were briefly reviewed (p. 29) and it was pointed out that the present day psychiatric hospital must offer much more than the negative and defeatist type of so-called custodial care which has all too often been provided in the past. Modern psychiatric nursing techniques are based on the primary assumption that each patient who enters the hospital, whether voluntarily or under some form of legal compulsion, does so in order to be *treated* for his emotional disturbance. Other considerations are often relevant—the patient may need to be protected from his own dangerous impulses, intolerable stress may need to be lifted from the relatives, the community may need to be safeguarded —but the fundamental purpose of hospitalisation must always be to explore all possible avenues of investigation and treatment which may make it practicable for the patient to return to the community. An atmosphere of protective benevolence is no longer adequate.

Certain specific types of treatment have already been examined in some detail and in Chapter 23 the role of social, occupational and recreational activities in the total therapeutic programme will be considered. But all these particular forms of treatment, valuable though each may be in numerous instances, do not in themselves provide a wholly adequate programme of care for the psychiatric patient. One other element is of vital importance—the atmosphere of the hospital itself, with all the innumerable details which contribute to this. The community of the hospital staff members and the relationships which they develop with each other and with the patients —these factors may in themselves be therapeutic and may exert a greater influence on the patient's behaviour and ultimate recovery than any of the special treatments which are administered to him. Concern with these attitudes and relationships has developed for more than humanitarian reasons, important though these undoubtedly are; therapy is now seen as incomplete if these matters are not the subject of constant, earnest study.

This means that psychiatric hospitals may develop exciting physical treatment programmes in special units and elaborate occupational and recreational activities housed in new and modern buildings, but may still miss out on a large part of their treatment potential if they fail to pay adequate attention to the therapeutic value of the patients' environment. Conversely, many psychiatric hospitals which are housed in old and inadequate buildings and which are severely understaffed—and many hospitals regrettably still belong in this category—may yet come close to the ideal standards of a truly therapeutic community.

The importance of the nursing staff in creating and maintaining this therapeutic environment can hardly be overstated. Even in the most advanced hospitals the amount of time spent by any patient in the various forms of treatment already considered will be only a fraction of his total day, almost always less than one-half and in many instances, especially in the case of very disturbed patients in so-called chronic wards, it may be a very small fraction indeed. Patients nevertheless are under care for 24 hours in every day and during the greatest proportion of this time their personal contacts will be with nurses. The psychiatrist may well be thought of, even by the nursing staff, as the glamour figure in the hospital organisation, but some patients may have no dealings with him for days or even weeks at a time. It is what the nurses say, what they do and, even more importantly, the attitudes they display—these are the things which create the environment which, if it is a helpful one, may play a major part in the recovery of patients.

SOME UNDESIRABLE EFFECTS OF PSYCHIATRIC HOSPITALISATION

Every patient admitted to a psychiatric hospital will, even in the most favourable circumstances, experience certain conditions which will have an unfortunate effect upon his basic illness. Even voluntary patients will encounter these difficulties, though they will tend to be much more marked in those patients who are admitted under some form of legal order. The fact that many of these situations can be regarded as inevitable should not blind us to their importance, nor should they be accepted as unmodifiable unless there is good reason for them to be considered as such.

Any psychiatrist can describe patients who have been maintained in reasonable touch with reality for a long period of time in the community but who, when hospital care has at last become inevitable for any one of a variety of reasons, have shown a rapid deterioration in behaviour and adjustment within a quite brief period following admission. Therefore, even though the hospital may be effectively furnishing protection for the individual or the community, and even though important physical or psychological treatments are being given, care must be taken never to lose sight of the pernicious influences which may at the same time be operating on the patient.

The Fostering of Dependence. A measure of personal independence is extremely important for all mentally healthy people. All of us have acquired this in relatively painful stages, beginning with the complete dependence of the infant upon its mother and progressing through the various hurdles of childhood and adolescence up to the mature self-reliance and self-confidence of the normal adult. For the psychiatric patient this process has almost certainly been even more complicated, because from our understanding of the causes of psychiatric illness we realise that he has been handicapped by uncertain and unsatisfactory personal relationships. Many persons reach adult life with major problems concerning dependence and independence (p. 144)—very commonly there is a thin veneer of independence hiding deep and unacknowledged longings for gratification of unsatisfied dependency needs. The fact that the hospital to some extent accepts this dependency is often a valuable aspect of treatment, yet an unchecked fulfilment of the patient's desire to lean on others will very likely prove in the long run to be a handicap to his recovery and his return to outside living, for which a good measure of independence is essential in our type of society.

The great danger comes from the fact that, in the short-term view, the excessively dependent and passive patient often presents no particular nursing problem and may in fact be easier to nurse than the more independent fellow who insists on sticking up for his rights, querying the reasons for his hospitalisation, criticising some aspects of ward routine and perhaps even trying to leave hospital. Some nurses may unwittingly encourage unnecessary dependence because it fulfils some need of their own to have people excessively reliant upon them, giving them a warm and comfortable feeling. Total dependence, however, is an immature way of relating to others and may well become a halfway house on the road to chronic illness; the task of the psychiatric hospital is to encourage independence and maturity. Once a patient has abandoned himself almost completely to reliance upon the hospital it will always be difficult, and may in some instances be impossible, to encourage him to take up independent living again—but if people are repeatedly denied the opportunity of making decisions, even small ones, concerning their own lives, they may gradually lose the capacity and the desire to do so.

The Destruction of Privacy. The ability to maintain a small segment of our lives as private and inviolate should we wish to do so is an essential aspect of civilised human behaviour. Though this certainly applies to some extent to both sexes, it is probably in our culture rather more important for women than for men. All hospitalisation involves some invasion of privacy. There is much less chance than in the ordinary community for a person to retreat temporarily to some place of physical isolation in order to gain relief from social pressures and, at an even more personal level, there is an essential disclosure of previously secret knowledge about the patient's past and a general loosening of conventional reserve. Much physical modesty may have to be sacrificed and for some women in particular this may be a shattering burden, with shame and embarrassment now added to the other difficulties experienced in adjusting to the hospital. The significance of any intrusion into personal privacy must always be realised, though urgent considerations of safety may at times demand this; there are furthermore some patients who cannot be allowed to be as private and seclusive as they wish because this behaviour is a crucial symptom of their sickness. On the other hand, in some psychotic illnesses inhibitions may already be loosened to some extent, leading to relatively shameless behaviour; it is essential for ward life to be so structured that this lack of modesty is discouraged. Nurses can easily, through thoughtlessness rather than indifference, lose sight of the fact that lack of privacy and any interference with normal feelings of shame concerning nakedness and excretory functions can quickly lead on to lack of self-respect and thus favour the development of intractable illness.

The Lowering of Personal Standards. No psychiatric hospital —in fact, no hospital of any kind—can ever hope to provide living standards which compare with those existing in the vast majority of the homes from which its patients come. Admittedly there is a small underprivileged group in any community to whom hospital care does represent more adequate shelter, better nutrition and greater material comfort than that to which they have been accustomed, but the size of this group is often grossly exaggerated by those people who wish to deny the inevitable existence of the many crudities in hospital life. There are still people who will say, against all the evidence, that we must not make hospitals too comfortable if we expect patients to leave them. (Occasionally patients *are* reluctant to face the outside world, but this is not the reason.) In a psychiatric hospital the details of routine living must have a most significant, even if unconscious, impact on behaviour; neglect of these aspects is not only contrary to humanitarian principles of patient care but will exert a specifically retarding effect on recovery and rehabilitation.

The number of these details is very great; some are of small consequence in themselves but in combination they produce a significant total effect. They include:

(*a*) the quality of the **food** and the manner in which it is served;

(*b*) the hygienic and pleasant nature (or otherwise) of **bathroom** and **toilet** facilities;

(*c*) the quality and attractiveness of hospital **clothing,** if circumstances are such that it is undesirable or impossible for some patients to wear their own clothes;

(*d*) the **furnishing** of wards, including cutlery, crockery, chairs and bedding, and most particularly the extent to which an effort is made to create a home-like and civilised atmosphere through the use of flowers, curtains and accessory furniture (p. 440).

The nurse may still at times hear the opinion expressed that one cannot provide patients with good clothing, or pleasant furnishings, because the primitive destructive impulses which may come to the surface in mental illness could lead to their speedy damage. Sadly one can still hear it said—or more frequently not said but implied in behaviour—that good meals, pleasantly served, will not be appreciated by psychiatric patients. Exaggerated stress laid on these very largely outmoded ideas has been one of the very important factors leading to the decline of the psychiatric hospital during the first half of this century; modern practice shows that these attitudes are almost totally unjustified and that in fact the provision of poor equipment and mediocre services fosters the very forms of behaviour which it is hoped to prevent. To a large extent *psychiatric patients, especially those with advanced illness, will adopt those forms of behaviour which they feel are expected of them by the staff.* Experienced and observant nurses are well aware that a female patient who has repeatedly destroyed ugly, ill-fitting institutional clothing will commonly adopt a completely different attitude towards an attractive dress which she has chosen herself, which arouses favourable comment from other patients and staff and which she keeps as one of her own possessions.

Any attempt made to normalise the physical environment of the psychiatric hospital will inevitably make it a more therapeutic institution and the nursing staff must constantly be striving to find ways in which this can be done within the limits laid down by essential considerations of safety and expense. In fact much can be achieved in this direction, with little or no financial outlay, by imaginative and sympathetic nurses who are not too much bound by traditional prejudices and who have no exaggerated fears of their patients' primitive impulses.

The Diminution of Individuality. Satisfactory and efficient management of a ward—or a hospital—must inevitably involve the sacrifice of some part of the individuality of each person concerned in the organisation. It is equally inevitable that the greatest sacrifices in this respect will be demanded from the patients, those members of the ward group who have little or no outlet outside the hospital where they can live—as the doctors and nurses do—individual, unique lives in their own fashion and according to their own preferences. They have little or no choice of the food they eat, the recreations which they indulge in or the hours they keep, and precious little chance to select companions with whom to spend their time. Every element in hospital life which discourages and minimises the differences between individuals, and which facilitates regimentation and passive conforming to the wishes of those in higher positions, must be regarded as a step towards chronic illness.

It is understandably easy for the busy nurse, beset by many pressing responsibilities from all sides, to fall into the tempting trap of thinking of the conforming and obedient patient as the " good patient ". These patients, barely asserting their individuality at all in the most obvious cases, are in the short-term view relatively easy to nurse—yet it is likely that she will be nursing them for a long time. On the other hand the patient who retains, or attempts to retain, a large segment of his own unique personality will be in many ways a rather more awkward person to have around, but in the long run he is likely to be a much more rewarding therapeutic prospect. One of the most valuable single indicators of a psychiatric nurse's capacity is her ability to run a ward or a small group, maintaining the consistent measure of control which encourages high morale and increases the safety of her patients, yet at the same time paying as much regard as possible to the individual differences which they show. No two patients are ever exactly alike; each one requires individual care up to the limits of time, tolerance and ability. To achieve some approximation of this, in a busy and perhaps understaffed ward, is an indicator of real maturity in a nurse.

The Abolition of Freedom. Residence in a psychiatric hospital, like residence in any other hospital, inevitably involves some surrender of personal liberty. Restrictions are placed on the patient which to some extent must be regarded as an essential part of the hospital's function; certainly a significant group, anxiously struggling to control their own frightening impulses, appreciate the limits which the hospital places on their behaviour. Such restrictions imposed on medical and surgical patients are only rarely of primary importance, though they may have a good deal of secondary significance; to a psychiatric patient, often burdened for many years with complex feelings about control stemming from his own childhood, this situation may mean a great deal. The nurse must never permit herself to forget the fact that loss of liberty is a potentially humiliating and threatening situation for the great majority of people; losing sight of this awareness can quickly lead to the mentality that sees a generally restrictive attitude as being inevitable and even actively desirable. In some psychiatric hospitals, for example, patients who have been granted freedom of movement within the grounds are referred to as " privilege patients "; surely it is more reasonable to see freedom of movement as a natural right, any curtailment of which is always viewed as a highly significant matter with its own repercussions on the individual and on the community.

Many of the occupational and general activity programmes which are playing an increasingly important part in the life of the psychiatric hospital demand a relaxation of the traditionally restrictive concepts of custodial care and a much greater concentration on the assets of patients rather than an exclusive focus on their handicaps, special symptoms and dangerous potentialities. There are still many people who regard all psychotic patients as potential murderers and rapists—extreme fears which are only justifiable in a tiny handful of the hospital population. Excessive preoccupation with these anxieties led, amongst other things, to the traditional rigid segregation of all male and all female patients, except on certain licensed and intensely supervised occasions of modest revelry. Fortunately this attitude has now broken down in an increasing number of hospitals, and it has been found that there are many advantages and no particular problems in the provision, for example, of mixed dining and recreation facilities. Where disturbed male patients are encouraged to participate in female occupational therapy sessions their behaviour has been found

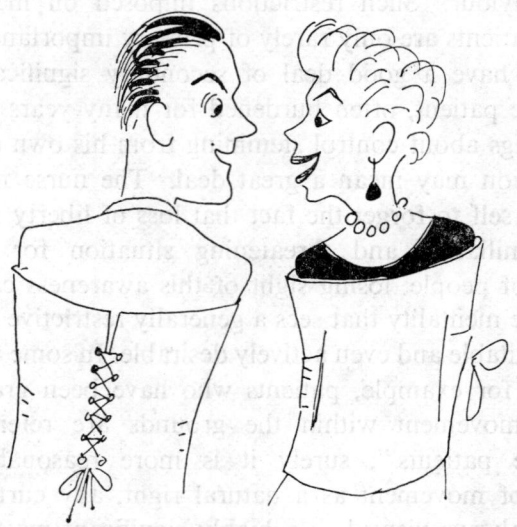

FIG. 30
The traditional rigid segregation of male and female patients.

to be capable of a much greater degree of control and maturity than had previously been suspected; in fact, the very idea of male and female occupational rooms has become outmoded. Some very disturbed patients are now being managed without incident in mixed wards in general hospital psychiatric units. Uninhibited sexual behaviour or obscene language, freely indulged in behind the doors of the chronic ward, may completely disappear in a more rational environment which permits normal conversational and social interchange with the opposite sex. Those people who steadfastly maintain the correctness of a completely segregated environment are often those who are most surprised and perturbed by the frequency of homosexual and masturbatory practices in the wards.

THE PSYCHIATRIC HOSPITAL

There is still a certain amount of controversy about the extent to which psychiatric hospital wards should be unlocked and the patients given unrestricted freedom of the grounds. The universal trend is towards much more liberal policies in this regard and in those hospitals which have become completely " open " the general opinion has been that, after an initial adjustment period, patient behaviour has been more predictable and on the whole more manageable. Other hospitals favour the principle of the open door policy, but make out a good case for the retention of a few wards providing maximum observation in a closed or semi-closed environment. Many observers have found that the incidence of disturbed behaviour is less in open wards and that staff at all levels express a greater interest and contentment in their work, though they may take longer to adjust to the change than the patients. These experiences have shown that there can never be any excuse for a return to the traditional, time-worn rituals of purely custodial care. If one's system of restrictions is tight enough it is easy to run a ward in which all unpleasant possibilities are completely forestalled; unfortunately it is almost certain to be a ward from which few patients are returned to the outside world.

THE CONCEPT OF THE THERAPEUTIC COMMUNITY

The concept of the psychiatric hospital as a therapeutic community implies that every single aspect of the hospital's structure and function, and the attitudes and behaviour of each one of its staff members, shall be regarded as having a potentially therapeutic effect on the patients under care. These communities represent a relatively new development in the psychiatric scene and there are still many unsolved questions relating to their organisation.

Some of the factors involved in the creation of such an environment will be obvious from what has gone before. It is clear that the nurse's task must include an attempted reversal, within the limits already discussed, of the unfortunate consequences of the five aspects of hospitalisation previously

described. There are therefore **five questions** which the nurse should repeatedly be asking herself, which may be put in this way: " How far can I, having due regard for the safety of my own and other patients, and within the limits set by my superiors, manage this patient so as to :
1. Foster his movement towards independence?
2. Grant him the greatest possible amount of privacy?
3. Maintain or improve his usual personal standards?
4. Make maximum allowance for his own individuality?
5. Interfere as little as possible with his freedom?"

The answers to these questions will never come easily, for reasons which have already been suggested; they will vary to some extent in each hospital and with each patient. But it may well be that it is some very small detail of the nurse's attitude to these problems which sets in train recovery mechanisms which have far-reaching effects, and she must be constantly on the alert for opportunities to make constructive moves in these directions.

The concept of the therapeutic community has in fact been developed in considerably more detail than this by certain creative psychiatric hospital administrators during the past 20 years. There are now many responsible psychiatrists who suggest that the whole social structure of the psychiatric hospital of the past has been anti-therapeutic; these people believe that some of the problems which have been described in this chapter cannot be really tackled without a radical revision of our whole idea of the distribution of power within the hospital. The traditional general hospital, for example, functions on almost entirely authoritarian lines—that is to say, power is wielded quite dictatorially, even though benevolently, from the top level of the administration, gradually being transmitted down through the ranks to the patient lying in bed, whose only task is to respond passively to the various instructions he is given and who plays no part whatsoever in determining his own treatment or in guiding the hospital's day-to-day procedures. It is perhaps arguable whether, even in the general hospital, this pattern always works as well as is commonly believed, but there can be little argument that its wholesale translation to the sphere of the psychiatric hospital is almost entirely inappropriate—and in the early years of this century and before, in the heyday of the large mental hospital, patterns of organisation were built up which were almost exact copies of the general hospital, even though the patient population and the type of problem which resulted were so vastly different.

Supporters of the therapeutic community in its most developed form, of whom **Maxwell Jones** is the best known, believe that it is essential for the environment of the psychiatric hospital to be as similar as is possible to the social organisation which exists in the community outside—which means that it will be very unlike a hospital as the term is usually understood. The power structure of such a unit is deliberately modified in order to allow patients and relatively junior staff members to share authority; this usually involves the development of patients' committees which, although potentially subject to the veto of the senior staff, have a good deal of say in the running of the hospital and in the determination of the limits of permissible behaviour for patients. In some hospitals this procedure has gone so far as to be dignified with the name of **patient government,** and it is said that in these units patients are participating in the democratic process to the fullest possible extent.

An essential feature of such a system is that the freest possible channels of **communication** are maintained within the unit so that decisions are made, not in any authoritarian fashion, but after the expression of all points of view. This emphasis on the importance of communication is an extremely healthy part of the climate of the modern psychiatric hospital; there are grounds for believing that many difficulties encountered in the older type of hospital, both with the patients and with the staff, were due to a lack of understanding at all levels about what was being done and why. Many units now include as an essential part of their day a large group meeting at which free and open expression of feeling is encouraged concerning the problems and tensions which both patients and staff are experiencing. Procedures of this type naturally involve a considerable blurring of the usual sharp status distinctions between patients and nurses; if the former are to be encouraged to be themselves and to express their hostilities and anxieties, then nurses (and doctors) have to be prepared to accept a good deal of outspoken comment of a type never heard in a general hospital ward. General hospital nurses, for example, may therefore be initially quite distressed in such an environment when they find that their role as nurse does not permit them to stand on their dignity and to retreat behind their position of authority in the way to which they have been accustomed. Nevertheless a good deal of experience suggests that this breaking down of the usual rigid barriers leads ultimately to a clearer understanding by the staff of their true role in the unit and it is believed that, if both staff and patients come to see each other in this more realistic way, all groups will benefit. The patient at the same time is being made aware of the effect of his behaviour upon other people and is thus given some degree of social insight. The nurse must appreciate, however, that while nearly all psychiatrists would agree that this type of group meeting represents an important development in patient care, there is considerable difference of opinion as to whether these procedures are simply auxiliary ones, opposing the otherwise antitherapeutic effects of hospital treatment and assisting the patient to develop new and more effective roles, or whether they are of absolutely fundamental importance in bringing about changes in underlying personality problems, and thus the single most important factor in the treatment provided by the hospital. Some aspects of this topic are also considered in the section on group psychotherapy (p. 336).

There is also a move in some quarters for the nurse to discard the traditional uniform of her profession and to carry out her duties in ordinary civilian clothes. We believe that there are many points both for and against this transition, which is mentioned here only to point out the fact that a number of experienced people are convinced that the most effective function of the psychiatric unit can only be brought about by the complete breaking down of the usual conventions associated with hospitals. These administrators feel that the typical nursing uniform is a real barrier to the development of realistic and effective nurse-patient relationships.

At whatever level of complexity the theory is developed the fundamental principle remains the same—to create a hospital environment which, in all its aspects, will hasten the patient's recovery by encouraging the emergence and development of mature, socially adjusted forms of behaviour. The hospital's function " should be to retrain the patient within a therapeutic community to meet the numerous stresses of an ordinary community ".[1]

CONCLUSION

We do not consider it too early to introduce the junior nurse to the basic principles outlined in this chapter; many of the problems she should be able to see for herself from the beginning of her ward training. But it will require the judgement and maturity which come from practical experience, together with a full course of training, to enable her to make any sort of major decision affecting the management of patient groups, and even then her attitudes must develop within the policy of the hospital, the medical superintendent, psychiatrists, matron and senior nurses. A casual reading of the preceding material should not lead her into hasty criticisms of the practices of those in authority over her; it is too easy for her to assume, for example, because supervised bathing is an ordeal for almost all newly admitted female patients, that women should invariably be allowed from the beginning of their hospital stay to bathe in private—a preventable suicide may quite possibly be the result. Yet it is to be hoped that this chapter has quite

[1] Baker, A., Davies, R. L. & Sivadon, P. (1959). *Psychiatric Services and Architecture*. Geneva: World Health Organisation.

clearly shown that an excess of supervision is unnecessary and in very many instances may be positively harmful. Throughout the period of her apprenticeship the trainee nurse should be observing, studying and attempting to understand patients' reactions to certain specific hospital situations, but moving to alter these only in minor ways where there is clearly no possibility of any unforeseen result.

The climate of the psychiatric hospital is changing fairly rapidly and it is probable that during the next 10 or 20 years there will be further substantial alterations in the role and responsibility of the nurse. There is by now a good deal of evidence to suggest that the traditional, authoritarian pattern of hospital or ward organisation is not in the best interests of the psychiatric patient and that maximum therapeutic benefit involves a much greater degree of participation by the patient in the running of the hospital than has previously been thought desirable. In any progressive change in the hospital structure the nurse is in a very real sense the key figure, for reasons which have been outlined; without her co-operation the idea of a therapeutic community is totally unworkable. It is in our view no overstatement to say that the ability to assist in the creation of a therapeutic hospital environment and to participate actively in its functioning is the ultimate goal of nursing training.

20

METHODS OF OBSERVING AND RECORDING BEHAVIOUR

For the nursing of psychiatric patients to be adequate it must be based on detailed, trained observation. Moreover, really effective nursing plans arise from a relatively long-term study of the individual patient which can determine the exact areas in which he needs help and the type of help which is best suited to his particular problems. The psychiatrist will usually have fairly definite aims and goals for the patient which, at clinical conferences or in other ways, he will make known to the nurse; these plans however are likely to be of a fairly general kind and in psychiatry, more than in any other branch of nursing, a mere slavish following of someone else's directions is quite inadequate. Implementation of the psychiatrist's ideas will depend on an intelligent translation of them into action by the nurse, and in fact her observations may be very important factors in modifying his own views. In any event, whatever the psychiatrist thinks and directs, the nurse must understand the patient herself, for only on this basis can productive co-operation be established.

Many senior psychiatric nurses with years of practical experience behind them appear at times to be intuitive—that is, they seem able to sense a patient's feelings before he expresses them, or predict his behaviour before it occurs, yet when asked to explain the reasons behind their judgements they are often unable to do so. It is therefore sometimes said, in a hopeless and pessimistic spirit, that there is little that can be done to train a nurse in the art of appreciating the significance of disturbed behaviour; those who hold this view put forward the theory that it is experience alone, or perhaps some inborn gift, which counts. Whilst extensive practical work is obviously an essential feature of any training programme, it is nevertheless true that, from her earliest days in the wards, the junior nurse can and should acquire under supervision techniques of skilled observation which will greatly shorten the otherwise tedious trial and error methods which have all too often been used in the past.

THE INVESTIGATION OF MENTAL STATE BY OBSERVATION AND CONVERSATION

Everyone meeting another person for the first time gains a definite general impression. As her knowledge increases the nurse will realise that she must not be misled by superficialities of behaviour and that this first impression must be carefully analysed; what may be dismissed by the untrained observer as eccentricity, queerness or viciousness will have a great deal more meaning to the experienced nurse. A satisfactory nurse-patient relationship begins with skilled observation and is further developed through the medium of conversation which leads to mutually understandable communication between the two parties. It is only through these techniques that the patient will come to develop trust in the nurse and this, as has been said elsewhere, is an essential beginning to any therapeutic work. The nurse's attitude is therefore of prime importance; only in a setting where the patient feels that an attempt is being made to understand him with genuineness and warmth will he begin to reveal his essential self. Throughout her training the nurse must be constantly refining the techniques of observing and chatting to patients without making them feel uneasy, so that in an unobtrusive manner she can gather information which can then be employed constructively in planning their treatment programmes.

Naturally the nurse's observations must be as objective as possible. An **objective observation** is one in which the observer's view of a certain piece of behaviour is not significantly coloured by her own personal emotional reactions. It is probably impossible to be completely objective—in fact too great an objectivity may be associated with a machine-like approach and an aloof clinical detachment which the patient may interpret as hostile and frightening. The nurse must react to patients as people and not as things and therefore to some extent she must respond with her own feelings; yet, on the other hand, too great a degree of emotional involvement will blur her capacity for detached judgement of what she is observing and will lead to a totally **subjective observation,** which is almost completely personal and therefore unreliable. As an elementary illustration of this, doctors do not ever treat their own close relatives and nurses are not asked to care for their own family members during a serious illness, because in each instance the degree of emotional involvement is likely to be so great that it will blur and distort impartial judgement. In the ordinary clinical situation the nurse must be aware of her own feelings and must seek to understand the reasons for them if she senses that they are in some way affecting her viewpoint on a patient in her care. That is to say, the observation of the patient by the nurse can never be divorced from a simultaneous observation of herself; the nurse's own feelings and the effect which she is having upon the patient may even be the underlying cause of the behaviour she is reporting.

Spontaneous behaviour is often more revealing than the somewhat guarded reactions which the psychiatrist sees during a planned and structured situation in his office; important unrehearsed responses will often be noted by the nurse during the patient's varied relationships with the staff, with other patients, with family, friends and strangers. There are no particular times at which observation can safely be relaxed; at all hours of the day and night, in all situations and for as long as the patient remains in hospital, useful information may be gained which can assist in the understanding and subsequent modification of his behaviour. While valuable knowledge may at times be gained from an isolated incident, the most helpful observations of all are those which reveal some consistent trend in behaviour.

The nurse's views of a patient will be substantially affected by the amount of knowledge which is gained about his previous personality and about the factors which have influenced him to become the kind of person that he is. Many of her early contacts, therefore, will be directed towards eliciting this kind of information through the medium of ordinary conversational interchange. Patients will often reveal to nurses significant aspects of their past history which they have either deliberately withheld from psychiatrists, or which they have not thought important enough to mention. The nurse may also be in the best position to assess the effect his illness is having upon his existence and to judge the extent to which his symptoms are limiting his participation in life. Here as always a purely surface study may be deceptive; the patient himself may not always say what he means or understand what he says.

It should not be understood from what has been said that it is necessary or desirable for the nurse to obtain a formal history of the type taken by the psychiatrist. Nor should her conversation with patients take the form of numerous questions requiring definite answers; most patients understandably will resent this. On the contrary, the contact between nurse and patient should be primarily in the form of random conversation, used initially in the establishment of a warm and friendly relationship but proceeding almost imperceptibly from that point to more significant areas. Of course conversation between nurse and patient, although random and seemingly casual, is never meaningless; chatty interchanges of whatever kind may have a deeper unrecognised significance for the patient. This is not to underrate the value of spontaneous warm feeling shown by the nurse, but she must be aware that even apparent trivialities in her conversation may have a significant effect, for good or ill, upon certain patients; if a seemingly insignificant remark has an effect quite different from that which might reasonably be anticipated, she must attempt to examine the possible reasons why this particular comment was " loaded ". The skilled nurse will not only be able to direct casual conversation into channels which she knows to be important from her previous study of the patient; she will also be aware of certain sensitive areas which must be avoided or in which she must tread with great care.

All this is designed to achieve a greater and deeper understanding of the patient's personality, past history and present symptoms. Because of the comparatively small number of psychiatrists in a large hospital doctors inevitably place a good deal of reliance on the trained observations of the nursing staff; their reports are essential for him to have adequate knowledge of the patients and of great assistance to him in confirming or disproving impressions and diagnoses. Frequently the nurse's observations will be instrumental in leading to a greater awareness of what the patient is really thinking and a more valuable understanding of his deeper unrecognised (unconscious) feelings.

THE SYSTEMATIC RECORDING OF INFORMATION

The enthusiastic nurse will tend, in the first instance, to acquire rather uncritically a mass of information, only some of which has any particularly significant meaning; she should not be dismayed by this, because with increasing experience she will learn to select those features which throw the greatest light on the problem. In training and systematising her observations she must have some way of organising the information she obtains which will help her to limit the accumulation of unnecessary and irrelevant material.

It is also desirable that the nurse should write down her findings or discuss them with a colleague, though she must learn to arrive at conclusions which are based primarily on her own investigations. Expert guidance is of great assistance, as is increasing theoretical knowledge, but in the long run it is unhelpful and sometimes dangerous for the nurse to accept another person's interpretation of the situation without testing it out or seeing the truth of it for herself. Even if many of her earlier observations are incorrect, as they undoubtedly will be, they are essential steps on the road to competence and maturity; if she always relies on the views of others she will place a severe limitation on her own capacity to learn.

In all psychiatric hospitals there will be an agreement between the psychiatrists to use some type of scheme in the assessment of a patient's personality and attitude, collecting the information which is known to be of value in coming to a conclusion about his illness, treatment and future outlook. Other team members will usually employ a somewhat similar scheme. In her own thinking, therefore, the nurse will be well-advised to follow the same sort of plan; she will then understand more easily what the others are saying and the result will be a more productive co-operation between the various members of the staff. Moreover, without such planning, reports are difficult to write, they may contain a mass of unnecessary material, conclusions tend to become confused and the whole thing will lack clarity for the person to whom the report is directed. It is also personally valuable for the trainee to have a scheme in which to assess her patients' behaviour in order that she can apply in a systematic fashion to different types of psychiatric illness the theoretical knowledge that she derives from her lectures and reading.

The following headings are suggested as a guide to the nurse in organising her observations—like any guide it may be altered, enlarged or curtailed, according to the requirements of her training school and depending on certain special problems and local conditions. (It should be read in conjunction with Chapter 6, where the types of abnormality encountered in psychiatric patients are considered in detail.)

General Appearance.
>Physical condition—weight, signs of physical ill-health, bodily deformities.
>Facial expression—anxious, blank, cheerful, hostile, preoccupied.
>Mannerisms—whether within normal limits or of a bizarre kind.
>Posture—any unusual positions.
>Personal hygiene—care of clothes and of the body generally.

Activity.
>General level of activity—overactive or retarded.
>Unusual forms of gait.
>Spontaneity—or lack of it.
>Special patterns of activity—stereotypy, catatonia, compulsions, and many others.

General Behavioural Patterns.
>Conventional and socially acceptable—or unexpected and unpredictable.
>Hostile, causing disturbance to other patients, or showing self-directed hostility.
>Occupation—purposeful or meaningless.
>Withdrawn or sociable—preferring to be alone, afraid of others or enjoying their company.
>Attitude towards the hospital—co-operative or antagonistic.
>Ability to take initiative.
>Behaviour in specific situations:
>— on the ward, with other patients, with the staff;
>— with the opposite sex;
>— at occupational or industrial therapy;
>— in social situations;
>— with visitors, family and friends;

Behaviour in specific situations:
— at meals: appetite and manners;
— at night: normal or insufficient sleep; difficulty in getting off to sleep, easily roused, waking early, causing disturbance at night, sedation required.

Speech.
Rate of speech—accelerated, retarded, unexpected pauses, mute.
Form of speech—logical or showing evidence of thought disorder, circumstantiality, perseveration, use of neologisms, aphasia.
Abnormal content—ideas of reference, delusions, hallucinations, obsessions, phobias, hypochondriacal concerns.
Special preoccupations—unusual subjects, repeated reference to some particular topic or person such as a family member, an incident in development, or a current stress.
Persons with whom patient usually converses.

Mood.
Excitement, elation.
Depression, evidence of suicidal preoccupation.
Anxiety, tension, apprehension.
Disinterest, apathy, inappropriate or incongruous emotional response.
Sudden changes in mood, lability.
Episodic or sustained hostility, passive aggression.
Guilt, shame.

Memory.
Retentive or forgetful.
Blank periods, amnesia, loss of recent or remote memory.
Confabulation.

Attention.
Level of consciousness and awareness.
Ability to concentrate and calculate.

Inattention, preoccupation.
Inability to understand simple communications.
Disorientation—for time, place or person.
Confusion—subjective or objective.

Intelligence.
Estimate of basic intelligence, degree to which intelligence is used appropriately.
General standard of education.
Evidence of deterioration from previous intellectual standard.
Special interests and talents.

Judgement and Insight.
Accurate or unrealistic judgement.
Attitude to illness—illness completely denied, attributed to physical causes, realistic or unrealistic attitude to hospitalisation, plans for future.

It is important for the nurse to become familiar with such a plan, to think of it during her everyday contacts with patients and to refer to it from time to time so that it becomes in the end a largely automatic way of considering abnormal behaviour. It is not of course intended to suggest that it should become fixed as a static scheme in her mind, for it would be futile for such a plan to become the beginning and end of all observation. All sorts of details which are not covered in the above table may be of importance in particular instances. But it is only when something like this has been mastered that the nurse can go on to expand her powers of observation and find new ways to improve her understanding of behaviour.

This detailed study of the patient should not be regarded by the nurse as something terribly advanced, to be learnt only when she is completely proficient in making beds, taking temperatures and giving out medicines. Observational skills, plus the development of meaningful conversation with the patient, should begin to be developed from the moment that the nurse commences duty. Every single task which she performs on the ward is done either in conjunction with or near patients; opportunities to establish communication are always present and should be seized as soon as possible. Some of the routine jobs inseparable from nursing can be made less dreary and more interesting if she uses them as an opportunity to observe and to get to know the patients with whom she is associated. With a large number of patients and perhaps too few nurses these techniques are essential for patient welfare, quite apart from their extreme importance in developing the alertness and sustaining the interest of the nurses themselves.

NURSES' NOTES AND RECORDS

However significant the nurse's observations of her patients may be, a large part of their value will be lost if accurate and complete records of her findings are not kept. The traditional type of nursing record unfortunately often contains little really significant information. All too commonly one finds only stereotyped behaviour charts and conventionally repeated phrases which have little real meaning; this pattern appears to have developed in an effort to save the nurse's time, but it is quite obvious that much time is in fact wasted in this way.

Nursing notes are already in use in many psychiatric hospitals and provide information of great value without in any way interfering with the nurse's other duties. The following may all be regarded as legitimate **purposes** of such notes:

1. To give the psychiatrist information about the 24-hour behaviour of the patient.

2. To indicate the patient's relationships with other significant people.

3. To pass on useful information to other nurses.

4. To serve as part of the official record of the patient; nurses' notes may be of great importance in planning current treatment, in subsequent research and may in some circumstances be a significant legal document.

OBSERVING AND RECORDING BEHAVIOUR

5. To assist the trainee nurse by stimulating her interest in the particular problem under consideration and to provoke her to additional reading.

6. To provide psychiatrists and senior nursing staff with a basis for teaching; the notes may be used in group discussions to help trainees to evaluate situations in an objective way and to analyse the factors which affect the nurse-patient relationship.

When nurses' notes are used regularly by the hospital and are referred to in case conferences, nurses will take pride in doing them well and will know that they are making a significant contribution to the welfare of their patients.

The following **10 principles** should be observed in the preparation of nursing notes:

1. Care must be taken to convey the precise meaning intended; description of behaviour and conversation must be accurate.

2. Statements should be as objective as possible.

3. Notes should be brief—the quality, not the quantity, is important.

4. Information should be concrete—generalisations are usually valueless.

5. Simple descriptive English should always be used in preference to technical terms.

6. Direct quotations can be most valuable, especially in reporting delusions and hallucinations.

7. The form of the notes should be flexible, depending on the type of patient being studied.

8. Notes should be written at least once weekly, with special incidents described as they occur.

9. Notes must be dated and signed; they are valueless if they lack a proper time sequence and if the writer cannot be identified.

10. Any relevant material produced by the patient himself should be included—for example, writings, sketches and paintings.

NURSING PLANS

The nurse should from time to time undertake a more detailed study of certain individual patients. Her aim in doing this is to arrive at a set of conclusions concerning the desirable part for the nursing staff to play in the patient's treatment and rehabilitation; to achieve this she will need to consider his current mental state, the history of his illness and certain factors from his past life and personality. Suitable patients for this type of study should be selected after consultation with the ward medical officer or senior nurses. Background should be obtained where necessary from the official records —the psychiatrist's and social worker's interviews, psychological test results and so on—but the main bulk of the information should come from her own observation and conversation along the lines already suggested, other material being used to check and expand her own views rather than as a primary source.

This material also requires organisation along fairly definite lines and the following scheme is suggested for the purpose; only when written down in some planned way will the nurse's views be clear in her own mind.

1. **History of present illness**—including reference to any apparent situation of stress which existed at the onset.

2. **Developmental history:** childhood, family situation, schooling, occupational and marital history.

3. **Previous personality,** noting any abnormal attitudes or personality traits which were in existence prior to the onset of the illness.

4. **Detailed description** of the patient at the present time— that is, relevant observations of the type described earlier in this chapter. Mention will be made of symptoms and signs shown in the areas of thinking, feeling and acting; his social adaptation to hospital routines and to other patients will be noted.

5. **Nursing problems** presented by the patient—for example, inadequate personal hygiene, abnormal attitudes to other patients and staff, relation of his behaviour to reality, aggressiveness, extreme dependence, abnormal sexuality, and so on.

6. **Possible solutions** for these problems—the ways in which staff attitudes and activities can best help the patient.

7. **The significance of the patient's behaviour**—to himself, to his family, to the community, before and during hospitalisation and after discharge.

8. **Difficulties in rehabilitation** and possible solutions for these—for example, economic, social, educational and personal problems.

Having assembled her material in this way, the nurse will have a much clearer idea of the specific benefit which might be expected to follow from nursing procedures in the particular case; she will have a more definite notion of the problems posed or likely to be posed in the nurse-patient relationship and may well have very distinct clues as to the sort of role which it will be most profitable for her to adopt.

We are not suggesting here that nurses from their own observations should develop their own personal theories of patient care and follow these regardless of the views of other team members. Ample stress has been laid elsewhere on the absolute necessity for co-operation and the place of the psychiatrist as leader of the therapeutic team. What we do believe is that the nurse will be a much more effective member of this team and that the trainee will learn more speedily and with greater understanding if she thinks for herself about selected patients under the general supervision of the psychiatrist, rather than follow passively and uncritically along the lines which he suggests. While her own training and background are nowhere near as detailed as his, her special closeness to the patient provides her with unique opportunities for observation and understanding, the importance of which she should not underrate.

GROUP OBSERVATION

We have so far been concerned with the nurse's observation of the individual patient. This must always form the basis of her opinion, but there are many occasions on which she will obtain valuable knowledge from the observation of patients in groups, and in some wards this may have to be her chief source of information. The patient's responses to the community life which is inevitable in a psychiatric hospital may be of great significance.

Observation of groups, like that of individuals, must be subtle and unobtrusive if it is to be meaningful. She will derive the greatest benefit if she can herself participate to the fullest possible extent in the group's activities; failing this, her observation is likely to be conspicuous and will probably in itself greatly distort the patients' reactions and lead to artificial and misleading responses.

From her observation of group interaction the nurse will learn many significant details about her patients' needs and problems. The impression which she has of a patient may, for instance, be substantially modified when she notices the people whom he chooses as his associates. Some of these contacts may appear unusual to her and in seeking the reason for them she may be led to understand new aspects of his personality. A significant aspect of her assessment of a patient will be the status which he has in the eyes of his fellows and the attitudes which others show towards him.

Group interaction is of great value to all psychiatric patients and the nurse must be constantly on the look-out for opportunities to draw the reluctant ones into some type of group activity. It is most important to do this at the patient's own pace, and on many occasions this may need to be a very slow one. His reaction to the nurse's attempts to involve him in group activity may be extremely significant; she may learn a lot from noting the types of group behaviour which cause him to withdraw and the circumstances which lead him to isolate himself and abandon communication with others. In a group previously unsuspected aspects of a patient's personality may be revealed; participation with others may arouse specific healthy or unhealthy reactions which throw a new light on his problem and his management.

CONCLUSION

The observation of psychiatric patients by the nurse, both as individuals and in groups, will present a constant challenge to her ingenuity and initiative. Throughout her training—in fact throughout her whole life as a psychiatric nurse—she will be developed and refining new techniques for the understanding of psychiatric illness through the medium of ordinary observation and conversation. Through the use of nurses' notes and nursing plans she will gradually improve her facility in systematising and recording these observations; these tasks, which appear so difficult to the young trainee, will gradually become natural skills with the passage of time. Florence Nightingale wrote in 1859: " the most important practical lesson that can be given to nurses is to teach them what to observe—how to observe—what symptoms indicate improvement—what the reverse—which are of importance—which are of none ". She went on to say " the vagueness and looseness of the information which one receives . . . would be ludicrous if it were not painful ", and added a warning to nurses, " . . . if you cannot get the habit of observation one way or other, you had better give up being a nurse, for it is not your calling, however kind and anxious you may be ".[1]

[1] Nightingale, Florence (1952). *Notes on Nursing*. London: Duckworth.

21

THE RELATIONSHIP OF THE NURSE TO THE PATIENT'S RELATIVES

AMONG the people who accompany the patient to the hospital and who visit him there are frequently those with whom he has lived and in whose company he has grown up. They all share different parts of his life; they may have been associated with the development of his illness and may to some extent have affected its course. The fact of his illness will also have had a significant impact on them. The nurse's knowledge and understanding of a patient will be greatly modified by her contact with his relatives and these things in turn will affect his progress in hospital and his future when he returns to the community.

Nurses have more opportunity than anyone else in the hospital environment to meet relatives, to talk to them and to understand their attitudes. Getting to know them is therefore an essential part of the nursing care provided for the patient.

THE EFFECT OF THE RELATIVES ON THE PATIENT

All the matters which have been considered in the previous chapter concerning the observation of behaviour can be re-examined in terms of understanding the patient's relatives. The ways in which they act towards the patient and speak to him help the nurse to realise the sort of feelings that they have about him and his illness. Only in the light of this information can she assess how best they can be called upon to assist him in his progress towards recovery.

One of the difficulties experienced by psychiatric nurses in their association with the patient's family is to maintain a reasonably informative level of conversation without being involved in deep and complicated psychological discussions. Even more than with the patients themselves, observation and conversation with the relatives can easily become an intrusion. The experience gained by the nurse during her training tends to lessen her own inhibitions about discussing emotional problems, but this does not apply to the majority of the population who do not find it easy to change overnight, to discard reticence and abandon their reluctance to talk about intensely personal

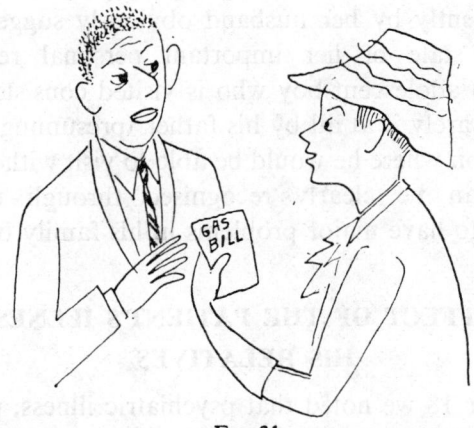

Fig. 31
The effect which visitors have upon his emotional state.

matters. Nevertheless all the information which can be obtained from those people who are close to him at home (or in the community) becomes extremely valuable when added to the information gained by other members of the hospital team and from direct interviews by the psychiatrist with the patient himself. From the relatives, quite informally, the nurse will learn a good deal about his activities, his habits, his dreams and desires, his interests and his achievements, as well as the pattern of his relationship with other people. She will need to note the closeness of the relationship between him and each one of his significant visitors and also to see something of the effect which particular visitors have upon his emotional state. It should be noted how he behaves while preparing for visitors, how he acts during the visit and after they have departed.

It is often extremely significant to observe which of his relatives visit the patient while he is in hospital or accompany him to the outpatient clinic, for it is commonly and correctly said that the individual who goes with the patient to the psychiatrist or to the psychiatric hospital probably plays a significant role in his illness. The fact that a young married woman in hospital is visited very regularly by her mother but only infrequently by her husband obviously suggests at once the current state of her important personal relationships. Similarly, an adolescent boy who is visited consistently by his mother but rarely if at all by his father (presuming that father is in a position where he would be able to visit without extreme difficulty) can be clearly recognised through this simple observation to have major problems in his family background.

THE EFFECT OF THE PATIENT'S ILLNESS ON HIS RELATIVES

In Chapter 18 we noted that psychiatric illness, particularly if it involves hospitalisation, poses certain domestic, economic and social stresses (p. 380). Furthermore, many of the reactions to illness noted in that chapter will affect the family as well as the patient himself. Families too may use **denial** mechanisms in an attempt to cope with the problems posed by illness—in most instances, except where psychiatric disorder is very acute and obvious, the family will have struggled for quite some time to avoid the realisation that one of their number is emotionally disturbed. This pattern may even persist during and after hospitalisation, some relatives, particularly those closely involved in the development of the illness, refusing to admit the seriousness of the patient's disturbance. An irrationally optimistic attitude may be maintained which may seriously interfere with his treatment and rehabilitation; this behaviour is especially noteworthy in the families of some schizophrenic patients.

When once the fact is faced that some member of the family is " sick ", all sorts of anxieties are stirred up in the remaining members. Feelings of hopelessness or helplessness may prevail in view of the fact that all efforts to assist him at home have been in vain, and in these circumstances unwarranted **pessimism** may be expressed concerning the probable outcome of his illness. Many relatives have a deep sense of **guilt** about the patient's hospitalisation—guilt that he became sick in the first place (because they vaguely perceive that they have contributed to his illness), further guilt that they have sent him off to the unknown perils of hospital, yet more guilt that in some ways life may seem easier at home without him. Sometimes hospitalisation has only been achieved after fairly consistent pressure exerted on the patient by his family and in such circumstances he may feel rejected and may convey this feeling to them, increasing their degree of guilt. In other instances unhealthy family pride is hurt by the fact that one of their members requires psychiatric help and this hurt pride may lead to further rejection of the patient, even if he does not in fact require hospital treatment. Rejecting attitudes may develop from an awareness of the inconvenience which his illness is causing or likely to cause in the future. These feelings of anxiety, guilt and rejection are frequently present even though they are not consciously recognised by the individuals concerned.

The presence or absence of such unconscious feelings will determine the ways in which relatives deal with the new situation. Sometimes they display active **aggression** against the hospital and its staff members; in other instances there is an excessive **dependency** on the hospital, by means of which they attempt to abandon all personal responsibility for the patient and his future. Attempts will also be made by some relatives to deal with their own anxiety and guilt by paranoid **projection,** by means of which they shift the " blame " for the patient's illness from inside the family to some factor outside the family circle. Often the hospital or some particular member of the staff is held, quite irrationally, to be responsible for his failure to benefit from treatment.

A further complication may develop out of the fact that the family has to " get by " without the sick person while he or she is in hospital. Mother may have to seek employment, father may need to engage a housekeeper or place the children with relatives or in foster-homes; an adolescent daughter may suddenly be required to shoulder a major share of the responsibility for the care of younger children. The way in which these problems are managed may be so efficient that considerable difficulty arises when the patient tries to get back into the family circle. This is of course particularly true when hospitalisation has been greatly prolonged; it is usually very difficult to persuade families to accept back into their ranks patients who have been away for two or more years. It is therefore important for the rehabilitation of hospitalised psychiatric patients to ensure that relatives maintain as much contact as possible with the patient so that, from both his own and his family's point of view, he is still regarded as one of their number. It has been shown in several hospitals that the patient who becomes almost completely cut off from his family stands a very poor chance of discharge and successful readjustment to society.

THE NURSE'S ATTITUDE TOWARDS THE PATIENT'S RELATIVES

Families take up a good deal of the nurse's time, especially in the beginning. Life in hospital tends to become an everyday affair to the nurse, but the patient and his relatives will view the matter quite differently and their anxieties will be reflected in numerous questions about hospital routines and treatment procedures. Many relatives behave in ways which sorely tax the understanding and the accepting attitude of the nurse, particularly in those instances where she can see their behaviour having a bad effect on the patient. Some appear to have an almost endless supply of questions; some will ask the same questions over and over again because their anxiety is so extreme that they do not take in the answers, or they forget them. They may express dissatisfaction in all sorts of ways with the service provided by the hospital and at times they may be openly irritable with the patient and with the nurses. In other instances they seem to have no realistic expectation of the hospital at all, demanding miracles from the staff and insisting on the rapid return to normality of a patient who has clearly been sick for years. Other relatives are excessively grateful to and dependent upon the hospital staff; this last reaction, whilst often easier for the nurse to handle, is in many instances as much an expression of anxiety, hostility and guilt as the more annoying behaviour just described. The understanding of these attitudes may prevent further difficulties being posed for the patient and may lessen the problems he already faces or will face upon his discharge. All this takes time, patience, tolerance and alertness.

No time is more satisfactory for the establishment of good contact with relatives than during the admission procedures (p. 438). Here the behaviour and the attitude of the nurse have an immediate effect which may extend for a considerable period into the future. Her desire to help will usually be conveyed more by her manner and her general approach than by the actual words she uses. She should be creating for the relatives, as well as for the patient, an initial contact marked by unhurried courtesy, kindness and sympathetic understanding. Whilst admitting the patient she should commence to be a source of support, reassurance, comfort and help to the family and should at this point begin to lay the foundations of a useful future relationship. The effort which she expends on daily chores about the ward, keeping it clean and tidy and as attractive and home-like as possible, will affect the physical and mental comfort of the patient's family, who are deriving their first impression of the hospital at this time. Their impressions will also be coloured by what they observe of the relationship of the nurse to other patients and to other staff members with whom they see her engaged in conversation.

The physical comfort of visitors and the psychological effect which this has upon them can easily be overlooked in a busy hospital. The nurse should be concerned about where relatives will wait to visit a patient or to see his psychiatrist or social worker, how long they wait and what they see and hear while waiting. Only a little planning and foresight should be necessary to ease their anxieties by offering them diversions during any such waiting periods—magazines and newspapers, turning on the wireless or television, suggesting where they can have a cup of tea (or producing one), providing a suitable companion for conversation.

While the visitor is actually with the patient the nurse should make an opportunity for casual but systematic observation of the relationship between them. The more the relatives are personally involved during the process of visiting the more will they be able to allay their own anxieties and be of real support to him. There are endless possibilities here—it can be suggested that they help by mending, sewing on name tapes, going to the canteen and so on. It can be suggested that visitors read aloud to him, play cards or word games or join in discussion with his associates. The encouragement of simple activities is particularly important when it appears that concentrated or confused conversation by the relatives about his family, home or business affairs is distressing to him.

It is often possible for the nurse to introduce relatives of different patients to one another and such contacts may be a great source of direct or indirect support to these families and therefore in the long run of benefit to the patient. Where a patient does not have relatives to visit him, or is far from his own home, the nurse can often be instrumental in seeking the aid of voluntary visitors. She should note as early as she can those patients who receive few or no visitors and draw the attention of other staff members to this fact so that, if possible, contacts can be made by the social worker which may improve the situation.

Reassurance can frequently be offered to relatives by drawing their attention to improvements in the patient's condition. For instance, it is usually comforting for them to be informed if his appetite has improved and if he is gaining weight, or if he is now sleeping throughout the night without sedatives, or if he is asking for information about his workmates. With some relatives, too insecure to seek information directly, the nurse has many opportunities to take the initiative, asking for example for writing-paper to be brought to the patient as he is now wishing to write to his friends.

A younger nurse may have difficulty here in that some older relatives feel that their own background enables them to understand the patient much better than she does; in some cases she may find herself being openly criticised for her lack of experience—such situations require more than her usual amount of understanding and patience. Some relatives can be so difficult that the nurse may find herself contriving ways of avoiding them and there is often the temptation to spend one's time during visiting hours with the more pleasant and obviously more grateful families. It is clear however that this course of action will tend to lead to a further isolation of the "difficult" relatives from the hospital organisation and in the long run will react unfavourably on the patient's progress.

The nurse should not lose sight of her potential role as a health teacher in the patient's family. For a start, her own appearance, physical health and emotional state will all have great impact upon the relatives. Friendly and seemingly casual discussions about food, cooking, current ideas on nutrition and dental care, the amount of sleep required (and on these and many other matters the family may have some quite extraordinary views)—all these topics can be opened up by the nurse, not only to gain a knowledge of the patterns of behaviour at home, but in an attempt to improve the situation to which the patient will be returning.

RELATIVES AND OTHER STAFF MEMBERS

The nurse must clearly understand where her role with visitors begins and ends and how it is related to the tasks of other members of the team. Maintaining her own role may be extremely difficult in those hospitals where the ratio of psychiatrists to patients is low and where few psychiatric social workers are available; relatives in such circumstances will tend to rely more completely on the nurse for information and the demands upon her will consequently be increased. Many questions may be directed towards her concerning the causes of the patient's illness, its probable outcome, or the form which his treatment is likely to take. All these are subjects on which the family must be referred promptly to the psychiatrist. The nurse however should make it her business to be aware of the psychiatrist's plans and to discuss with him wherever possible the various problems which arise out of the relationship of the patient to his family. She should be in a position to reinforce what has already been discussed between the relative and the psychiatrist and in some instances may be able to support his views by the elaboration of certain details with the family. Except on practical matters she must refrain from passing an independent opinion.

Some relatives are reluctant to disturb busy doctors or are unwilling to become too involved in discussions which they see as likely to implicate themselves; others fail to understand (or do not wish to see) their own vital role in the patient's illness and treatment. It is an important part of the nurse's job to make them aware of the availability of the psychiatrist and the social worker and to make sure that they have adequate opportunities for contact with them.

Finally, the nurse should be well informed about available social services and about voluntary as well as official agencies which exist in the community for the benefit of the psychiatric patient. Where voluntary lay groups such as rehabilitation clubs come into the hospital the nurse should encourage active participation in these organisations by the family where this seems appropriate.

CONCLUSION

In all sorts of ways the contact which develops between the nurse and the patient's relatives can affect the patient's subsequent behaviour. (He will of course note this relationship—his reaction may be one of puzzlement or anxiety or may lead him to see his family in something of a new light.) Through discussions with her fellows and with senior staff members, and by writing down her own observations and referring back to them, the nurse will gain a further realisation of the subtle and complex influences which affect one person's relationship with another. The understanding and handling of these situations should be a constant challenge to her powers of discovery. Furthermore, when the nurse by her example and conversation succeeds in bringing to a family and to other visitors a greater awareness of the patient's disabilities and creates increased tolerance of them, not only then is one particular patient affected but a little bit more knowledge is spread through the community about mental health and the problems of psychiatric illness.

22

NURSING CARE IN SPECIAL SITUATIONS

MANY general aspects of the nurse's role in patient care have been looked at in this book. In this present chapter we consider some problems posed for the nurse in certain special situations which she will encounter with considerable frequency on any psychiatric service.

ADMISSION PROCEDURES

When a patient is admitted to a psychiatric hospital as an emergency the atmosphere established by the nurse is important in creating in his mind the impression that she and the hospital are willing and able to care for him. More commonly, plans can be made to prepare his bed and surroundings for his arrival and this preparation alone may make him feel expected and welcome. Immediately the nurse should be able to demonstrate, frequently without words, her ability to help him. By taking care of his belongings, by making him familiar with his environment, by introducing him to everyone with whom he comes in contact—in all these ways she starts to give him a feeling of understanding and acceptance. These simple actions, right from the beginning, can favourably influence his opinion of himself and his illness. General home-making duties, which occupy so much of the nurse's time and effort, may make a great impact on him. He may not show this sense of acceptance and may not even be consciously aware of it, but if the nurse is quietly confident and inspiring she lays the foundation for a belief that he will improve with the care and support which is being offered to him. As far as is possible at this time she assists him to appreciate what this care will involve.

NURSING CARE IN SPECIAL SITUATIONS

Some patients on admission, because of the acuteness of their illness or the overwhelming nature of their problems, may be unable to understand or accept the help which is given. Many junior nurses therefore find it difficult to see that they are making any contribution to the patient's psychological care. They may initially be dismayed by his apparent failure to respond to the warmth of their welcome and may find it difficult to accept delay in seeing the result of their labours.

The attitude of the nurse to the patient's relatives at the time of admission has already been discussed (p. 433).

We have mentioned only the *attitudes* required of the admission nurse. There are also extremely important detailed *procedures* which need to be undertaken at this time; as these will vary to some extent from one hospital to another they are not specified here.

AIMS FOR THOSE WHO NEED LONG-TERM HOSPITAL CARE

Goals which are unrealistic have no place in psychiatric nursing. They will place intolerable burdens on the patient and may actually hamper his adjustment; moreover they will tend to frustrate and discourage the nurse. In the present state of psychiatric knowledge it is inevitable that a certain group of patients will fail, for one or another reason, to respond to available treatments and will require long-term, even if intermittent, residence in hospital (p. 31). Many of those who might in an earlier time have come into this category are now being cared for in outpatient clinics, day hospitals, geriatric centres, sheltered workshops or working settlements, and in many instances are being kept away from institutions altogether by adequate community services.

For the truly long-stay patient a rather different type of programme needs to be initiated which understands his assets and uses them to the full in order to ensure his most satisfactory and contented adjustment to hospital life. For these people the psychiatric hospital becomes home in every sense of the term and it should resemble home as closely as possible—in appearance, in atmosphere and in function. Attention must therefore be given to both the physical and the psychological environments in which the patient is going to live.

The Physical Environment. The nurse must be constantly mindful of those small details in the physical environment which make life easier and more comfortable for her patients. She will be much rewarded when she uses her ingenuity to create a pleasant atmosphere even in basically unfavourable surroundings, such as in old buildings with large rooms. Every effort should be made to take away a forbidding, regimented appearance; for example, long lines of beds in dormitories can be broken up in various ways, being arranged in small bays with the use of different coloured bedspreads and small tables interspersed between them. Any touch of colour from soft furnishings, flowers, books, magazines and small personal possessions may be beneficial. Chairs placed in small groups are conducive to informal discussions and more friendly relationships. Furthermore, since chairs are now receiving scientific attention regarding their height, size and shape, special thought must be given to those used by the aged and physically handicapped, so that they may be made more comfortable and yet more independent. Although modern functional furniture may be attractive by the nurse's own standards, and relatively easy to maintain, she must remember that for many of her older patients it may seem too stream-lined and impersonal and not at all " like home ".

It is a worthwhile goal to maintain as far as possible the orientation of all patients who require long-term care. Clocks should be placed in prominent positions in the ward, large calendars should be available, and there should be easy access to newspapers, radio and television. Frequent alterations in the disposition of furniture in the ward may lead to confusion and difficulty. Orderliness, neatness and, within limits, lack of change are important to these patients. It is helpful for things to be kept in the same place and the nurse should see that they are always returned. Floors should never be highly polished or slippery; any material spilt should be quickly mopped up to avoid accidents; small mats must be avoided. Special attention should be given to bath-rooms, where accidents happen very commonly; patients should not be able to slip on bath-mats, and the nurse should ensure that the necessary fittings work easily. If it seems necessary and appropriate she might recommend the installation of hand-rails in bath-rooms and lavatories and perhaps seats in baths. Wheel-chairs and mechanical lifting devices may be used with great benefit. The maintenance of equipment and supplies is primarily the nurse's responsibility and it is essential for her to see that vital services are kept in proper working order.

Patients should be arranged in the ward so that those most in need are nearest to bath-rooms and toilets.

Living routines should be as simple as possible although some variety and change are desirable within the limitations set by the patient's condition; here again imagination and originality are required of the nurse.

The Psychological Environment. The problem here is to create an environment which is safe in the psychological sense of the word, yet which permits and encourages the patient to function in an individual way, utilising the remaining assets in his personality. Here, as in any other situation, the nurse needs to be dependable, consistent and supportive, accepting the patient's changes of mood and his inconsistencies, tolerant of any slowness and difficulty in comprehension on his part, yet persisting in her efforts to foster his independence and never relaxing in her desire to see him consolidate any progress. She will try to lead the patient to make small choices for himself, to select what he would like to do out of the various possibilities available. She will help to minimise any tendencies towards withdrawal if she quietly brings into their conversation everyday happenings which help him to keep in touch with reality. She must be prepared to remind him of the same things day by day, even hour by hour, if this seems helpful to him. Every effort must be made to keep him in touch with his surroundings —by frequently naming the hospital, talking about local geography, discussing the date, the day and the season, the time of day and the whereabouts of people known to him. At the same time the nurse must become aware of the extent to which the patient's judgement is unreliable so that she can prevent him making foolish mistakes. She may need to see that he does not lose his belongings or give them away; it may be necessary to supervise his money, his tobacco and his fruit so that he does not misplace them or use them all at once.

Effort and personal participation by the nurse will be required to see that the patient does, if practicable, the things that he might do at home, that are familiar to him, and which are part of the pattern of everyone's daily life. She should try to get him to see his illness, if he is aware of it, in its proper perspective and not as the only thing that matters in the world. In these patients it is common for various types of socially unacceptable behaviour to appear and, in advanced cases, the patient may be untroubled by this or even unaware of it. The nurse here has a problem in interpreting this behaviour to other patients and in preserving the all-important human dignity in those circumstances where living may be reduced to fundamentals. Courtesy and respect, here as elsewhere, are important; for example, the patient should be called by his correct title and not by some pet name. She will need to accept exaggerated patterns of behaviour, to tolerate endlessly repeated stories of the past and to adapt to sudden changes of mood. Understanding is easier if she realises that some of the patient's behaviour represents the result of defensive mechanisms which he employs in an attempt to cope with insoluble conflict, intellectual deterioration or failing memory.

Every opportunity must be taken to stimulate mental activity. The nurse must never lose sight of the undesirability of segregated living and should be alert for the chance to arrange meetings and chats with persons of the opposite sex. She can do much to encourage outside visits and trips away from the hospital, whether for a few hours, a week-end, or even for an annual holiday. Every effort should be made to include the patient in a group where, in however limited a way, he can share experiences with others and derive support from them.

The nurse will need to become aware of those things which cause anxiety in each particular patient; she will try to discover any factors which increase his disorganisation, so that she can lessen them as far as she can. It is important for the individual, and vital for the harmony of the ward, for her to be able to anticipate patients' reactions to certain situations and forestall these wherever possible. The pace of life usually needs to be slowed down to fit their capacities: quiet unhurried skills are essential features of the nurse's role.

Occupational, recreational and social therapies are perhaps more important with this group than with any other. In some instances the patient may find a secure niche in one of the service departments of the hospital—in the laundry, in the carpenter's shop or in the canteen. Patients may revive old skills in handicrafts or develop new ones, particularly if special hobbies and interests are considered, and if they are presented with a definite object in view. Making gifts for family members or articles to be used in the ward may increase the capacity to participate. Some of these patients may benefit from involvement in hospital industrial programmes (p. 464) and in some instances these activities may lead to a remarkable rise in the patient's overall level of competence and a general improvement in his behaviour.

Habit Training. Regressive behaviour may be very conspicuous in some chronic psychiatric disorders, whether these be of schizophrenic or organic origin. Patterns of eating, elimination and sexual conduct can return to a quite uninhibited level, though this behaviour is not always as " accidental " as it seems and may arise as a response to conflict in the patient's life or in the ward about him; some patients, like very small children, may wet or soil their clothes as an expression of hostile feelings. Overcoming this deterioration in habits will not only aid the patient but will certainly make the ward a more pleasant place in which to work.

In all these areas of activity new habits can be learnt by teaching, by continued supervision and by reward. A daily timetable is drawn up for activities, with set times for patients to bathe, dress, feed and go to the toilet; gradually the patient is encouraged to use his own initiative in carrying out the task. Progress may be surprisingly rapid in such a group, the theoretical basis of which is **operant conditioning** (p. 341). Similar principles are involved in the institution of training programmes for the mentally retarded (p. 311).

Biological Needs and Physical Care. The nurse must ensure that these patients are adequately nourished, obtain sufficient rest and sleep, get sufficient fresh air and exercise and that their personal hygiene is of a high standard. In the serving of meals small amounts may need to be given at frequent intervals and fluids of high caloric value may be necessary to supplement the diet. Foods which are easily handled and eaten will be required for some patients, and allowance must be made for the fact that some items in the hospital diet may be unfamiliar or disliked and that some choice is important. Monotony in the diet must be avoided if appetite is to be adequate. Every use should be made of those aids which might enable the patient to continue feeding himself if this is proving difficult for him—drinking vessels which are easy to handle and to lift, feeding cups, drinking straws and special cutlery. Water supplied after meals will help to prevent food particles remaining in the mouth and will lessen the possibility of constipation. Regular weekly weighing is of value to check nutritional state and general health.

Many of these patients will require regular rest periods during the day. At night they will be reassured by seeing the nurse constantly in the vicinity; staying with the patient where this is necessary and possible, talking and listening to him, may lessen his worries and fears and may diminish the incidence of nocturnal incontinence. Patients whose confusion is more severe at night may easily fall out of bed and a low bed may prevent many unnecessary injuries. Care should be taken if bed-rails require to be used, as the cage-like effect which the patient can experience in these circumstances may in fact increase confusion and fear. The care of any confused patient, by day or night, will be easier if the nurses in attendance on him change as little as possible.

Unless physical illness intervenes only a few patients will need to remain in bed; if bed care becomes inevitable, the period must be kept as brief as possible. Any prolonged confinement to bed increases the risk of bed-sores, permanent muscle contractures, pneumonia and thromboses, as well as aggravating any physical weakness present. Getting the patient up, walking him about and encouraging simple exercise should be feasible in nearly every case, though fatigue must be avoided. The nurse will find that, even though these chores are time-consuming, the results in the long run are very rewarding, not only because the condition of her patients is improved thereby, but also because the ward will be a more attractive and more satisfying place in which to work.

Physical activity should thus be maintained as fully as possible for as long as possible. Simple uncomplicated surroundings will reduce risks to a minimum. The greatest degree of freedom should be allowed which is consistent with safety, though some of these patients may have a tendency to wander away and precautions may need to be taken to guard against this if some risk seems to be involved. Some patients will even require protection from common physical dangers such as fire. Where physical handicaps exist, with limitation of hearing, vision or movement, special attention will need to be paid to the impact of these on the patient's psychological adjustment. The nurse must also be alert to notice those patients who might be helped by spectacles, false teeth or a hearing aid and should see that these are provided when necessary and make sure that the patient uses them.

Frequent examination of bodily condition is called for, remembering that these patients may not be able to verbalise clearly, if at all, any physical complaints. Old people in particular tend to bruise very easily; every care must be taken to prevent falls, as fractures can be easily sustained and will greatly complicate the patient's condition. The nurse must be constantly aware of the possibility of physical illness and of her responsibility to see that changes in the patient's physical condition do not go unreported. Alterations in body temperature, pulse rate or respiration, the development of a cough or skin rash, increased or decreased urine output or bowel function must all be noted. More than the usual amount of attention will require to be given to general cleanliness and to care of the hair, nails, skin and clothes. The patient's choice of clothing may need gentle supervision to ensure that it is adequate and suitable.

The nurse should avoid producing monotonous, stereotyped reports about patients requiring continuous care. Frequently little information of value concerning them is passed on to other staff members, so that others do not hear of small changes in attitude and response which might aid the formulation of plans for future care. The nurse should also not overlook the families of these patients (p. 432); she should attempt to involve them wherever she can, but if no relatives or friends are available she may seek to establish the patient in a continuing relationship with a suitable voluntary worker.

It is inevitable that deaths will occur among this group of patients and the nurse will then be called upon to maintain the dignity which should surround the ending of life. She will have to console and help the relatives, make arrangements with the Minister and perhaps in some cases be the patient's only companion in his last hours. Too often in hospitals nurses exaggerate the effect of death on other patients and seek to conceal the happening. If she is secure in the knowledge that everything possible has been done, then a mature acceptance of the inevitability of death will allow the nurse to help other patients cope with this without exaggerating or prolonging the attendant sadness.

THE SUICIDAL PATIENT

The thought of suicide raises anxiety and apprehension in most normal people. Until quite recently our culture has looked on suicide as a crime and in various epochs people who have committed "self-murder" have been denied proper burial and have had their possessions confiscated; now we know that it is evidence of sickness and not of wickedness.

Many patients in a psychiatric hospital pose some degree of suicidal risk. The highest incidence of self-destructive behaviour is in those patients diagnosed as having depressive illnesses but suicidal preoccupation and attempts are by no means rare in patients suffering from schizophrenic illnesses, some forms of neurotic reaction and in organic disorders associated with depression. Some general comments on suicide have already been made in Chapter 11 (p. 249).

The psychiatric nurse is required to assume a good deal of responsibility for the protection of patients in hospital from self-injury. Her own attitudes to this task may well be influenced by her own upbringing, past experience and religious training. When a clear indication exists that a patient harbours suicidal thoughts the psychiatrist will issue definite instructions to the senior nurses which will be passed on to those more junior; juniors however must accept responsibility for the reading of reports and must keep themselves up to date with important information about the patient. Moreover, even when definite suicidal precautions are not laid down for a particular patient, the nurse must be aware that there is some truth in the statement that "every depressed patient is potentially suicidal", even though she is meant to be alerted and not alarmed by this phrase. She will also realise that some hallucinated patients may be directed to commit suicide by their voices; others in a state of confusion may make suicidal attempts in an effort to escape from terrifying visual hallucinations. Patients with delusions of persecution or ideas of reference may act impulsively in a suicidal manner.

Routine precautions against the risk of suicide will tend to vary according to the type of hospital, the type of ward, and the characteristics of the group of patients under care at the time. It is the nurse's responsibility to understand and implement any restrictions which may be imposed concerning bathing, smoking and the use of sharp instruments. Hospital policies on these matters must also be clearly conveyed to the patient's relatives, and they may need to be given concise instructions about certain articles which should not be brought into the hospital and handed to the patient, at least for the time being. All these precautions will be even more important on night duty, when fewer staff are available. At the same time it should not be forgotten that suicidal acts take place in many areas other than the wards or grounds of psychiatric hospitals; in the outpatient clinic, in the day hospital, or in her work in the community, the nurse must be continuously sensitive to the possibility that depressed patients may harbour serious suicidal impulses.

Over and above these generalised precautions the nurse's powers of observation and deduction will be of vital importance in the individual case. The care of the potentially suicidal patient is one of the most difficult situations which she will encounter; she is required to be eternally watchful, without making this supervision objectionable and a further stress for the patient. Training and experience will teach her to recognise the varying degrees to which patients can become withdrawn, sad, despairing, hopeless and finally absorbed in morbid thoughts of self-destruction. The prime responsibility of the nurse is to provide trained, accurate observation, together with meticulous reporting. It cannot be too often stressed that the best way to know what is really going on is by the sharing of activities with the patient, rather than by aloof scrutiny without participation. Living and working with him she will take note of his appearance, his posture, his general behaviour and his change of mood; she will be alert to the occurrence of any unusual elements in his conversation. She will carefully note any suggestions, direct or indirect, that " life is not worth living " or that " I'd be better off away from it all ". Certain changes in the patient's behaviour may be ominous—she will carefully investigate anything which suggests that he may be hiding sharp objects or collecting harmful tablets. She will be wary of any patient who spends any substantial period of time in secluded, unfrequented places such as bath-rooms and kitchens. Her observation will be especially keen in the early morning, when suicidal attempts are not infrequent, and at times when the majority of the staff are busily engaged elsewhere or are changing shifts. It is also worth noting that the process of admission into a psychiatric hospital may markedly increase the patient's depression and, by adding to his feelings of worthlessness and hopelessness, may heighten the risk of suicide at this time.

Her attitude towards the patient and her relationship with him may have a substantial preventive value. Any attempt made to rouse him from a state of self-preoccupation will be a step in the right direction and the provision of occupation and recreation is extremely important. Successful participation in ward activities, with increased interest in things outside himself, will be helpful. Moreover, her own relationship with him should be such as to suggest, quietly and usually indirectly, that she wants him to live, that she considers him worthwhile and that she realises that it is only his illness which causes him to entertain such thoughts. When precautions appear to be further aggravating the patient it may be helpful for her to point out that these are taken because of the staff's interest in his well-being.

The situation is made even more complicated by the fact that there are a substantial number of patients who talk of suicide, sometimes in a very flamboyant way, yet who appear to have little or no genuine self-destructive intent. For some of these patients such communications represent an appeal for more attention, or a desperate cry for help; there may also be a significant punitive component, the patient (usually unconsciously) finding gratification in his ability to create anxiety or guilt amongst the staff. Yet any nurse who adopts the position that people who talk about suicide never commit it will sooner or later receive a very painful shock; there are some very tricky situations indeed in which behind the most flagrantly exhibitionistic talk and gesture there lurk strong suicidal drives. Snap judgements in these matters are always dangerous, and a proper appraisal of such a patient will require close observation and careful study, prior to some type of staff meeting at which his needs, personality patterns and current conflict situations can be fully examined.

Whatever the patient's past record, one day the decision has to be made to relax constant observation in the interests of his progress; he must take up again the responsibility for maintaining his own life. This decision is not of course one which is ever made by nursing staff alone, though it is to be hoped that their views will always be considered. The nurse must not take the following statement to indicate any wish to diminish the importance of suicidal precautions, both generally and in particular cases. Nevertheless it is true to say that it would almost certainly be possible to run a ward or a hospital in such a way that no patient had any chance of making a suicidal attempt. Such a completely restricted environment, however, would almost certainly be one in which few patients would ever get better.

When a patient has made a suicidal attempt without success the nurse must give careful thought to her subsequent manner of approach to him, taking care not to avoid him, yet avoiding equally any show of exaggerated concern. She should be guided by his own wishes as to whether the subject is to be discussed between them; if he does want to talk about it then she should listen carefully, making only those comments which show her understanding, reinforce her willingness to help and prove that it makes no difference to their relationship.

If suicide is successfully completed in the hospital then the nurse will have to examine her emotions concerning this with great care. She may feel guilty, angry, helpless and discouraged, all at the same time. She will need to think carefully about the part she herself played in caring for the patient, trying to learn from the episode and neither seeking simply to justify her behaviour nor accepting the result as inevitable. Nevertheless she must be realistic about the extent of her responsibilities and understand that, once the crisis has been met and consolation and assistance offered to distressed relatives, it will be necessary to offer support and reassurance, not only to other patients, but perhaps also to her colleagues.

THE AGGRESSIVE PATIENT

The manifestations of aggression in patients range all the way from a display of dissatisfaction and dislike up to intense anger and hatred shown in assaultive behaviour. Its recognition is easy when it is expressed by swearing, obscenity, abuse or sarcasm or by physical violence directed at other people or at clothing and equipment. It is somewhat more difficult to see when expressed passively (p. 124) or is turned by the aggressive person against himself—the person who " tears his hair with rage ". The nurse however must guard against confusing aggression with healthy self-assertion; a tight control exercised over a group of patients may, under the guise of preventing aggressive behaviour, stifle in some measure even normal activity and useful expression of emotion.

The nurse should try to recognise those factors which are creating or exaggerating her patients' aggressive impulses. Some of these can be understood from a consideration of diagnosis—for example, the epileptic patient may be aggressive either before or after his seizures; the mentally retarded person may become angry if he is urged beyond his capacity; the hallucinated or delusional person may become violent as a response to his abnormal experiences. Certainly no patient becomes aggressive without a reason, though the reason may not be easily apparent to the nurse and may even be completely hidden from the patient's own conscious awareness.

Aggressive behaviour usually tends to increase, both in the individual patient and in the ward as a whole, if action is not taken to deal with it. Usually there is a period of incubation which the alert nurse will try to recognise, after which she will guide her actions by the level of tension which she senses to be existing. Various factors within the ward can be of great importance, not only physical difficulties such as overcrowding, uncleanliness and general disorder, but also factors in the psychological environment. Aggression tends to be more common when patients are uncertain of what is happening, when they fail to understand what is expected of them, and particularly when they feel that unnecessary restrictions are being imposed. Irritating personalities, either among patients or staff, will aggravate the situation; many observations suggest that outbursts of aggression in a ward are very likely to occur when there are differences of opinion between the nurses themselves and when staff tensions and dissatisfactions are high.

If the nurse knows which patients tend to become disturbed it is often possible to draw them away from the group to another part of the ward, or to a quieter room, where there are no distressing influences. Occupation, recreation and socialisation will be vital in helping to direct the excessive energy created by emotions into useful and constructive channels. Relaxation and physical tiredness may be induced by exercise and movement; vigorous activity out of doors, such as games, walking or gardening, can be valuable. In some patients aggressive impulses may subside if they can be diverted to occupations which they find interesting, which absorb their attention and concentration and which are creative and satisfying. Social activities, whilst important, may need to be limited if the patient is showing little control, gradually being re-introduced later with carefully selected companions.

Visiting may promote aggressive feelings in some patients. The nurse should be aware of this problem if it exists and if

NURSING CARE IN SPECIAL SITUATIONS

necessary pass on information to the psychiatrist so that restriction of certain visitors, or of the length of their visit, can be recommended.

Some angry patients are better if left alone, but it may be difficult for the nurse to assess when and for how long; usually a short period is sufficient.

If all these precautions fail more definite measures may need to be taken to check or control aggressive behaviour. Whatever the procedure, it is important to tell the patient what is being done and why—any suggestion of unnecessary domination must be avoided. In most circumstances a "no touch" technique is best adopted—especially if the nurse is uncertain herself, when she will certainly transfer this uncertainty to the patient. Any suspicion of manhandling will invariably increase the patient's violent tendencies. Long leisurely baths may be soothing and relaxing if the patient can be encouraged to take them. A small percentage of patients, openly aggressive or destructive, may require segregation in a single room to prevent their being a danger to themselves or to other people. The room reduces the number and variety of stimuli to which the patient is exposed and should be in a quiet area—simply furnished, with restful colours, containing no hazards nor harmful objects, properly ventilated, well lit but able to be darkened to induce rest. The term **seclusion** refers to the segregation of the patient in a *locked* room. The law requires that such a decision must be entirely the responsibility of a medical officer, by means of a written order. In an extreme emergency the nurse may have to place a patient in seclusion on her own initiative, but she must immediately notify the doctor and obtain written permission for her action.

More definite **restraint** is today brought about almost invariably by the use of drugs, usually of the tranquillising groups (p. 366); these may be ordered intramuscularly or even intravenously in an emergency. Physical controls such as camisoles, leather belts and hand-cuffs have now joined the chains and leg-irons of Pinel's time as museum pieces. Should any form of mechanical restraint ever be used a medical prescription is again necessary to conform with legal requirements.

In all her dealings with the aggressive patient the nurse must be quiet and relaxed in her manner, flexible and capable of accepting strong emotions and refusing to be upset if criticised or rejected. Such attitudes may require enormous control and understanding, particularly in those rare instances when a patient unexpectedly becomes violent towards her, requiring immediate action on her part. It is at these times important to summon adequate help; the senior nurse should be available to assume responsibility and medical assistance should be requested immediately. Many patients, however openly aggressive, may in fact be terrified by the destructiveness they perceive inside themselves and may be powerfully influenced by the nurse's calm in dealing with their anger and reassured by her capacity to assume control.

Reports about patients who have been aggressive must be comprehensive and honest. Too frequently it is found that a patient's aggressive behaviour is exaggerated and only the occasional incidents of violence are reported. This creates a false impression and leads to apprehension in those reading the report. Nurses should also be careful in their conversation with their colleagues to avoid building up a legend about the aggressiveness of a particular patient; unreasonable anticipation that he is dangerous may lead to his being neglected, or to his being subjected to excessive repression, both of which may only add to the strength of his angry impulses.

EMERGENCIES IN THE PSYCHIATRIC HOSPITAL

Some of the emergency situations which may arise while caring for psychiatric patients have already been mentioned. Whenever the mental state is extremely disordered, such as in extreme confusion or grave depression, the possibility always exists that a crisis may arise calling for rapid action on the nurse's part.

NURSING CARE IN SPECIAL SITUATIONS

Various physical events in the patient's life may require immediate action; some of these occur more frequently in the psychiatric hospital than elsewhere. Such situations include burns and scalds, fractures and sprains, accidental or self-inflicted wounds, choking, poisoning, sudden unconsciousness and so on. The procedure in these cases will be essentially similar to that carried out when a mentally normal person creates such an emergency, but the nurse will find that mental disturbance can mask or in other ways make more difficult the detection and management of the first-aid problem. In a psychiatric hospital, perhaps even more than elsewhere, it is an essential part of the nurse's task for her to know at all times the location of emergency equipment—to know where to turn for the telephone, fire extinguishers, drugs, dressings and bandages, instruments, suckers, oxygen cylinders and fittings.

Some of the above accidents may be prevented or minimised by a knowledge at all times of her patients' whereabouts, and by having a real understanding of their present mental state.

Two special problems remain to be considered.

Fire. This can be a grave danger in a psychiatric hospital, particularly where there are old and inconvenient buildings and most especially where there are locked sections. Every nurse must know the plans existing in her own hospital which are to be put into effect in case of fire and must know how to raise the alarm. The safety of the elderly, the bed-ridden and the very grossly mentally disturbed patients will be her first consideration and prompt, efficient action and attention to the directions of her superiors may prevent grave loss of life. She should think first of people and their safety, then of any substances which may increase the fire danger such as inflammable liquids and gases, lastly of property and personal possessions.

Unauthorised Departures. As soon as a patient is found to be missing from the ward or from his usual place of occupation an immediate report must be submitted to senior staff. Sometimes the psychiatrist or one of the executive nurses will notify relatives and police, or will authorise the nurse to do so.

Accurate reporting can greatly simplify the task of all concerned and can in some instances prevent a tragedy. The nurse should be able to report where the patient was last seen and by whom, and may be able to give information as to the probable route of his departure from the hospital. It is of great value if she can give an account of his clothing. Other useful information will be that bearing on his current mood and behaviour and any clue as to his intention which may have been dropped during his conversation with her or with other patients.

The prevention of alarm in other patients is important, as a mood of anxiety and even aggression may be quickly created in the ward by such an incident.

Whether the patient returns of his own volition or is brought back by others, the process of receiving him into the hospital again will be important and it will be desirable for the nurse to act naturally and to try, usually without any direct inquiry, to understand the reason why he saw fit to leave. If her study of the situation leads her to conclude that some oversight or carelessness was responsible for the incident then it is obviously important that a lesson is learnt from the occurrence.

23

OCCUPATIONAL, RECREATIONAL AND SOCIAL THERAPIES

THE use of occupation, recreation and social activities as essential elements in the treatment of the psychiatric patient is by no means new; many of the 19th century reformers were well aware of the value of such procedures within the psychiatric hospital. In fact it has been known throughout the history of mankind that all human beings require to participate in these three segments of life if emotional equilibrium is to be maintained and if pleasure and satisfaction are to be achieved. With the development of interest in the psychiatric hospital as a therapeutic community, there has however been a renewed emphasis

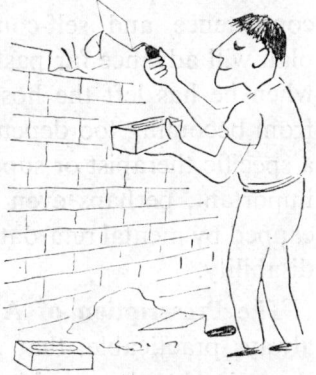

FIG. 32
The brick layer . . .

on the importance of these activities and the present day psychiatric nurse is required to know a good deal about the techniques which can be employed to ensure maximum participation by her patients in the life of the hospital. Many psychiatric illnesses are characterised, at least for a time, by withdrawal, disinterest and apathy, and it is frequently by means of therapies of the type described in this chapter that patients are first brought into some reasonable contact with their environment. The all-important nurse-patient relationship may well be first established within the framework of such an activity, just as the relationships between patients themselves may grow and mature in the same circumstances.

GENERAL PRINCIPLES

Activities as Therapy. Therapeutic goals must be operative at all times, whatever form the activities take and whatever procedures are involved in carrying them out. Even when the patient seems likely to remain permanently in hospital, activities must be used in such a way as to improve his adjustment to hospital life and to develop and maintain those assets which he still has. The aim must be to bring him to the highest possible degree of physical, mental, social and economic independence. Though it may initially be important for a patient to concentrate on one particular activity in order to gain some degree of competence and self-confidence, a reasonable occupational plan will advance far past this and will look ahead to the days when he has left the hospital behind. He must be prevented from becoming too dependent upon a particular activity or on a specific therapist or supervisor. Therapeutic goals are just as important, perhaps even more so, when the patient is handicapped by mental retardation, organic brain damage or physical disability.

The Prescription of Activities. It is desirable, though not always practicable, that patients should be referred for these therapies by the psychiatrist, either with a prescription of a general kind or, better still, with a specific request for some particular type of activity for a particular reason. Far too much in the past there has been a completely non-specific use of these treatments for so-called " diversion ", mainly perhaps to stop patients thinking about the total lack of purpose in hospital life; these attitudes were part of the older concept of custodial care and are giving way to a growing awareness of the extent to which rational planning of the patient's day can positively assist in reversing psychiatric illness. In the past the patient has often been obliged to conform to the standardised activity programme available in the hospital, rather than any effort being made to tailor a special regime to meet his requirements, for which task a good deal of imagination and creativity may be required. In this context his current problems, past experience and likely future will all be taken into account.

Therapies Adapted to Needs. Therapy will always have maximum success when it meets the patient's needs, whether these are conscious or as yet unknown to him. His needs may be obvious in particular circumstances such as following a leucotomy operation, or after a cerebral vascular accident, but the same principle applies whatever the patient's diagnostic label may be. Primarily one seeks to find activities which will meet his emotional needs—tasks to provide a sense of achievement, to furnish outlets for suppressed or repressed emotions, to permit him to use leisure time constructively and even creatively, to cultivate neglected social skills. Attention should at the same time be given to satisfying his physical requirements, both through providing adequate physical outlets and in the direction of improving his health and fitness. It is also important to provide activities which fit vocational needs, realistic occupations which later will be useful at home or in employment. It may be desirable for both male and female patients to improve work habits and skills, though other activities may obviously vary according to both sex and age.

Creation of a Therapeutic Environment. Activity programmes must be used to create an environment similar to that of the outside community, yet containing the essential elements of supervision, support, tolerance and permissiveness which make allowance for the patient's emotional disturbance. Most activities can be used to aid the patient's socialisation and to assist him in the development of new personal relationships; at least one activity involving group participation should be included in his programme.

CHOICE OF ACTIVITY

It is always important to discover in the first instance what the patient himself would like to do. One should carefully evaluate any attempt on his part to take the initiative and if he wishes to move in what seems a healthy direction then he should be offered support in this. The nurse should refrain where possible from guiding and directing him along specific paths which *she* feels are good for him; she should aim, through intimate knowledge of each individual patient, to discover his special abilities and interests and help him to utilise these. A patient with some particular skill may be able to guide and teach others and this may be helpful, not only for the entire group, but for the patient himself. Yet concentration for too long a period on one particular activity which was already familiar or which has become familiar in the hospital can gradually become a defence against genuine social participation and turn into a means of retreating from reality.

Some patients may be unable or unwilling to exercise any choice and their potential can only be guessed; therefore a certain amount of trial and error may be unavoidable, especially in the early stages. Except in very special instances it is not advisable to push the patient when he is unwilling; rather should every opportunity be taken to find some task, however small, in which he will participate spontaneously and through which some entry can be gained to his inner world. Even when some gentle direction of activity is inevitable, it may be that choice can still be encouraged in small ways—for example, a patient may have to be persuaded to take up knitting, but may then respond to an invitation to choose the pattern and colours for herself. Stimulation of interest may with some patients be an almost constant task and the nurse's powers of observation must be ever alert to detect some flicker of enthusiasm showing through the defensive armour of indifference and inertia.

In addition to the selection of occupation in accordance with age, ability and degree of handicap, the following questions should be in the nurse's mind when thinking about a particular activity for any patient.

Will it benefit him? How much? Is he capable of doing it? Intellectually? Physically?

Will he need guidance and assistance? How much? Will it be possible to provide it?

Is it related to his previous experience?

If so, can this be used to help others at the same time as it helps him?

Is it sufficiently interesting? Can it be made more so?

How can routines be varied and made more attractive and enticing?

Should payment for work be considered? If so, when and how?

How long should this activity last?

Is this all he can manage? Or can it be added to or varied?

How does he appear to react to this task?

Is he getting more attention than others? If so, is this reasonable?

Special problems will be posed by certain patients with particular types of disturbed thinking or behaviour. The **overactive patient** often wants to direct everything himself, to be busy all the time, and he may request and may in fact need rapid changes of occupation. In some circumstances it may be essential for him to work and play alone, at least for part of the time, so that he does not have too much of a disruptive influence on others. Whatever task he is doing he requires plenty of material and plenty of space in which to operate and he will usually do better with equipment which is large and which requires little fine concentration. His tasks should be well within his capacity in order to reduce the possibility of frustration.

A **quiet withdrawn patient** on the other hand tends to respond best to simple repetitive activities which should be colourful and stimulating but which do not make too much demand upon him at first.

The range of activity available for patients in a psychiatric hospital of any size is, or should be, almost limitless. Support and assistance may come from surprising areas if the possibility of help from such a quarter is envisaged. Some of these activities are set up by special departments in order to meet patients' needs; others involve their participation in the ordinary working life of the hospital. There are dangers, though not inevitable ones, in the latter group of tasks; the risk is always present that a patient may assist a hospital staff member in the first instance for a purpose which is directly therapeutic, but with the passage

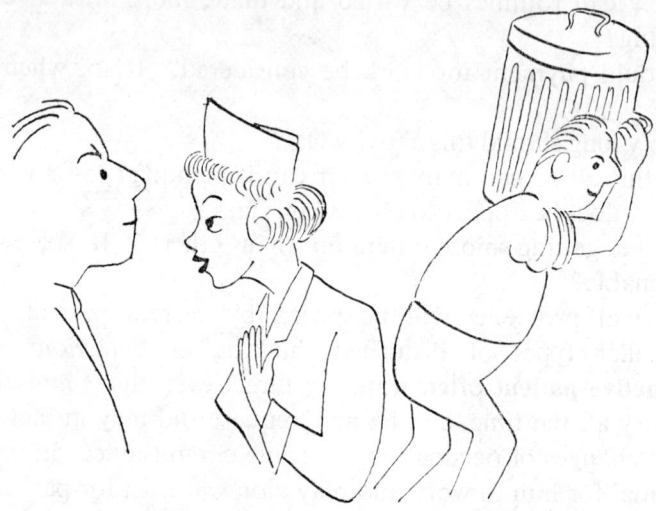

Fig. 33
A poorly paid member of the hospital team.

of time this aim can very easily be lost sight of and it comes about that he turns into an invaluable, poorly paid or unpaid member of the hospital team. It should be part of the nurse's job to review periodically those patients who are assisting in ward domestic tasks or who are spending large parts of their day away from the ward working with members of the staff, in order to ensure that a continuation of these activities is in fact in the patient's best interests and that more could not be done to rehabilitate him towards more normal living outside the hospital. The dreadful danger of institutionalisation is nowhere more real than in these circumstances.

Provided that this sort of scrutiny is regularly carried out, then all of the following activities may be regarded as legitimate parts of the programme which the hospital can offer to its patients.

Activities within the Ward:
- bed-making
- helping with meals
- knitting and sewing
- reading and writing letters
- hobbies — for example, stamp-collecting
- ward cleaning
- assisting other patients (with feeding, dressing and grooming)
- reading aloud to other patients
- radio and television (in small doses)
- games, either in pairs (draughts, chess) or in larger groups

Activities with the Hospital Staff:
- carpentry
- electrical maintenance
- laundry work
- typing and office administration
- plumbing
- painting
- gardening and construction work
- assisting hospital drivers

Craftwork:
- leather-work
- lampshade making
- metal-work
- toy making
- weaving
- cooking
- millinery
- basket-work
- wood-work
- pottery
- floral art
- cake-decorating
- book-binding
- painting, finger-painting, drawing

Artistic and Educational Activities:
- literature group
- music appreciation group
- language study
- hospital choir
- puppetry
- formal education
- poetry group
- art appreciation group
- play-reading
- work with hospital magazine
- quizzes
- correspondence courses

Social Activities:

concerts
dances

films
picnics and barbecues

Sporting Activities:

of any type depending on climate and season (see next section).

Many hospitals are now developing specific industrial programmes, occupying patients in process work of various types under contracts which are negotiated with local employers or public utilities. These factory-type activities may be carried out in detached units, sometimes known as **sheltered workshops,** but some may even be done in the wards themselves. These programmes, when they are practicable, tend to have many advantages over the traditional mental hospital occupational programme; patients are likely to develop more satisfactory work habits when they are engaged in such clearly meaningful and practical activities, and the payment they receive for their services further encourages this. Some patients may learn under supervision more adequate ways of coping with work stresses than they had ever previously known. Their self-esteem rises, their thoughts become more and more directed towards the outside world, and some may become suitable for discharge from hospital and the taking up of a routine occupation after perhaps many years of hospitalisation. Some others may develop previously unsuspected supervisory skills working in such an atmosphere. At the very least, industrial employment within the hospital may be one of the most satisfactory ways of preventing deterioration in the long term or permanent resident, such programmes also being suitable for some mentally retarded adolescents or adults who require continuous care (p. 443).

PHYSICAL EXERCISE AND RECREATION

Physical fitness is a worthwhile goal in itself for the hospitalised psychiatric patient and it is part of the nurse's responsibility to see that the highest possible level of activity is maintained

OCCUPATIONAL AND SOCIAL THERAPIES

consistent with the age, physical and mental state of her patients. Movement and exercise will induce a healthy tiredness and will thus tend to lead to sound sleep, often reducing the need for hypnotic drugs. Increased flexibility and co-ordination are promoted, posture is improved and the proper functioning of bodily systems is aided. In children and adolescents growth and development are stimulated and in the elderly patient exercises will help to prevent or to minimise stiffness and deformity.

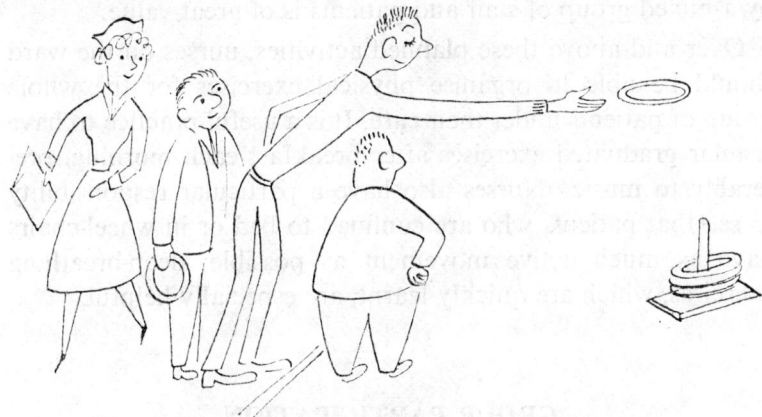

FIG. 34
Harmful rivalry should be avoided.

Planned exercises and sports on any major scale will usually be instituted and carried out by the recreational therapist, but the nurse will be regularly required to assist in these activities and in some hospitals may have to fill many of the roles normally assumed by such a person. Sport will enable some patients to participate in the hospital programme who would not otherwise be able to do so effectively, and will provide a valuable method of discharging aggressive tensions and of dealing with anxiety. Competitive games can be advantageous, provided that harmful rivalry is avoided and that patients selected to compete are those with roughly comparable abilities. Sports should be varied to maintain interest and it is helpful to provide coaching from outside instructors if these are available.

For those patients who are disinterested in the idea of exercise for its own sake, physical fitness can often be maintained through certain social and recreational activities. Ballroom dancing is of value here (quite apart from its role in helping to overcome shyness and anxiety in the presence of the opposite sex), as well as folk-dancing and square-dancing. Other patients, particularly in country hospitals, may enjoy and benefit from hikes and expeditions of various kinds. In all these activities, just as in the more formal sports, participation by a mixed group of staff and patients is of great value.

Over and above these planned activities, nurses on the ward should be able to organise physical exercises for the whole group of patients under their care. It is a useful practice to have regular graduated exercises after breakfast each morning, preferably to music. Nurses also have a particular responsibility to see that patients who are confined to bed or in wheel-chairs have as much active movement as possible; deep-breathing exercises, which are quickly learnt, are especially helpful.

GROUP PARTICIPATION

Nearly all the activities mentioned in this chapter can be used, not only for their own intrinsic value, but as a means of encouraging patients to work and play with others in groups. They provide opportunities for them to experience the ordinary give-and-take of living and will aid their capacity for making meaningful communication in a social situation. The induction of certain patients into participation in group life is a task, however, which in some instances will call for the utmost skill and sensitivity from the nurse. The patient's emotional state will always govern the size of the group he is able to join and the degree of co-operation which can be coaxed from him. Consultation with the psychiatrist may be required to determine whether he is in fact ready to join a group and how much support he should have in it; if he fails in one type of group, is it perhaps too early for him to be involved in group life or might a different sort of group be the answer? There are also some patients who, by reason of deep-seated personality characteristics, have always found group participation an intolerable strain and if this has become a completely fixed way of living then, with the psychiatrist's concurrence, it may be inevitable that such a person be allowed to continue his social isolation to some extent in the hospital.

Even when patients willingly participate in some type of group activity numerous problems may arise. Some will need almost constant gentle support to overcome their feelings of inadequacy in the situation; others will need to have subtle checks applied to prevent them dominating the group to the detriment of its other members. Others again may use the group as a place to hide, failing to make any real contribution to the group life.

The ultimate goal in encouraging this form of participation is to have the person relating easily and confidently in a mixed group of people—mixed sexes, mixed interests and mixed aims. Such a goal is of course not always practicable, particularly with chronic patients who have already suffered the consequences of long-term hospitalisation; however, even these individuals will have their mental and physical deterioration halted or much lessened by as active as possible a group life. In the vast majority of cases it should be possible to allow free social interchange between male and female patients without anything but the most minimal supervision.

If the nurse herself participates in some of these group activities this can be a very striking influence in changing a ward from a pattern of custodial to one of therapeutic care; however skilled her observations, aloof supervision from the sidelines has a strongly custodial flavour and, as has been pointed out in Chapter 20 (p. 426), the observations themselves will not be as meaningful and spontaneous as they would be if she were joining in. As a participating observer she is much better able to assess the reactions of patients and to decide upon alternative procedures for those who are proving outsiders in the group.

Obviously participation by nursing staff in patient activities is a tricky subject which can have its own difficulties and complications. Necessary limits are set by the fact that hers is a professional role, any major departure from which will be a threat not only to her patients but to herself (though one can of course be a professional and still have a warm emotional involvement). The possibility also exists that participation in patient activities can be unwittingly employed by the nurse to meet her own needs rather than those of the patients. Once again she will be helped by a certain degree of self-knowledge and by a realisation of her own pattern of defences and her motivations in particular situations.

It need hardly be stressed that, with these therapies as with all others, the nurse, even when not directly involved, needs to play a warmly supportive role and to take a sincere interest in the tasks which the patient is undertaking. Such an interest greatly aids the patient's acceptance of the therapeutic programmes; he tends to be more confident in undertaking them, less apprehensive and far more inclined to view them as part of his treatment. The nurse's actions in this regard will also exert some influence on the relatives, who may thereby grasp more easily the purpose of the patient's activity programme and may even, in appropriate circumstances, be prepared to become involved. Many nurses will find that, within reasonable limits compatible with a private life of their own, they derive interest and satisfaction from participating during off-duty times in patients' clubs, concerts and social evenings; occasional visits of this kind will reinforce the idea that these activities are worthwhile and therapeutic. In any event, many of these programmes require the staff's support and example, at least in the early stages.

PATIENTS' CLUBS AND PATIENT PARTICIPATION

Chapter 19 has stressed how desirable it is that the patient should assume maximum responsibility whilst in hospital for directing his own life, within the limits set by his illness and by hospital regulations, and the establishment of patients' clubs is one important way of ensuring this. Clinical evidence suggests that it is beneficial for patients to have a situation in which they can express their opinions (many of which may be very valuable) and take an active, constructive part in some aspect of hospital life. The essential feature of clubs or committees such as these is that a good deal of responsibility is placed in the patients' hands, even though many or most of them will require periodic or even constant gentle supervision from the staff. The possibilities are numerous: reception committees for new admissions; welfare clubs for visiting and entertaining patients who have no relatives or friends; social clubs; sports' clubs; music clubs; drama clubs; book clubs. Some of these, particularly if dealing with chronic and regressed patients, may need a good deal of active staff participation. Some hospitals bring in from the community volunteer workers to assist in the organisation and running of some of these clubs; quite apart from the special skills which such people may provide, some patients may find it easier to develop relationships with these individuals than they do with the more authoritarian figures within the hospital.

Some clubs are open to recently discharged patients and offer them support until they are properly established on their own feet; in other instances there are special **ex-patients' clubs** (p. 479).

CONCLUSION

Nurses must recognise that occupational, recreational and social therapies should be taking place throughout the day on every day of the week; they are not necessarily activities

PSYCHIATRIC NURSING

for which patients have to leave the ward and go to a special room or department. In some circumstances several patients assisting a nurse to make beds in a dormitory can be occupational therapy of the best kind, though it can quickly degenerate, as has been indicated earlier, into an immoral use of cheap labour. Recreation should not be some rare phenomenon which the patient attends if he has nothing better to do; every patient needs some form of recreation from the earliest days of his admission. Working with the special therapists, discussing problems with them, or working by herself with patients, the nurse should be learning all the time and adding to her own experience and ability. On numerous occasions, if she takes the trouble to look, she will be surprised to find quite exciting talents hidden beneath the external shell of illness and she must be ever alert to prevent herself making snap unfavourable judgements about the potentialities of patients in her care. A man's occupation on admission may be listed as " bricklayer "—but it may be that he derives substantial therapeutic benefit from learning to play the violin.

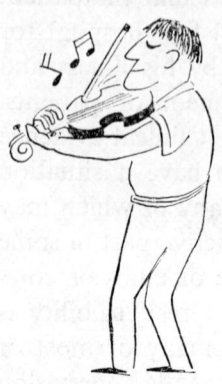

FIG. 35
... Who learned to play the violin.

24

CONVALESCENCE AND REHABILITATION

THE last decade has seen a greatly increased interest in the problems of convalescence and rehabilitation; many studies have examined the process of recovery from illness, both in general and psychiatric hospitals. This is a natural development from therapeutic, rather than custodial, patterns of hospital care (p. 29) and a psychiatric service is incomplete if it neglects to deal with the difficulties which can arise at this time.

Convalescence is defined as " the gradual recovery of health and strength after a sickness ". **Rehabilitation** involves the restoration of a handicapped person to the highest physical, mental, social, vocational and economic levels of which he is capable. Our concept of total care must extend past any simple notion that treatment has been successful just because the patient has been returned to work; rehabilitation is directed towards " living again ", which means far more than the old idea of just " working again ". The hospital's treatment programme cannot stop at the front gate, but must follow the patient back into the community.

The difficulties inherent in this approach are apparent when it is remembered that the vast majority of cases of psychiatric illness result, at least in part, from disturbed personal and social relationships, often located in the family structure. This means that special attention must be given to the environment to which the patient returns, for it is likely to be the same environment in which his illness developed. No one would suggest that a patient convalescing from typhoid fever should go back to a situation where he was exposed to exactly the same possibility of infection, yet a very similar process may be involved in returning, for example, a schizophrenic patient to participate in the family tensions which were essential causative factors in his illness.

A fully adequate rehabilitation programme will therefore pay a good deal of attention to the person's domestic environment. Most frequently attention to the family members is given by means of supportive interviews, usually conducted by the psychiatric social worker, in which attempts are made to resolve their own anxieties about the patient so that they can integrate him most satisfactorily into their midst. The nurse, however, should be aware that some hospitals are now developing programmes aimed at involving the significant relatives of patients in the treatment programme in a much more ambitious way. Sometimes, for example, the mother of a schizophrenic teenage girl, or the wife of an alcoholic man, may herself receive quite intensive psychotherapy from a member of the hospital staff. The purpose of this is twofold —not only is the relative's anxiety or disorganisation modified, but it is hoped that reduction of her personal problems will lessen the tension on the patient. Programmes are even being developed which aim to take the whole family, or as many members as possible, into group therapy; this research development arises from the idea that individual episodes of psychiatric illness frequently represent the end product of a so-called "sick family" and that the logical approach is therefore to the primary source of conflict.

THE STAGES OF ILLNESS

It is customary and convenient to divide the course of any illness into three stages. In the earliest stage the illness is developing but is not yet clearly recognisable. This is followed by the acute stage, where the symptoms are clearly revealed and treatment is commenced; as this begins to take effect there is a gradual shading into the third stage, that of convalescence. These phases are usually clearly visible in diseases such as pneumonia, measles and appendicitis, but in psychiatric disorders the period of convalescence is still commonly one of continuing treatment directed towards persisting facets of the illness. Removal of the symptoms of psychiatric illness is still only half the battle; phobias, depression, confusion due to drugs—all may fairly readily be brought under control in many instances, but the patient still has to make important alterations to the unsatisfactory living patterns and personality defences which contributed to the development of his sickness. If this is not done, the nurse will frequently note that return to the outside world leads to a rapid flare up of the original symptoms. The point is therefore emphasised that reduction of distress is not in itself evidence of really effective treatment.

It follows that rehabilitation, commonly seen as the last phase of an illness, actually begins and should be planned from the first contact which the patient makes with the hospital. This highlights from a different viewpoint the extreme importance of the environment provided by the hospital; psychiatric symptoms may well be brought under control regardless of the situation in which treatment is given, but a programme for a seriously ill person which is designed to permit more effective functioning in the future will only be possible in the setting of a therapeutic community (p. 407). Moreover, rehabilitation needs the range of skills which can only be provided by the various members of the therapeutic team; more than ever at this time treatment demands co-operative teamwork.

PROBLEMS OF CONVALESCENCE

With convalescence the time has approached for the patient to make a whole series of adjustments—he has to adjust to himself and to the fact that he has been ill, he has to leave the hospital and return to his family, his work and his social community. Just as hospitalisation produced conflicts and separation anxieties (p. 380), so may convalescence produce stresses of a different kind. This is a time of transition from dependence on the hospital to the re-establishment of his own identity, security and independence. Not always does he progress in smooth, easy stages; his readjustment may ebb and flow depending on various factors both within his own personality and in the outside world. The " road back " may be in many instances an extremely rough one.

The sick person is usually beset with anxiety concerning his symptoms (p. 387); his interest is diverted from external things on to himself and he becomes dependent upon the hospital and its staff, often in a quite infantile way. As his symptoms are reduced his attention will be increasingly directed away from his inner world on to the world about him. Occupational and social activities may appear in a new light as possible sources of real gratification. Yet many patients still have to outgrow the dependency which they have established, particularly if hospitalisation has been prolonged. For many individuals the hospital has been making the decisions, providing for them and protecting them from hostile forces in the outside world or from dangers within themselves. Because the patient's anxieties have been lessened, the hospital is often seen as a benevolent parent whom he can trust; he may have the feeling, conscious or unconscious, that as long as his relationship with the hospital continues he will be safe. Clearly this problem will be at its worst when the hospital structure has been such that the patient has been almost completely deprived of his initiative and robbed of his willingness and capacity to make his own decisions (p. 400).

Convalescence can thus be seen as a weaning period during which the patient has to advance towards independence while simultaneously wishing to hang on to the source which has been gratifying his dependency needs. Anxiety, anger and guilt may arise in much the same way as they did at the original time of weaning (p. 39). The patient may make intermittent progress towards independence, then regress for reasons which are not immediately apparent. At this point his activity programme is of great importance, and will nearly always require substantial modification from that which was in operation when he was more acutely ill; his daily round should involve him to an increasing extent in new relationships in which he can test out healthier patterns of living and learn more mature and socially acceptable forms of behaviour. A full evaluation of his previous capacities, recognising whether or not these have been reduced by his illness, is essential for intelligent planning. New skills—for example, dancing —may be taught at this time which will open up fresh avenues of adjustment after leaving hospital. Some housewives (often forgotten because they are not usually bread-winners) may be greatly helped by special training in home-making techniques.

At the same time convalescence should provide new opportunities for healthier and more stable identifications. The attitudes and behaviour of the staff, perhaps now more than at any other time, should give the patient personal experiences designed to correct previous faulty impressions about the feelings of other people towards him. The nurse's warm interest in his future plans should indicate to him that someone is concerned for his welfare and for him as an individual—and for many patients this may be a constructive and meaningful experience.

Just as a person with a fractured leg is supported and encouraged while he takes his first faltering steps, so must the psychiatric patient be constructively supported as he tentatively feels his way back towards independence. Many patients are unfortunately over-confident at this time, using mechanisms of repression and denial (p. 93) to avoid facing the fact that they have suffered a serious illness; for many of these the future, because of their unrealistic attitude, will provide shattering blows. While it is certainly not part of the nurse's duty to attempt to break down such defences by frontal assault, she should certainly on the other hand avoid reinforcing them and should accept any opportunity to support the realistic idea that life will have many problems for every patient after a period of psychiatric hospitalisation. Likewise she should not let her enthusiasm for his future outrun her judgement, a state of affairs which may lead her to encourage impossible or unlikely goals which he is contemplating for himself; if he is to pursue aims beyond his capacity this is almost certainly going to be a recipe for failure, frustration and possible return to hospital.

There may be many difficulties in the patient's family. Frequent visiting may have minimised these, but does not in itself provide any complete solution. When the patient comes out of hospital he has experiences to report which have not been shared by his relatives; at the same time things have been happening in his family group when he has not been a part of it. His relatives, often not facing the issue squarely and having a completely unrealistic picture of what hospitalisation might accomplish, may form a very rosy picture of his homecoming based on the fantasy that he will be a completely new person; such a hope is almost certain to be rapidly dispelled, with anxiety and confusion all round. They may have formed an idealised picture of him, remembering during his absence only the better things about him; the same process may work in reverse, the patient having a quite false idea of what life is really like in his family group. They may have many anxieties about their ability to look after him, because their memories are coloured by their experiences with him prior to his admission. Moreover, the patient who saw hospitalisation as evidence of rejection by the family is likely to return home harbouring bitter feelings. Yet another difficulty arises when he has been away for a sufficient period of time for the family to have adjusted themselves to the idea of being without him; his return may then create a whole new series of problems, of which the family members may or may not be consciously aware (p. 432).

The patient's return to work may also be a stress situation requiring fresh adjustments. In the first instance he may even have difficulty in accepting the routine which is part of an ordinary working day, and this is often best tested within the hospital or by attaching him to a **sheltered workshop** (p. 464). He may no longer be capable of handling his former position, and in these circumstances he must face the necessity of learning a new job, which may carry less status and earn him

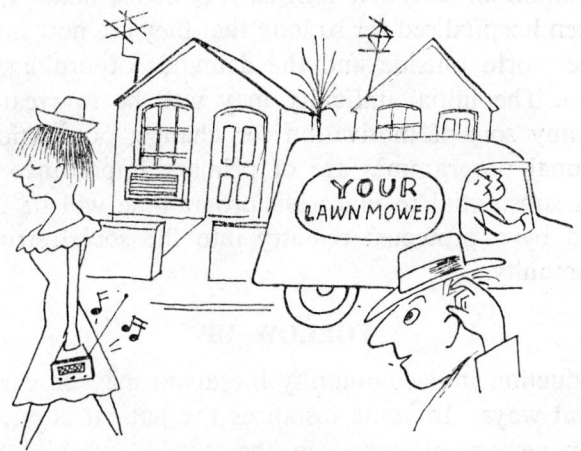

FIG. 36
Unfamiliar with the demands of ordinary living.

less money than his previous occupation. Vocational guidance and the efforts of rehabilitation officers are often essential at this stage. Pamphlets and books relating to employment opportunities may stimulate interest if they are freely available in the ward. The provision of a new job does not however necessarily lessen anxiety, guilt and anger if he feels that he has been downgraded; these emotions may well be reflected in his behaviour both at home and at work. Even if his old position is still open the patient may find that, during his absence, relationships between himself and his fellow employees have changed. Sometimes the knowledge that a man has had a psychiatric illness will lead his colleagues to avoid him or distrust him. One of the gravest anxieties faced by the patient about to leave hospital is centred around the questions which he may be asked about his illness and his treatment; some hospitals quite specifically try to help the patient meet this situation, sometimes encouraging him to act in little plays which dramatise the problem so that he will feel more confident when it arises in real life.

Somewhat different issues arise when one considers the rehabilitation of chronic, long-stay patients, some of whom have been hospitalised for so long that they are now unfamiliar with the world outside and the demands of ordinary living. (Fig. 36). The initial difficulty may well be to create in the patient any sort of motivation for change; occupational and recreational programmes are of primary importance here (p. 464). A substantial re-education programme will be required, followed by a protected re-entry into the social structure of the community.

FOLLOW UP

Introduction into community life again may be carried out in several ways. In some instances the patient is encouraged to commence employment in the outside world while still living in the hospital, this situation being continued until he feels secure enough in his work and social skills to live independently. This scheme has been successfully used for both acute and chronic psychotic and neurotic adults and for some mentally retarded persons. The nurse must be actively involved in this process—seeing the patient off, perhaps cutting his lunch, welcoming him back and taking a warm interest in hearing what he has been doing. Signs of progress, here as elsewhere, should be met by favourable comment. In other instances the patient leaves hospital and takes up residence for some time in a protected environment, usually run by a governmental or semi-governmental agency, variously known as an **after-care hostel, halfway house,** or by some similar term. These places are run more like a home than a hospital but are usually supervised by a trained person. Support and guidance are provided while the patient is finding his feet.

Yet another way of achieving this transition is by discharg-

CONVALESCENCE AND REHABILITATION

ing the patient from the hospital wards proper and admitting him to a **day hospital;** he is now living in the ordinary community at nights and week-ends, but still continuing treatment and supervision for a substantial part of the time. (Many patients of course are now being treated throughout their illness in a day hospital setting, for it is hoped that in this way effective therapy can be given whilst avoiding the pernicious effects of complete separation from the family and total dependence upon institutional life.)

Whatever the actual method of transition, there is now a general realisation that there are few if any patients whose contact with the hospital should terminate immediately after discharge. Quite apart from its other functions in establishing early diagnosis and in some instances preventing hospital care altogether, the hospital **outpatient department** has an invaluable role in providing continuing support for those people whose inpatient treatment has been completed but who still require supervision and in some instances further active therapy. In such a department, either attached to the psychiatric hospital itself or in a general hospital or community clinic, the once hospitalised patient may have a drug programme supervised, he may receive supportive interviews from the psychiatrist or social worker or may in some instances be involved in active psychotherapy. The role of the social worker in such a setting is a particularly vital one (p. 500), and she will also have a good deal to do with the **ex-patients' club** which is now a feature of many psychiatric services, through which patients gain regular social experience in a not particularly stressful setting while gaining self-confidence. At any age, but particularly with elderly people, an introduction to Church or other community groups may be very helpful. These continuing programmes are even more important when the patient lacks supporting relatives or helpful friends, or when he is a migrant lacking real roots in society. They serve to bridge the gap, still too often a very large gap indeed, between the life of the hospital and the life of the outside world.

CONCLUSION

Treatment does not stop with the last electrotherapy session, when drugs have produced their maximum effect, or when an apparently successful leucotomy operation has been carried out. The therapeutic attitude, and the utilisation of all possible treatment skills, must carry over into the period of convalescence; in many instances it is during the rehabilitation programme that the effects of devoted, individualised nursing care will be most noticeable, and at this time the nurse may well obtain her greatest degree of personal satisfaction. It is usually not too difficult to modify a patient's acute distress to the point where he is able to leave hospital, but in very many instances it is only careful planning, in which the nurse is closely involved, which will keep him in the community and ensure his continuing improvement. Furthermore, the successful rehabilitation of even one chronic and institutionalised patient, often a seemingly hopeless task at the beginning and always demanding great reserves of patience, persistence and enthusiasm, may provide for some nurses the greatest reward which their profession has to give.

25

THE NURSE IN THE COMMUNITY

AT various points in earlier chapters it has been indicated that the modern psychiatric service, whether or not it is based on a psychiatric hospital, is showing an increasing tendency to extend its activities into the surrounding community. As this change is occurring, so is the psychiatric nurse becoming involved in activities outside the gates of her parent hospital or clinic. Like many other trends in modern nursing, this too was foreshadowed by Florence Nightingale, whose vision clearly included the development of nursing as a community service in addition to its role with patients receiving hospital treatment. Certainly throughout the history of nursing there have been many individuals in the profession who have carried out important tasks in community care programmes of various kinds.

THE JUSTIFICATION FOR COMMUNITY PROGRAMMES

There is increasing recognition of the fact that psychiatric services must be planned to meet the many needs of the population they intend to serve, rather than providing a hospital programme and then sitting back and seeing what happens. A variety of research findings and clinical experiences have made us realise that what *has* been happening has led to certain undesirable consequences, which must now be reviewed.

1. Systematic surveys of the amount and type of mental illness present in the community, in the United Kingdom, North America and Australia, have indicated that there exist many more emotionally disturbed people than was previously recognised. Moreover, only a small proportion of these individuals have in fact received specialised help. It is clear, therefore, that the traditional type of psychiatric service fails to reach many of those who might benefit from it.

2. Psychiatric services in the past have tended to talk, rather critically, of " patients unsuitable for our treatment ", as if nothing could possibly be wrong with the treatment provided, only with the patients who couldn't or wouldn't avail themselves of it. Now a shift in values and a considerable lessening of self-satisfaction have altered our attitude towards the gap between what some patients need and what is actually provided for them, so that currently more and more people talk somewhat anxiously and self-critically about the fact that " our treatments seem unsuitable for some of our patients." In the past, when a patient was discharged from hospital and recognised as needing continued supervision, but was reluctant or flatly refused to attend the hospital outpatient department, a common reaction might be " well, that's that . . . there's nothing more we can do ". But if a hospital service is failing to meet the needs of such a patient, for whatever reason, and with accumulating evidence that such patients run a significantly higher risk of readmission in the future, the contemporary trend favours actively seeking him out and attempting to provide an after-care programme on terms which are acceptable to him.

3. Increasing clinical experience has led to the inescapable conclusion that a very large proportion of patients, by the time they come or are brought to a psychiatric hospital, have a pretty fixed and well-established illness, with the inevitable result that both patient and staff might end up somewhat dissatisfied with the results of treatment. There are of course special reasons why some psychiatric patients tend to postpone treatment for as long as possible (p. 388), but it has perhaps been too readily accepted in the past that nothing could ever be done about this. But the staff of an arthritis clinic, for example, would very soon become dissatisfied with the situation where a large proportion of their patients attended for the first time with advanced muscle contractures, and this is not too dissimilar from the situation existing in many orthodox psychiatric services. It has become apparent, therefore, that a psychiatric service should try to detect people who might benefit from psychiatric help at

an earlier stage of their illness—but to do this, an active reaching out into the community is required.

4. It is recognised that individuals with psychiatric problems only fairly rarely turn to psychiatrists in the first instance, for they commonly believe their problems to be due to something else, if indeed they acknowledge the existence of a problem at all. The "front line troops", therefore, in the detection and early treatment of psychiatric illness, are persons such as general medical practitioners, public health nurses, school teachers, baby health centre nurses, probation officers, clergymen, policemen and many other professionals whose daily work involves contact with human beings in some form of distress or manifesting abnormal behaviour. Recognition *and* management are both clearly important, for if these persons were simply taught to detect individuals with psychiatric disturbance, and then send them all on to the psychiatric unit for sorting out, the clinical services of the latter would immediately be overloaded, so large is the proportion of any population who might benefit from psychiatric help. Those persons working in the community, therefore, require not only continuing education in the recognition of psychiatric disturbance, but also on-going consultation with psychiatrically trained professionals so as to enable them better to manage the numerous persons with emotional problems whom they encounter during their everyday activities.

5. Going even further into what might be called a "public health" approach to psychiatry, many psychiatrists have become concerned with those factors in personal and community life which might predispose the individual towards the development of a psychiatric illness, or which might precipitate a predisposed person into the development of frank neurosis or psychosis. For many years, for example, there has been good evidence that the relationship between mother and child is of crucial importance in the formation of strong ego functions, capable of withstanding later stressful situations without too much disruption (p. 149), and it has therefore been argued

that psychiatrists and those who work with them should be vitally interested in any factors which may improve or interfere with the mother-child relationship. Psychiatrists and psychiatric nurses, for example, were in the forefront of those who advocated that children admitted to hospital should, wherever possible, be able to be visited by their mothers on an unrestricted basis, so as to minimise the chance of problems arising due to separation (p. 386). This is but one of many examples of a theoretically preventable stress which would seem to have relevance to the later development of psychiatric illness, and which therefore should be a matter of serious concern to all members of a psychiatric service.

6. Much has already been said (in Chapter 19) about some of the possible disadvantages of being an inpatient in a psychiatric hospital. Moreover, it has become increasingly obvious that a period spent in hospital is only an episode in the overall management of a psychiatric illness, in the great majority of cases, and that therefore both pre-hospitalisation and post-hospitalisation programmes may be vital aspects of the patient's total care. Those patients who are treated throughout in the outpatient department or day hospital, never requiring full scale admission, also need an extension of the hospital's supportive functions into the community if treatment is to be truly effective. Finally, there is a small group of patients who may be treated, for one reason or another, on an entirely domiciliary basis, without ever knowing where the psychiatric hospital is or what it looks like. Many of these patients will be managed essentially by the general practitioner, but with the domiciliary service of the hospital playing an active supportive and advisory role, and in treatment programmes such as this the psychiatric nurse has an invaluable contribution to make.

THE ROLES OF THE COMMUNITY PSYCHIATRIC NURSE

The developments and changes in attitude which we have listed in the previous section clearly expand the scope and horizons of psychiatric nursing. Having moved from what was once a largely custodial role into her present position as an active member of the therapeutic team, the nurse now finds herself in the middle of yet another development—the carrying of clinical services of various kinds into the community, together with the development of new and important educative and consultative roles. Though there is a good deal of overlap between these various functions, they can be more easily described by a somewhat artificial separation along the following lines:

The Domiciliary Role. As indicated in the preceding section, the after-care of discharged patients is now recognised as a task which may require a very active participation by members of the hospital staff, not least from the psychiatric nurse. For a variety of reasons some patients, once they have been discharged from inpatient care, are reluctant to maintain their contact with the hospital; they may fail to keep their outpatient appointments, may attend only irregularly, or they may refuse to obtain or to take the drugs prescribed. These individuals are particularly likely to need to return to hospital at a later time for further inpatient treatment, so that the psychiatric service has very legitimate reasons for wishing to keep as many of them as possible under reasonable after-care supervision. The nurse may be required to visit some of them in their homes, in which situation she will need to acquire some of the social worker's skill (p. 502); during her visit it may be necessary for her to observe the patient's condition, to form an opinion about his present mental state, and she may talk to the relatives in order to hear their opinions and help to increase their understanding. She may assist the patient to make contact with his old employer, or to find a new job, or may assist his entrance into a suitable local club or sheltered workshop. For some of these patients, particularly those in the older age group, she may need to provide help with basic nursing, ensure that they have suitable occupation and recreation, and perhaps arrange for the hospital to make available to the family various mechanical aids which may to some extent ease the relatives' burden. She may find it necessary to give advice on dietary matters or on questions of personal hygiene. In much of this work she carries a new and exciting responsibility because, though her work will always be in some measure under the supervision of a psychiatrist, who may from time to time see the patient himself, many of the decisions will be hers and hers alone, even in quite important matters.

Much of this work involves her in activities which are far removed from the traditional concepts of nursing. At first sight it may seem somewhat unspectacular to go out on a domiciliary visit, dressed in ordinary street clothes, for the express purpose of accompanying a patient to an important interview about which he is anxious, or to ensure that he is taken for a drive so that he gets some variety in an otherwise very monotonous life. But there is a good deal of evidence to suggest that these supportive tasks, and the increased morale of those who receive such support, are important factors in enabling some patients to maintain themselves in the community when under other circumstances they might have needed to return to hospital, perhaps even for permanent care. To prevent this is not only a gain for the hospital—much more importantly, in the great majority of instances it is certainly in the patient's best interests too.

The nurse in her domiciliary role will take a particular interest in the clubs and social groups available to the patients in her area. Patients who have been discharged to convalescent homes, hostels or boarding houses are still likely to need some supervision from her, and in some of these instances her supportive domiciliary role may well be combined with, or blend into, a consultative and educative role to the staff who are in charge of these institutions. The same judicious mixture of functions may also be involved in her interest in sheltered workshops, craft centres and social agencies of various kinds; here too she will probably show a primary concern for her patients who are attending these organisations, but it may follow naturally from this that she is of real assistance to the staff in helping them to work along more generally therapeutic lines, even though in some circumstances they may hardly realise that she is doing this.

So far we have spoken only of patients who are well-known to the hospital and have been treated in one of its clinical services. There are, however, other patients who, for a variety of possible reasons, have never attended the hospital at all but have been managed throughout their illness by the hospital's domiciliary team, in which the nurse inevitably plays a vitally important part. The psychiatric service now recognises an obligation to provide appropriate treatment, where possible, for persons in the community whose anxieties and prejudices are too strong to permit them to come to the hospital and ask for help, or who are for whatever reason unable to do so, *e.g.*, because of extreme physical disability. When the general practitioner or some other person notifies the hospital of the existence of such a clinical problem, a visit by one or more members of the domiciliary team is usually arranged; the nurse may well be the first person to see the patient, followed shortly afterwards by the psychiatrist, and in any event a large part of the supervision of the patient's treatment is likely to fall to her. A bedridden man, for example, handicapped by serious physical illness with the superadded complication of severe depression, may well be regarded by the psychiatrist as suitable for domiciliary care throughout his illness. In such a case the nurse will be an indispensable member of the therapeutic team, supervising his medication and reporting his response and possible side-effects, supporting the family and interpreting his illness to them, as well as carrying out the many possible tasks which may be indicated as part of his after-care programme, as previously described.

The Consultative Role. As already indicated, the nurse may consider on her visits to convalescent homes or other community agencies that there is an important task to be done in providing assistance to the staff members of the institution over and above the direct service that she may be giving the patients themselves. This is more difficult than it sounds, and indeed much harm can be done, and much discredit brought on the psychiatric service to which she belongs, by a brash and uninvited intervention in the affairs of another agency or institution. The nurse may, for example, have excellent reasons for believing that some of the policies pursued in a particular hostel are not in the best interests of the patients, perhaps not even in the best interests of the staff. Yet it is a highly unusual organisation which recognises its own limitations, even though these may be glaringly obvious to outsiders, and it is certainly unlikely that such an agency will welcome the unsolicited advice of others, however well-intentioned this may be; almost inevitably it will be construed as criticism, with the result that the nurse and other members of the psychiatric service are no longer welcome as visitors.

The nurse must therefore recognise that in the great majority of instances a good deal of preparation is required, commonly involving other members of the team, before she can be truly effective in her consultative role. In the case of a convalescent home, for example, she may consider that the physical and mental condition of the patients, and the personal satisfactions of the staff, would be greatly improved by the introduction of a supervised, graduated activity programme, which might well reduce the incidence of incontinence, insomnia and restlessness. To suggest this, without preparation, would very likely be seen as an insult by the staff members concerned. Her aim, therefore, is to get them to see this for themselves, so that if all goes well they may eventually *ask* her to assist them in the development of such a programme. But to reach this point she will certainly be required to demonstrate her competence, to show that she is trustworthy, and in particular to prove by her actions that she has truly come to help, and not to criticise—simply to state this is not enough, human nature being what it is, and the establishment of this image of herself may be a time-consuming process, requiring a good deal of patience. The nurse must recognise, as all persons in similar situations must recognise, that the outsider with professional skills is often seen as " threatening " by any organisation, whatever its nature and purpose, and she must learn to approach her goal in stages, taking whatever opportunity she can to demonstrate, by example rather than words, that they can feel safe and comfortable in talking to her and asking for her help.

In other instances the nurse may see the opportunity to provide help of a consultative kind, but be unable to take any action until the agreement of those in authority has been

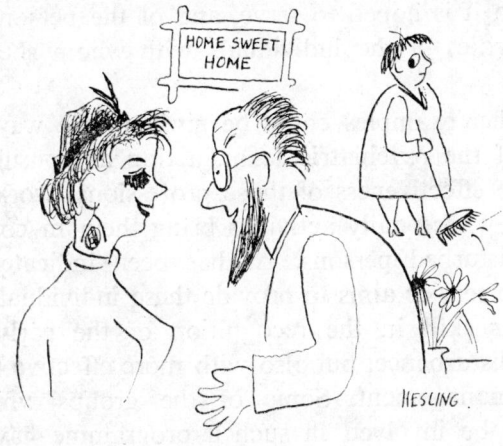

Fig. 37
The nurse may be a most effective consultant in a geriatric setting.

obtained. She may for example, through her contacts in the community, be invited to pay periodic visits to the local Baby Health Centre, for discussions with the nursing staff about some of the difficult mothers and problem babies on whom the clinic sisters are asked to give advice. Even such an invitation, however, might have unfortunate consequences if it later emerges that she is making visits to the clinic without the knowledge and approval of the senior administrators who are responsible for the functioning of the clinics in this particular area. In matters such as these, of course, the nurse will not be expected to act on her own, nor would it ever be desirable for her to make definite arrangements to undertake consultative activities without discussion with her own senior colleagues in the psychiatric service; negotiations with senior administrators, for example, are likely to be undertaken on her behalf by her supervising psychiatrist, if the programme is considered to be a desirable one. The point is emphasised here, however, to ensure that the nurse realises that in community psychiatric work, as in so many other human activities, " good intentions " may fall disastrously short of their desired goal, if they are not linked with a thoughtful understanding of the structure of the organisation it is hoped to serve, and of the personal feelings and sensitivities of the individuals with whom she comes in contact.

Many other examples could be given of the way in which members of the psychiatric team, acting as consultants, can improve the effectiveness of those professional workers in the community whose daily activities bring them in contact with mentally disturbed persons. As has been indicated, such a consultation service aims to provide these individuals not only with greater skill in the recognition of the early signs of emotional disturbance, but also with more effective techniques for their management. Some of the groups which might legitimately be involved in such a programme have already been mentioned (p. 483). It at least some of these situations the nurse, given proper training and supervision, may be a most effective consultant, sometimes *more* effective than some of her colleagues because she may be seen as rather less threatening. A community organisation providing supportive services to geriatric patients may, for example, welcome a nurse as a consultant, when a psychiatrist might be quite unacceptable to them.

The Preventive Role. It is only relatively recently that psychiatry has begun to concern itself with deliberate attempts to prevent psychiatric illness. Some of what has already been said in this chapter is directly related to what is commonly known, in public health terms, as **tertiary prevention**, that is, the prevention of the disability that may be caused by illness, coupled with an active rehabilitation of those affected and the greatest possible fostering of their remaining skills and abilities. The consultative role is intimately concerned with **secondary prevention,** the detection of illness at the earliest possible time, in the belief that the most effective treatment can be given while the disturbance is still in an acute, fluid stage, before it has become a relatively fixed and stable pattern of maladjustment.

To a greater or lesser extent, psychiatric services are also concerning themselves with **primary prevention,** that is, the attempted modification of those factors in individual or community life which may increase the risk of mental illness in those exposed to them. In practical terms, this is usually inextricably linked with secondary prevention, but is certainly worth considering as a special and most important task. If the nurse visits a baby health centre as a consultant concerned with the early recognition and management of mothers whose problems with their babies seem to be stemming directly from emotional disturbance, she also has another important and potentially even more far-reaching opportunity in this setting —to influence generally, through her nursing colleague attached to the centre, the relationships between mothers and their babies. It has been indicated in Chapter 3 that there is a good deal of evidence that the anxious, insecure mother may in some circumstances make it difficult for her child to develop trust and confidence in himself and the outside world; lacking this trust, perhaps saddled thereafter with a good deal of unsatisfied dependence, the clinical evidence suggests that he may as an adult be more liable to develop a psychiatric illness if exposed to various precipitating factors. It is logical, therefore, to suggest that anything that reduces a mother's anxiety, which gives her more confidence in her ability to handle her baby and to provide for his needs, may lead to that baby becoming in later life a more stable, less vulnerable adult. These things are hard to prove with statistical certainty, and for this reason are often criticised by some psychiatrists and nurses, who suggest that they are based more on wishful thinking than on scientifically valid evidence. At the very least, however, there would seem to be ample reasons for believing that the promotion of mutually satisfying relationships between mothers and children is a worthwhile end in itself, quite apart from the somewhat more speculative idea that this will be valuable in primary prevention.

Psychiatrists interested in prevention also concern themselves with many human crisis situations, for there is fairly definite evidence here that a small but significant percentage of persons involved in crisis are thereby predisposed towards subsequent mental disorder. A number of studies, for instance, have shown that the health of widows is significantly likely to deteriorate in the year following their bereavement, this deterioration including the development of a small but definite number of frank mental illnesses. Other evidence suggests that it is likely that the provision of more effective supporting services for widows would reduce the incidence of these sometimes serious consequences. The details of such interventions in crisis would take us beyond the scope of this book; suffice to say that here is another example of the extent to which the contemporary psychiatric service is looking beyond the ordinary limits of known mental disorder, and searching for ways in which groups of human beings known to be at particular risk may be managed so as to minimise the likelihood of later psychiatric illness. Many of these tasks will require, now or in the not too distant future, the participation of the psychiatric nurse.

CONCLUSION

As the psychiatric service moves out to assist those who are reluctant psychiatric patients, or those who might not yet generally be regarded as in need of psychiatric help, the tasks of the psychiatric nurse are acquiring a new and rich dimension. She is certainly unfitted to participate in such programmes without acquiring a basic education about human behaviour and psychiatric illness, and without developing fundamental

THE NURSE IN THE COMMUNITY

clinical skills and experience in understanding human relationships, as has been described elsewhere in this book. Many of these new tasks present a great challenge; no longer are nurses on their own home ground, that of the hospital, working within the comfort and familiarity of a relatively clearly defined role. Meeting the patient in *his* own environment, working with colleagues in the community on a basis of partnership, learning to relate to a wide variety of professional and volunteer organisations, some of whom do not in the beginning see the relevance of the psychiatric nurse for their own work—all these things make special demands on the nurse's own personality, her flexibility and tolerance, yet undoubtedly increase her status as well as the range and depth of the satisfactions that she may derive from the practice of her profession.

26

PSYCHIATRIC SOCIAL WORK

BOTH social work and nursing are old professions, with origins deriving from those groups in the Middle Ages who cared for the acutely ill, the poor, the socially isolated, the chronically sick and disabled. Each has a modern history commencing in the middle of the nineteenth century, and each has experienced major changes during the past 25 years in both educational programmes and employment opportunities. While the two professions have tended to develop along their own routes, it is currently imperative, in the light of our present views concerning the management of psychiatric illness, that they should be able to communicate and work with each other, understanding and respecting the special contribution which each can make to the team approach. Nurses and social workers increasingly work side by side in psychiatric hospitals, general hospital psychiatric services, outpatient and community clinics, health centres, centres for the aged, nursing homes, baby health centres, and in the homes of patients in the community. In these working alliances their shared aims are not only therapeutic, but also have a major preventive component.

Each profession however has its own series of special tasks, and thus a special contribution to make to the common goal. Understanding will be fostered if the nurse can appreciate some of the specific skills and viewpoints of the social worker. These she has acquired through a university education of four years' duration, during which she has taken courses in subjects such as developmental psychology, social systems, concepts of family and society, and has studied issues such as stress and reactions to stress, including ways of coping with both physical and psychiatric illness. A great deal of emphasis is still placed on the satisfactory completion of field placements and practical work under the close supervision of an experienced social worker. Following graduation, in addition to the numerous career possibilities in some type of psychiatric facility, social workers may elect to work in general hospitals, in family or youth agencies, with migrants or old persons, or in a wide variety of community programmes.

UNDERSTANDING THE PATIENT AND HIS FAMILY

One of the psychiatric social worker's more visible roles is as a member of the team working on an inpatient ward. Here she has a particular responsibility to contribute to the team's understanding of the causes of the patient's illness, through an assessment of the factors which made it necessary for him to come to hospital. She will try to understand as much as she can about the patient's social and cultural network, through the provision of answers to questions such as: what family does he have? Does he see the members of his family, or some of them, as helpful or non-helpful? Where did he work and what is his complete work history? Are there other persons in the community whom he sees as supportive? What are his social achievements? Does his life style seem to be chronically unsatisfying, or does his recent situation represent a temporary crisis? Rarely is it sufficient for her to confine her interviews to the patient alone, even though she will certainly be building a special relationship with him; she will also want to interview relatives and special friends (sometimes referred to collectively as " significant others ") in order to hear their views on the nature and origins of his illness and to appraise as best she can their attitudes and feelings towards him.

Through interviews of this nature she will be building up a **social diagnosis** or **social history.** Some of the nurse's own information and observations concerning the patient may well be very valuable to her in this task (p. 416). The social worker's own special contribution stems from her assessment of the patient's adequacy or inadequacy in relation to his social situation, and the way in which she enables other team members to see him from this perspective. When decisions are made concerning the patient's treatment and management, therefore, she will be able to help other members of the team to see that certain recommendations may, for example, be acceptable to the patient but totally unacceptable to his immediate family as matters stand at present, or it may be that a recommendation which is clearly likely to be of benefit to the patient will have potentially disastrous consequences for one or more of his relatives.

Because it is generally accepted that the period of hospitalisation should ideally be kept as brief as possible, the social worker will also be preparing the patient for re-entry into the community, right from the beginning of his hospital experience. At the same time, she will need to be preparing the significant members of his social network for his return. She will set aside time for the parents or spouse to enable them to ventilate their feelings about the sick person—feelings which will range from genuine concern and anxiety to frustration, resentment and angry bitterness, and will sometimes involve all these conflicting emotions at once (p. 432). Her aim is to assist them towards a greater understanding of the patient's problems, a greater tolerance of any residual disabilities, and thus a greater willingness to become involved with attempts to resolve the problems and to provide supportive care where this is indicated. In the process it may be necessary for them to acquire an understanding of the extent to which their own attitudes and behaviour may have contributed to or magnified the patient's problem. They may also need to work through some of their irrational fears about the stigma of psychiatric illness, to gain a deeper understanding of the patient's needs, and examine a range of possibilities concerning his future life style, some of which may at first be very hard for them to accept.

SOCIAL CASE-WORK

All the types of activity just described, based on the social worker's particular skills in interviewing and the understanding of relationships, are forms of **social case-work**, often continuing through and beyond the hospitalisation period to facilitate the patient's reintegration into a less stressful and more benign social environment. As a result of her endeavours, family members may come to recognise the magnitude and importance of their own problems and may become motivated to engage in marital or family therapy, at which the designated " patient " may or may not be present; they may thus achieve important and beneficial changes in their own attitudes to themselves and in their interpersonal relationships, so that in the long run an entire family group and not just one particular person comes to function more effectively and contentedly.

Two examples may illustrate the type of problem and the manner in which it is approached:

(1) A 17-year-old girl was admitted to hospital suffering from a severe neurotic depressive reaction. She had withdrawn from social contacts and was unable to concentrate at school, which she wanted to leave although until recently she had been a very successful student. She had difficulties in both eating and sleeping and was extremely argumentative with all her family members, particularly her mother with whom there was rapidly developing a mutually antagonistic relationship. The social worker was asked to assess the family situation, to evaluate any problems which might be relevant to the patient's complaints and to offer assistance to the parents in understanding their daughter's illness. Weekly sessions with both parents quickly revealed a good deal of chronic conflict in their marriage, coupled with great resentment towards their daughter; as the social worker continued to offer support and clarification of some of the principal issues, the couple were enabled to gain greater insight into their difficulties and became more confident in themselves and developed a greater understanding of the girl's behaviour. Their previously overprotective

attitude towards her gradually subsided and they were able to support her moves towards greater independence. Later some therapy sessions were held involving the whole family, including the patient's 11-year-old sister and nine-year-old brother, at which patterns of communication within the family were discussed and the norms of family behaviour frankly reviewed. The result was a clear improvement, not only in the presenting patient's symptoms, but in the gratifications derived from relationships within the family and the functioning of the family as a whole.

(2) A married man aged 26 was admitted to hospital for treatment of an almost completely disabling phobic illness. He had married young, while still a university student, and now had three children under the age of five; his wife claimed to be happy about this, although he said that he found the situation very difficult. Both parties denied, however, that there were any major problems in the marriage, and it was not until the social worker interviewed the wife that the real issues began to emerge. After having been shown a good deal of kindness, encouragement and understanding she was able to talk about massive dissatisfactions in their married life—in particular their feeling of being burdened by three unplanned children, with consequent disruption of the patient's career aspirations and their desire to find a more suitable home. Weekly joint sessions enabled this young couple to ventilate their anger towards each other, discuss their problems constructively for the first time and begin to assume responsibility for their own and the children's lives, whereas previously they had been on the surface passively accepting of their " fate " yet ineffectually and inwardly rebellious about it. Gradually the patient's symptoms subsided, although they had previously been completely resistant to a variety of different treatment approaches. The husband returned to full-time work as a statistician but was able to make a constructive job change, his wife began to work part-time, and both started to plan on a shared basis the day-to-day management of their family problems and finances, working towards the future purchase of an appropriate house.

In many instances the social worker's skills will be particularly relevant for those patients who are on their way towards more normal living as a result of good nursing and medical care during the acute stage of the illness. She gradually moves closer to these patients, offering where appropriate temporary financial assistance to help them get on their feet again, information and perhaps practical help in finding suitable accommodation, advice re unemployment, sickness or pension benefits, the role of intermediary with an old employer or guidance in seeking new (and perhaps more appropriate) employment. In these and other ways she helps the patient build a plan for his rehabilitation, and she may become a vital link between the newly discharged patient and the supportive services provided by the hospital (p. 479).

In all these activities the social worker makes constant use of her specialised **interview skills.** Above all she requires to be a good listener, able to promote the confidence and trust of a very wide range of people; she must be able to focus her entire interest and attention on the person currently in her office, in this way helping him to tell his story frankly, in his own fashion, thus allowing him to gain a clearer understanding of his present situation and what he would like done about it. At times she will comment on what emerges, at other times ask specific questions, and will certainly guide the interview in subtle ways so that relevant issues are not ignored or skipped over lightly. The patient or relative may need to be encouraged to " let off steam ", for this too may be necessary if he is to examine his problems more realistically. The overriding aim is *not,* despite much popular opinion to the contrary, to give specific advice, but rather to help him come to as clear as possible a definition of his problem and decide for himself what he should do, having looked squarely (perhaps with some prompting) at the advantages and disadvantages in the various possible courses of action, and with the added information which the social worker has provided about available resources and forms of assistance.

OUTPATIENT PRACTICE

In the outpatient clinic the social worker will plan to continue her contact with many of those patients with whom she first became involved during their inpatient experience; the adequacy of the relationship she has established will quickly become apparent once the patient is free to go his own way in the community. She will also become involved with many other new patients presenting to the outpatient clinic and will contribute to their management, often on a " crisis " basis in some type of walk-in or emergency service. Her skills and particular interventions may be of vital significance, for example, in patients presenting with acute psychiatric symptoms resulting from deteriorating interpersonal relationships or sudden catastrophic losses, in patients who have made suicide attempts or who have impulsively taken overdoses following a major domestic dispute. She will encounter patients who have previously been in treatment and who are now confronted with a new stress and who need to talk over their current situation before they can decide what to do. Her role and her techniques in this setting are not of course essentially different from those previously described, for here too she is aiming to help the patient, or the family, to cope on their own and take their own decisions. She has to recognise, however, that it is quite unrealistic (and potentially very destructive) to impose this goal on every single patient; for some individuals, conspicuously lacking in psychological and/or social and/or physical resources, further burdened by a harmful, stressful but basically inescapable environment, continuing and sometimes lifelong support will be required. Every psychiatric service, however progressive its orientation and methods, has its own share of such persons; the task of providing them with a reliable source of supportive gratification, a task which often falls to the social worker, is certainly not to be despised. Indeed the provision of such support with honesty and without patronising contempt, and without fostering the patient's dependence and further undermining his sense of competence, requires professional attitudes and skill of a high order.

THE SOCIAL WORKER IN THE COMMUNITY

Effective treatment and rehabilitation procedures require a sophisticated knowledge of the resources available within the community and its institutions which may be of assistance to patients with specific needs. The social worker therefore develops useful links with such facilities as vocational rehabilitation and employment centres, sheltered workshops (p. 464) and special training schemes, hostels providing totally or partially supervised accommodation, social and recreational organisations and so on. She can assess which of these various resources will be of the greatest benefit to the patient and his family, and then use her relationship skills with the patient and her prestige in the community to help him make the most of what these facilities have to offer to meet his needs in a way that is acceptable to him. Here as elsewhere this process contains within itself the encouragement of the patient's ability to achieve goals for himself, granted adequate assistance in the early stages.

The social worker's involvement in the community, however, is much more extensive than this. She will increasingly be found working within some type of Community Health Centre, usually separated physically from a psychiatric hospital though administratively connected with it. Here she is placed very strategically to provide the earliest and best possible management for people in crisis (p. 492), encouraging citizens to make use of the appropriate community resources, paving the way for definitive treatment where this is indicated, and mobilising supportive networks (in the family or elsewhere) for those who are clearly not coping on their own. The community clinic also provides a very effective base for the care in the community, rather than in hospitals or other institutions, of those who need long-term supervision and support. Here in particular she works side by side with the psychiatric nurse, their roles and functions clearly overlapping a good deal. The section on the roles of the community psychiatric nurse (p. 484) has therefore considerable relevance here, and should be revised in conjunction with this paragraph. The social worker too, for example, will be involved in home visits (which may have their own difficulties—Fig. 38), helping patients and their families to cope with new and different stresses, visiting patients who are housebound, and participating in a host of other supportive activities. The social

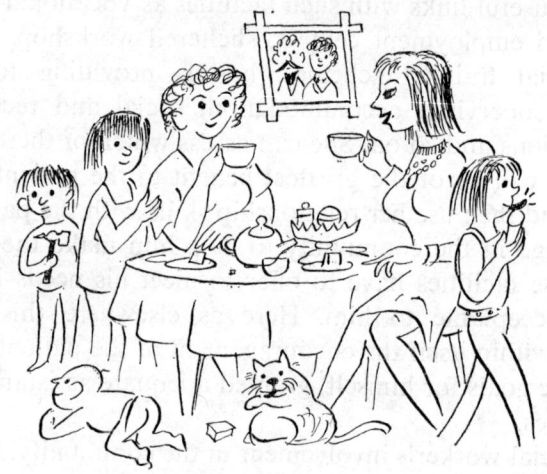

Fig. 38
Home visits can be trying situations.

worker and the nurse will, in favourable circumstances, develop a mutual respect for and reliance on each other's skills—for example, the nurse's comments on new or reawakened symptoms of illness, and her judgement of the patient's response to his present medication, may need to be blended with the social worker's perceptive comments on shifts in the dynamics of family interaction and her recognition of new strains emerging in the relationship between the patient and his immediate community.

The social worker may also be an important contributor to **research** on community issues; her investigations may for example reveal pockets of special need due to particular local circumstances or unusual deprivation. She may also be a most valuable consultant to other social agencies and thus help to bring about a greater coordination of effort in the attempt to find solutions to community problems.

GROUP WORK

Most psychiatric units or clinics use one or more forms of group activity as components of their therapeutic plan, so that it is usual to find all members of the team involved in some type of group work. Sometimes the groups are psychotherapeutic in the sense described in Chapter 16 (p. 336), others may have a more direct focus on practical problems, perhaps using role playing, work, drama or other activities. The social worker, who has usually had a special training in group dynamics, will frequently be found leading such a group (perhaps jointly with another team member), and her own background leads her to be particularly involved in those groups which aim to improve the members' capacity to cope when facing real life problems; the group may perhaps be largely composed of people facing similar problems—for example, imminent discharge from hospital—or common treatment experiences. Though such groups certainly make economical use of professional time, this is not their principal justification; much more importantly they give patients the opportunity, under skilled leadership, to pool their resources and experiences in trying to help others work out acceptable solutions to their own problems.

Social group work of this kind is also a valuable technique in community settings. The social worker may, for example, develop group programmes for adolescents in youth clubs or social agencies, for normal mothers wishing to discuss aspects of child-rearing, or for widows who are having major difficulties in coping with the problems posed by their bereavement.

Her group work skills will also be of vital importance in any contribution she may be able to make to **community organisation**. Social workers have recently played major roles on committees studying social problems, in pointing out gaps in community facilities (e.g., inadequate care for the children of working mothers) and by participating in research on various aspects of social welfare programmes.

CONCLUSION

The treatment of psychiatric patients is a matter of teamwork, the psychiatric social worker being the team member who particularly deals with the patient, not just as an individual, but as a member of family, social, community, work and social groups. She helps patients and their relatives to deal with outworn superstitions about mental illness and with the shame, fear and guilt which are so often attached to psychiatric hospitalisation. She functions as a practical support to the patient both before and after his period of hospital treatment and interprets his illness to his family, his employer and any other interested party. She aims to get him back, whenever possible, into the community as a functioning and productive member of it; she may assist many others to avoid hospitalisation altogether. In carrying out these tasks she makes a flexible use of her particular skills in the establishment of case-work relationships and in group work. She too, in her own special way and using her own special training, aids the patient in the rebuilding of his unsatisfying personal relationships.

27

CLINICAL PSYCHOLOGY

EVEN experienced nurses are at times confused by the terms **psychiatrist, psychologist** and **psychoanalyst.**

The **psychiatrist** is always a medical graduate, a physician who has directed his studies particularly towards an understanding of psychiatric illness—its causes, prevention and treatment; his chief interest is in the varieties of abnormal behaviour.

Psychology, on the other hand, is a science primarily directed towards the understanding of normal behaviour and only secondarily to the relationship between normal and abnormal mental function.

A **psychologist** is a university graduate, holding an Arts or Science degree which has included a special emphasis on psychology throughout four years. Some psychologists undergo special training in educational techniques and become **educational psychologists;** others study the ways in which a man's potentials may best be employed in his job and are known as **vocational psychologists.** In a psychiatric service the nurse encounters the **clinical psychologist,** who has usually completed additional university studies and gained further years of experience under the supervision of a senior psychologist before he is regarded as adequately trained.

The **psychoanalyst** may or may not have a medical degree, the unique feature of his background being that he has himself undergone a period of psychoanalysis (p. 327), usually of several years' duration, in order to learn through personal experience the technique of treatment and to enable him to recognise some of his own inner conflicts so that he may be a more objective therapist. He is the only person who is able to carry out psychoanalytic treatment in its strict sense.

The trained clinical psychologist possesses a detailed knowledge of normal and abnormal behaviour coupled with practical experience in the study of psychiatric patients. He thinks of people in terms of their capacities, their personality traits and their defences and he is concerned to discover the extent to which an individual's behaviour deviates from the normal, and in what way. He has a special training in the methods by which a scientific problem may be studied. He is equipped with knowledge of the uses and limitations of various measuring instruments known as psychological tests, by means of which he can examine and appraise intelligence and personality characterisics. He has training and skills in a range of treatment procedures which he may use himself or from which he may construct treatment programmes for other members of the staff to use under his supervision. The extent to which a psychologist will be involved in any of the functions to be described will depend, in some measure, on the role and policy of the hospital and its associated services—whether it treats children and adolescents, whether it is a teaching hospital, whether it is responsible for major clinical and research activities in the community, whether rehabilitation schemes have a prominent place in its programme.

DIAGNOSIS

Chapter 8 has stressed that the fixing of a particular diagnostic label to a patient is only rarely of much value in psychiatry. The much more important level of diagnosis involves arriving at an awareness of what the patient's symptoms mean in relation to his current problems and life history. In this sense " diagnosis " means " understanding ". The psychologist is able, through the employment of **psychological tests,** to provide information about various aspects of the patient's mental life, both conscious and unconscious, which will help the psychiatrist and the other team members to assess the significance of his illness and to plan his treatment programme.

Psychological tests are important because they are objective

CLINICAL PSYCHOLOGY

measuring instruments which reveal information which is relatively unbiased by personal impressions, hunches or beliefs. Certain tests, known as **intelligence tests,** are designed to estimate the patient's intellectual capacities. (The concepts of **intelligence quotient, chronological age** and **mental age** have been discussed in Chapter 14, to which reference should be made.) This knowledge may be helpful in a variety of ways. It may be found, for example, that the patient's aims in life are far higher than his abilities would permit and that consequently, should he pursue his unrealistic ambitions, he is doomed to failure and frustration. His intelligence will be one of many factors which will be considered in the selection of appropriate treatment, particularly should psychotherapy be contemplated, and it will substantially influence the type of programme planned for his rehabilitation. Intelligence tests can also be used to assess the presence or absence of intellectual deterioration; both organic and schizophrenic reactions may leave their own special mark on the person's intellectual capacities even in their quite early stages. Some persons on testing display an intellectual level which would be considered within the mentally retarded range, yet a further analysis of the test material may show that the person is not in fact retarded but is now functioning at that level because of a psychiatric illness of one of the above types, which has interfered with an originally average intellectual endowment. The intelligence quotient as measured by these tests will also be one important factor, though by no means the only one, in determining the most suitable management for a mentally retarded child. The intelligence tests most commonly used by clinical psychologists are the **Wechsler Adult Intelligence Scale (WAIS), the Wechsler Intelligence Scale for Children (WISC)** and the **Stanford-Binet Intelligence Scale.** It is not possible in this book to describe these tests, but the nurse during her training should endeavour to see some of the materials used and to know some of the questions asked, so that she may better understand the psychologist's aims and her patients' reactions to his procedures.

Tests of a different kind, known as **personality tests,** are designed to uncover otherwise hidden aspects of the patient's mental life and to provide some measurement or precise description of certain of his attitudes and characteristics. Some of these are called **projective tests** and are based on the belief that, if a person is asked to describe a vague ink-blot or picture, his spontaneous comments will reveal certain aspects of his mental life of which he is himself unaware. The test employing ink-blots is known as the **Rorschach Test** and the responses which patients give to these blots can be scored in a very precise fashion. The most common test employing pictures is the **Thematic Apperception Test (TAT);** the themes which the patient brings into the stories which he weaves around these pictures will have meaning in terms of his past life and conflicts. Other tests are of the **questionnaire** variety, in which the individual is asked to indicate whether particular statements are " true " or " false "—the following examples are taken from a test which contains in all 566 of such items:[1]

" Most people are honest chiefly through fear of being caught."

" I like to flirt."

" What others think of me does not bother me."

" I enjoy children."

" I forget right away what people say to me."

"A large number of people are guilty of bad sexual conduct."

All these tests will reveal information about the person's deeper anxieties, guilts and drives and will indicate the defences which he uses to counteract these; much useful knowledge may be gained even though he may not be particularly co-operative. They will offer evidence as to his feelings about significant people such as parents, marital partner, children and authority figures and will indicate his attitudes towards emotions such as love, hate, jealousy and fear. Previously hidden sexual problems

---

[1] Hathaway, S. R. & McKinley, J. C. (1943). *Booklet for the Minnesota Multiphasic Personality Inventory.* New York: Psychological Corporation.

may become clearly apparent. Knowledge of these matters obviously leads to the establishment of a diagnosis which is deeper and more meaningful than a mere label such as " phobic reaction " or " schizophrenic reaction, paranoid type ".

TREATMENT

The psychologist is not qualified to administer the traditional physical treatments, such as electrotherapy, nor can he prescribe drugs. His own special training, however, usually fits him to undertake psychotherapy either in individual or group treatment programmes.

He is also an increasingly important contributor to treatment activities other than psychotherapy, in particular those forms of treatment known as behaviour therapy (p. 340) which are derived from the principles of learning theory. He may devise a treatment programme to help a child or adult, through the learning of new patterns, to overcome an unrewarding habit such as a motor spasm (for example, writer's cramp) or a tic, or to deal with certain isolated fears of objects or situations such as social anxiety or travel in public transport (p. 215).

He is also equipped to devise programmes for the education of children with specific defects such as reading disability, and will also be concerned with the retraining of brain-damaged patients in such functions as speech, writing and motor co-ordination. He will be a vital contributor to any scheme to train the intellectually handicapped in simple habits or in particular skills which may fit them for employment. He may design graded activity programmes, usually implemented by the nurses, which aim to reduce incontinence, to offset the reduction in social information, skills and intellectual activities experienced by the socially isolated elderly patient, or to counteract the effects of long periods of hospitalisation.

TEACHING

For all members of the psychiatric team, and particularly for those in training, the psychologist is the person best equipped to provide them with information about the processes of normal personality development, as well as other theoretical aspects of normal and abnormal behaviour. The nurse who has a good relationship with the clinical psychologist in her team will find that he will be able to give her a great deal of assistance in the difficulties which she encounters, both in her studies and in her understanding of certain patients.

RESEARCH

Research is essential in any field of study if progress is to be made. There is no place for the persistence of ideas about psychiatric illness and its treatment which are based purely on hunches or intuition. But not only do we not as yet know the answers to many questions about psychiatry, we are still in some areas uncertain which are the right questions to ask. The psychologist is experienced in the use of the scientific methods which must always form the basis of research and he is frequently called upon to guide and contribute to the development of research in the psychiatric hospital. He studies such problems as the effects of electrotherapy on concentration and memory, the changes in symptoms and behaviour induced by drugs, and the relationship of treatment outcome to the expectations of the therapist. He is tending to be increasingly involved in studies of the effects of social factors on the mental health of the community. Considerable attention is being directed towards the detection of those individuals in the community who are at special risk (for example widows, socially isolated individuals and those in the culture of poverty), and in the assessment of the effectiveness of intervention programmes directed towards these people. Psychologists have also been instrumental in analysing the effects of staff attitudes and hospital procedures on patient behaviour.

The nurse will be asked to co-operate in some of these programmes and will find that such participation makes her own tasks more interesting and rewarding. In some research studies her observations have a unique value and she is often asked to record them in a systematic manner, a task which she should welcome as indicating very clearly her essential role as a member of the research team, as well as the treatment team.

CONCLUSION

In Chapter 2 (p. 26) mention was made of the desirable relationship between the nurse and the psychologist and both there and in this present chapter it has been indicated that each will benefit from the support of the other. Many psychologists work within the hospital in somewhat isolated offices and tend to be thought of by some of the patients as being " peculiar " people and their tests regarded with grave suspicion. The nurse can do a lot to play down these anxieties and to ensure that the patient as far as possible sees the psychologist as yet another ally for him in his struggle towards maturity. The psychologist is a specialist who is capable of making a unique contribution to the well-being of individual patients and to the morale and overall function of the hospital; here, as always, mutual understanding between the different members of the team must inevitably lead to more effective patient care.

RECOMMENDED READING

NOTE: This list of books and journal articles is obviously much more extended than that which usually accompanies a nursing text. It is supplied in this form because there are substantial grounds for believing that many trained psychiatric nurses and advanced students are anxious to read more widely, but lack experienced guidance as to what to read.

It is *not* intended that trainee nurses should read at all widely in this list, certainly during the early part of their experience; nevertheless some items have been marked thus (*) to indicate their particular suitability for senior students. Items marked thus (†) are works of reference and it is intended that they should be consulted only on specific points on which the nurse desires more knowledge or a different viewpoint.

In particular it is hoped that this list will be useful to the post-graduate nurse, perhaps trained in a time when nursing education was purely descriptive and stereotyped, who wishes to gain a further knowledge of present day concepts in psychiatric nursing.

General Texts on Psychiatry

ALDRICH, C. K. (1966). *An Introduction to Dynamic Psychiatry.* New York: McGraw-Hill.
† FREEDMAN, A., KAPLAN, H. I. & SADOCK, B. J. (eds.) (1972). *Synopsis of Comprehensive Textbook of Psychiatry.* Baltimore: Williams and Wilkins.
† GREGORY, I. (1968). *Fundamentals of Psychiatry.* Philadeplhia: Saunders.
† SOLOMON, P. & PATCH, V. D. (1971). *Handbook of Psychiatry.* California: Lange.
STAFFORD-CLARK, D. (1963). *Psychiatry Today.* London: Penguin.
TREDGOLD, R. & WOLFF, H. (eds.) (1970). *U.C.H. Notes on Psychiatry.* London: Duckworth.
† ULETT, G. A. (1972). *A Synopsis of Contemporary Psychiatry.* St. Louis: Mosby.

Psychiatric Nursing

ACKNER, B. (1964). *Handbook for Psychiatric Nurses.* London: Baillière.
ALTSCHUL, A. T. (1972). *Patient-Nurse Interaction. A study of interaction patterns in acute psychiatric wards.* University of Edinburgh Department of Nursing Studies Monograph, Number 3. Edinburgh and London: Churchill Livingstone.

RECOMMENDED READING

AXLINE, V. (1971). *Dibs: In Search of Self.* London: Pelican Books.
* BARNES, E. (Ed.) (1968). *Psychosocial Nursing: Studies from the Cassel Hospital.* London: Tavistock.
BROWN, E. L. (1962). *Newer Dimensions of Patient Care.* New York: Russell Sage Foundation.
BROWN, M. M. & FOWLER, G. R. (1961) *Psychodynamic Nursing: A Biosocial Orientation.* Philadelphia: Saunders.
BURR, J. (1970). *Nursing the Psychiatric Patient.* 2nd ed. London: Baillière, Tindall and Cassell.
BURTON, G. (1964). *Personal, Impersonal and Interpersonal Relations: A Guide for Nurses.* New York: Springer.
DENNIS, L. B. (1967). *Psychology of Human Behaviour for Nurses.* Philadelphia: Saunders.
HOFLING, C. K., LEININGER, M. M. & BREGG, E. (1967). *Basic Psychiatric Concepts in Nursing.* Philadelphia: Lippincott.
* JONES, M. (1963). What is psychiatric nursing? *Lancet,* **2,** 1108.
KALKMAN, M. E. (1967). *Psychiatric Nursing.* New York: McGraw-Hill.
MCGHIE, A. (1973). *Psychology as Applied to Nursing,* 6th ed. Edinburgh and London: Churchill Livingstone.
MATHENEY, R. V. & TOPALIS, M. (1965). *Psychiatric Nursing.* St. Louis: Mosby.
* SCHWARTZ, M. S. & SHOCKLEY, E. L. (1965). *The Nurse and the Mental Patient: A Study in Interpersonal Relations.* New York: Wiley.
* WEDDELL, D., BOGIE, H., THOMAS, B., GAZDAR, E. J., GLEESON, I. & ELLES, G. W. (1957). Nursing emotionally disturbed patients. *Nurs. Times,* May, June & July.
* WORLD HEALTH ORGANIZATION (1956). *Expert Committee on Psychiatric Nursing: First Report.* Geneva: W.H.O.

History of Psychiatry

ALEXANDER, F. G. & SELESNICK, S. T. (1966). *The History of Psychiatry.* New York: Harper and Row.
BOSTOCK, J. (1968). *The Dawn of Australian Psychiatry.* Sydney: Australasian Medical Publishing Co.
SCHNECK, J. M. (1960). *A History of Psychiatry.* Springfield: Thomas.
* WALK, A. (1961). The history of mental nursing. *J. ment. Sci.* **107,** 1.

Personality and Behaviour

† ARNHEIM, R. et al. (1971). *Developmental Psychology Today.* California: CRM Books.
† ARNHEIM, R. et al. (1972). *Psychology Today: An Introduction.* 2nd ed. California: CRM Books.
BOWLBY, J. (1968). *Child Care and the Growth of Love.* London: Penguin.
DAVIS, D. RUSSELL (1966). *An Introduction to Psychopathology.* London: Oxford University Press.
* ERIKSON, E. H. (1967). *Childhood and Society.* London: Penguin.
† KISKER, G. W. (1972). *The Disorganised Personality.* New York: McGraw-Hill.
† LIDZ, T. (1968). *The Person: his Development throughout the Life Cycle.* New York: Basic.
* MADDISON, D. C. & RAPHAEL, B. (1971). Social and psychological consequences of chronic disease in childhood. *Med. J. Aust.,* **2,** 1265.
† MORGAN, C. T. & KING, R. A. (1971). *Introduction to Psychology.* New York: McGraw-Hill.
PARKES, C. M. (1972). *Bereavement: Studies of Grief in Adult Life.* London: Tavistock.

STAFFORD-CLARK, D. (1968). *What Freud Really Said*. London: Penguin.
STARKE, J. G. (1973). *The Validity of Psychoanalysis*. Sydney: Angus and Robertson.
WINNICOTT, D. W. (1967). *The Child, the Family and the Outside World*. London: Penguin.

Clinical Syndromes

CROWCROFT, A. (1968). *The Psychotic*. London: Penguin.
DOMINIAN, J. (1968). *Marital Breakdown*. London: Penguin.
* FREEMAN, T. F., CAMERON, J. L. & MCGHIE, A. (1958). *Chronic Schizophrenia*, Chap. 10. London: Tavistock.
KESSEL, N. & WALTON, H. (1965). *Alcoholism*. London: Penguin.
LE DAIN, G. et al. (1971). *The Non-Medical Use of Drugs*. London: Penguin.
MADDISON, D. C. (1964). The positive diagnosis of neurotic illness. *N.Z. med. J.* **63**, 349.
MADDISON, D. C. & MACKEY, K. H. (1966). Suicide: the clinical problem. *Br. J. Psychiat.*, **112**, 693.
MADDISON, D. C. (1973). The management of depression in consultant medical practice. *Aust. N.Z. J. Med.*, **1**, 89.
† MENDELS, J. (1970). *Concepts of Depression*. New York: Wiley.
† POST, F. (1965). *The Clinical Psychiatry of Late Life*. London: Pergamon.
STENGEL, E. (1964). *Suicide and Attempted Suicide*. London: Penguin.
STORR, A. (1965). *Sexual Deviation*. London: Penguin.
WEST, D. J. (1968). *Homosexuality*. London: Penguin.

Child Psychiatry

FINCH, S. M. (1960). *Fundamentals of Child Psychiatry*. New York: Norton.
† KANNER, L. (1960). *Child Psychiatry*. Springfield: Thomas.
NURCOMBE, B. (1972). *An Outline of Child Psychiatry*. Sydney: University of New South Wales Press.

Mental Retardation

ADAMS, M. & LOVEJOY, H. (1972). *The Mentally Subnormal—Social Work Approaches*. London: Heinemann.
BENSBERG, G. J. (1965). *Teaching the Mentally Retarded*. Atlanta: Southern Regional Education Board.
CLARKE, A. M. & CLARKE, A. D. B. (1974). *Mental Deficiency—the Changing Outlook*. 3rd ed. London: Methuen.
GUNZBURG, H. C. (1973). *Social Competence and Mental Handicap*. 2nd ed. London: Baillière, Tindall and Cassell.
GUNZBURG, H. C. (1973). *Mental Handicap and Physical Environment*. London: Baillière, Tindall and Cassell.
KIRMAN, B. H. (1972). *The Mentally Handicapped Child*. London: Nelson.

Psychosomatic Disorders

ALVAREZ, W. C. (1943). *Nervousness, Indigestion and Pain*. New York: Hoeber.
BALINT, M. (1957). *The Doctor, his Patient and the Illness*. London: Pitman.
† ENGEL, G. L. (1963). *Psychological Development in Health and Disease*. Philadelphia: Saunders.
† LIEF, H. I., LIEF, V. F. & LIEF, N. R. (1963). *Psychological Basis of Medical Practice*. New York: Hoeber.

RECOMMENDED READING

MADDISON, D. C. (1960). Psychological aspects of surgical practice. *Aust. N.Z. J. Surg.*, **30,** 9.
MERSKEY, H. & SPEAR, F. G. (1967). *Pain. Psychological and Psychiatric Aspects.* London: Baillière, Tindall and Cassell.

The Provision of Psychiatric Services

BAKER, A., DAVIES, R. L. & SIVADON, P. (1959). *Psychiatric Services and Architecture.* Geneva: World Health Organization.
* BARTON, R. (1966). *Institutional Neurosis.* Bristol: Wright.
BESKIND, H. (1962). Psychiatric inpatient treatment of adolescents: a review of clinical experience. *Compreh. Psychiat.,* **3,** 354.
* CAPLAN, G. (1964). *Principles of Preventive Psychiatry.* New York: Basic Books.
† CAPLAN, G. (1970). *The Theory and Practice of Mental Health Consultation.* London: Tavistock.
† CLARK, D. H. (1964). *Administrative Therapy: The Role of the Doctor in the Therapeutic Community.* London: Tavistock.
FREEMAN, H. & FARNDALE, J. (1963). *Trends in the Mental Health Services.* Oxford: Pergamon.
FREEMAN, H. & FARNDALE, J. (1967). *New Aspects of the Mental Health Services.* Oxford: Pergamon.
GOFFMAN, E. (1968). *Asylums.* London: Penguin.
HOENIG, J. & HAMILTON, M. W. (1969). *The Desegregation of the Mentally Ill.* London: Routledge and Kegan Paul.
* JOHN, A. (1961). *A Study of the Psychiatric Nurse.* Edinburgh and London: Churchill Livingstone.
JOHN, A. L., LEITE-RIBEIRO, M. O. & BUCKLE, D. (1963). *The Nurse in Mental Health Practice.* Geneva: World Health Organization.
JONES, M. (1968). *Social Psychiatry in Practice.* London: Penguin.
LAMB, H. Richard (1971). *Rehabilitation in Community Mental Health.* San Francisco: Jossey Bass.
* MADDISON, D. C. (1966). The changing responsibility of the psychiatrist. *Med. J. Aust.,* **2,** 302.
MARTIN, D. V. (1962). *Adventures in Psychiatry: Social Change in a Mental Hospital.* Oxford: Cassirer.
PANZETTA, A. F. (1971). *Community Mental Health: Myth and Reality.* Philadelphia: Lea and Febiger.
PILOWSKY, I. & MADDISON, D. (eds.) (1969). *Psychiatry and the Community.* Sydney: Sydney University Press.
RAPAPORT, R. N. (1960). *Community as Doctor: New Perspectives on a Therapeutic Community.* London: Tavistock.
RINSLEY, D. B. (1963). Psychiatric hospital treatment. *Arch. gen. Psychiat.,* **9,** 489.
SCHWARTZ, M. S. & SCHWARTZ, C. G. (1964). *Social Approaches to Mental Patient Care.* New York: Columbia University Press.
STANTON, A. H. & SCHWARTZ, M. S. (1954). *The Mental Hospital: A Study of Institutional Participation in Psychiatric Illness and Treatment.* London: Tavistock.
WILMER, H. A. (1958). *Social Psychiatry in Action: A Therapeutic Community.* Springfield: Thomas.
ZINBERG, N. D. (ed.) (1964). *Psychiatry and Medical Practice in a General Hospital.* New York: International Universities Press.

Psychiatric Treatment

† FOULKES, S. H. (1964). *Therapeutic Group Analysis.* London: Allen and Unwin.
FRANK, J. D. (1961). *Persuasion and Healing: A Comparative Study of Psychotherapy.* Baltimore: Johns Hopkins.

LANGSLEY, D. G. & KAPLAN, D. M. (1968). *The Treatment of Families in Crisis*. New York: Grune and Stratton.
PARAD, H. J. (ed.) (1965). *Crisis Intervention: Selected Readings*. New York: Family Service Association.
SARGANT, W. & SLATER, E. (1972). *An Introduction to Physical Methods of Treatment in Psychiatry*, 5th ed. Edinburgh and London: Churchill Livingstone.
WENRICH, W. W. (1970). *Primer of Behaviour Modification*. London: Brooks Cole.

Occupational, Recreational and Social Therapies

FIDLER, G. S. (1969). The task-orientated group as a context for treatment. *Am. J. occup. Ther.*, **23**, 43.
MOSEY, C. A. (1973). *Activities Therapy*. New York: Raven.
SHANNON, P. D. (1970). The work-play model: a basis for occupational therapy programming in psychiatry. *Am. J. occup. Ther.*, **24**, 215.
SHANNON, P. D. (1972). Work-play theory and the occupational therapy process. *Am. J. occup. Ther.*, **26**, 169.
WEST, W. L. (ed.) (1959). *Changing Concepts and Practices in Psychiatric Occupational Therapy*. Iowa: Wm. C. Brown Book Co.

Psychiatric Social Work

FINK, A. E., WILSON, E. E. & CANOVER, M. B. (1964). *The Field of Social Work*. New York: Holt, Rinehart and Winston.
GARRETT, A. (1972). *Interviewing: its Principles and Methods*, 2nd ed. New York: Family Service Association of America.
KONOPKA, G. (1963). *Social Group Work: a Helping Process*. New Jersey: Prentice Hall.
SCHWARTZ, W. & ZALBA, S. R. (eds.) (1971). *The Practice of Group Work*. New York: Columbia University Press.

INDEX

Entries in italic figures indicate the main references

A

Abstinence syndrome. *See* Withdrawal symptoms
Acceptance, 20, 236, 307, 351, 438, 441
Accidents, 181, 186, 320, 441, 455
Acrocephaly, 302
Activity, 108-110, 251, 405, 419
  maintenance of, 445, 452
  programmes, 488
Addiction, 196-197. *See also* Drug dependence
Adjustment reactions, 159, 162, 284-285
Admission, 354, 378, 433, *438-439*
Adolescence, *54-64, 88,* 138, 192, 206, 225
Adoption, 294, 307
Adrenaline, 372
Adualism, 40-41
Adulthood, 65-69
Advice, 351, 499
Affect. *See* Mood
Affectionless character, 288
Affective reactions, 241-252
After-care, 8, 478, 482, 485
Aggression, 143, *145-146,* 177, 194, 246, 329, 331, 388, 393-396, 420, 431
  as symptom, 123-124, 204-205, 290, 419
  bodily effects of, 313, 314-315
  defences against, 102-103, 120, 143, 146, 389
  displaced, 393-394
  fear of one's own, 87, 141
  management of, 332, 451-454, 465
  origins of, 36, 39, 43, 45, 62, 145-146, 204, 386
  passive, 124, 210, 348, 395, 420
  towards staff, 329, 342-343, 348-349, 393-396, 410, 431
Agitation, 123, 244, 255
  management of, 270, 365, 368
Agranulocytosis, 369
Akathisia, 369
Alcoholics Anonymous, 373
Alcoholism, 2, 72, 135, 137, 172, *198-200,* 212, 225, 320
  acute organic reactions due to, 256
  chronic organic reactions due to, 263-264
  clinical picture, 198-199
  frequency of, 198
  treatment of 336, 373-375, 472
Allegron, 371

Alzheimer's disease, 160
Ambivalence, 109
Amenorrhoea, 243, 247
Amentia. *See* Mental retardation
Amitriptyline. *See* Tryptanol
Amnesia, *126,* 182, 262, 363, 420
Amphetamines, 371-372
  dependence on, *201-202,* 371
  psychosis due to, 137, *202,* 257, 371
'Amytal', 336, 365
Anaemia, 267
Anaesthesia, 258, 267, 326, 335, 359, 360, 363
Anal phase, 42, 147
'Anatensol', 368
'Anectine', 360
Anger. *See* Aggression
Animism, 50
Anorexia
  as symptom, 179, 180, 199, 202, 243, 247, 285, 289, 371
  induced, 371
  management of, 215, 249, 252, 364
  nervosa, 318
'Antabuse', 373
Antibiotics, 258
Anti-depressant drugs, 215, 248, *371-373*
Antisocial character disorders, 52, 150, *203-206,* 218
Anxiety, *84-89,* 340, 410, 447
  arising from illness, 314, 323-325, 380-383, 388, 389, 432
  aroused by loss of love, 86, 141, 194
  aroused by one's own instincts, 87, 122, 149
  as symptom, 122-123, 179-181, 222, 263, 376, 420
  bodily effects of, 85, 123, 179-180, 313-314
  castration. *See* Castration anxiety
  definition of, 85
  free-floating, 179, 188
  in childhood, 285, 290, 292, 323
  management of, 214, 357, 364, 368, 370, 465
  origins of, 84-87, 380
  types of, 88
Anxiety reaction, 179, 181, 199, 285
Apathy, 124-125, 222, 392, 420, 457
Aphasia, 110, 264, 420
Aphonia, 110, 168, 184
Apomorphine, 374
Appearance, 105-107, 262, 419
Appetite. *See* Anorexia

517

Apprehension, 254, 257, 356, 357, 368, 420, 454
'Artane', 270, 370
Arteriosclerosis, cerebral, *264-265*, 271, 275, 357
Artistic activities, 463-464
Association of ideas, 110
  disorder of, 110, 219-220
Asthenic build, 226
Asthma, 289, 316, 318, 320, 322, 357
Ataractics. *See* Tranquillising drugs
Atropine, 257, 359, 360
Attention, 127-129, 420-421
Aura, 272, 277
Autism
  early infantile, 291
  in schizophrenia, 220-221
Automatism, 273, 278
Autonomic nervous system, 317
'Aventyl', 371
Aversion therapy, 340, 341, 374

B

Baby health centres, 9, 489, 491
Barbiturates, 270, 372
  acute organic reaction due to, 137, 257
  cessation of, 275
  dependence on, 169, 201
  treatment with, 11, 215, 280, 356, 365, 372
Bathing, 237, 411, 448, 453
Bath-rooms, 402, 441, 449
Bed
  avoidance of, 445
Bed-sores, 445
Bed-wetting. *See* Enuresis
'Bedlam', 6
Behaviour
  abnormalities of, 108-110, 261, 403, 419-420, 442
  determinants of, 33, 77-103
  therapy, 215, 311, *340-342*
Belladonna, 257
Bereavement, 71, 86, 102, *141-142*, 193, 503
Bewilderment, 225, 254, 258
Binet, Alfred, 299
Blindness, 98, 184, 185, 445
Blocking, 110-111, 220
Blood counts, 258
Blood loss, 258, 326
Body build, 226
Body image, *41*, 138, 221, 290
  development of, 41
Bone disease, 357
Borderline intelligence, 301, 306
Bottle-feeding, 38, 298
Bourne, Harold, 231, 305

Bowlby, John, 40, 288
Brain abscess, 137, 304
Brain syndrome
  acute. *See* Organic reactions, acute
  chronic. *See* Organic reactions, chronic
Brain tumour, 129, 137, 180, 266, 269, 271, 275, 279
  fear of, 180
Breast, 206
  development of, 56, 58
  feeding, 38, 39, 69, 146
Breath-holding, 292
'Brevidil', 360
'Brietal', 360
Bromides, 11, 137
  acute organic reaction due to, 257, 259
Bronchopneumonia, 256

C

Cade, John, 370
Cancer, 319
  fear of, 97, 189
Cannabis. *See* 'Marihuana'
Cardiac arrest, 267
Cardiac disease, 357
  as cause of psychiatric illness, 137, 257, 267
  due to alcoholism, 199, 256
  emotional aspects of, 318, 324, 235
'Cardiazol' 355
Case-work, 497-500
Castration anxiety, *47*, 87, 88, 149
Catatonia, *106*, 109, 223, 419
Causes of psychiatric illness, *134-152*, 176-178, 226-228, 239-240, 244-245, 256-258, 263-267, 292-294, 301-305, 315-320
  complexity of, 17, 23, 133-134
  in adolescence, 59, 88
  physical, 133-134, *136-138*, 226-258, 263-267, 302-304
  precipitating, *136-142*, 176-177, 245
  predisposing, 48, 86, 135, *142-152*, 176-178, 239-240, 244
  psychological, 133-134, *138-142*, 227-228, 292-294, 304-305
  related to ego defences, 89, 103, 207
  related to learning theory, 340
Censorship, 81-82, 125
Cerebral vascular accidents, 110, 136, 265, 459
Chaplains, 24
Character neurosis, 158, 161, 174-176, 187, 373
  course of, 212-213
  patterns of, 196-210

INDEX

Charcot, Jean, 10
Cheese, 372
Chickenpox, 304
Child-birth
  difficult, 304
  psychiatric illness following, 3, 135, *139,* 211, 228, 258
  reactions to, 68
Childhood
  emotional disturbances in, 178, 263, *283-298,* 304-305, 371
  importance of, 143-152, 185, 328
Child psychiatry, 283-298
Chloral hydrate, 270
Chlorpromazine. *See* Largactil
Cholecystectomy, 138
Christian church, 3, 4, 13-14
Christian scientists, 4
Chromosomes, 302
Chronological age, 306, 507
Circumstantiality, 111-112, 420
Cirrhosis, 199, 264, 320
Clang associations, 110, 242
Clergymen, 483
Clinical psychology, 505-511
Clonic phase, 272, 277, 360, 361
Clothing, 107, 199, 242, 262, 359, 402, 419, 444, 456
  importance of personal, 237, 383
Clubs
  ex-patients', 469, 479
  patients' 469
'Cogentin', 270, 370
Coma, 129
  insulin, 231
Combat, military, *141,* 146, 181, 211
Communication, 150-152, 236, 337, 350, 422, 449, 466
  in psychiatric hospital, 409-410
Community, 405, 436, 471, 501-504
  agencies, 9, 501, 503
  health centre, 501-502
  meetings, 337, 408-409
  organization, 503-504
  psychiatric hospital and, 481-493
  protection of, 31-32, 396
  return to, 478
  separation from, 380-382
  services, 307-308
Compensation neurosis, 181, *186-187,* 264
Compulsions, *109,* 116, 172, 189-193, 207, 212, 419
  in childhood, 191-192, 289, 290
Compulsive personality, *192,* 210, 212, 246
Concentration, 127, 129
  disturbance of, 129, 179, 264, 290, 292, 420

'Concordin', 372
Concussion, 257
Conditioned reflex, 340, 374
Conditioning
  operant, 341-342, 444
  positive, 340, 341
Conduct disturbances, 285, 287-289
Confabulation, *126-127,* 264, 420
Confidentiality, 21, 339
Conforming, 43-44, 404
Confusion, *128,* 201, 225, 254, 258, 260-261, 262, 268, 272-273, 326, 362, 363, 445, 447
  objective, 128, 421
  subjective, 128, 264, 421
Confusional psychosis. *See* Organic reactions, acute
Congenital heart disease, 303
Conolly, John, 9, 15
Conscience, *52-53,* 84, 164, 205, 288, 317
Consciousness, 81, *127-129,* 254, 261, 273, 363, 420
Constipation, 243, 247, 249, 318, 369, 444
Consultation
  by nurse, 487-490
  service, 9, 483
Continuous narcosis, 364
Control
  in hospital, 405, 406
  intellectual, 90-91, 389
  self-, 65-66, 87, 251
Convalescence, 393, *471-480*
Convalescent homes, 487-488
Conversation, *414-417,* 427, 441
  with relatives, 428-430, 432-435
Conversion, *97-98,* 110, 184
Conversion reactions, 10, 109, 124, *184-187,* 194, 212, 217, 278, 289
Coping devices, *91,* 92, 93
Coronary occlusion, 318, 357
Corticotrophin, 257, 259
Cortisone, 137, 257
Craftwork, 463
Cretins, 304, 305
Crichton Royal Hospital, 14
Crime, 183
  as an expression of psychiatric illness, 175, 199, 205, 222, 274, 447
  in antisocial character disorders, 203-206
Crisis, 142, 492, 500, 501
Critical life periods, 138, 139
Criticism, 395
Crowds, fear of, 188
Cruelty, 178, 263, 287, 310

519

Cry, epileptic, 272, 277
Cushing's syndrome, 267
Custodial care, 29, 397, 405, 407, 467, 471
Cyclothymic personality, 210, 212, 246

D

Dancing, 466
Dark Ages, 3, 4
Day-dreaming, 220, 228, 391
Day hospitals, 8, 439, 479
Deafness, 98, 184, 239, 305, 445
Death, 363, 372, 391, 446
Death wishes, 96-97
Defaecation, 42-44
Defences. See Ego defences
Deformity, 52, 107, 138, 221, 419
Déjà vu, 127, 274
Delinquency, 62, 165, 172, 174, 197, 212, 288, 296, 337
Delirium, 159, 253. See also Organic reactions, acute
Delirium tremens, 118, 254, 256, 258-259, 264
Delusions, 112-115, 158, 202, 212, 222, 223-224, 236, 238, 239, 243, 247, 284, 335, 396, 420, 423
  behaviour influenced by, 223, 238, 240, 241, 448, 451
  dynamics of, 101, 1322, 390
  erotic, 224, 238
  hypochondriacal, 114-115, 120-121, 194-195, 221, 224, 244
  management of patient with, 235-236, 240-241
  nihilistic, 114, 122, 244
  of grandeur, 115, 238, 243
  of guilt, 113-114, 122, 244
  of poisoning, 38, 118, 238
  persecutory, 101, 113, 224, 238, 261, 379, 396, 448
  religious, 224, 238
  systematised, 113, 223
  unsystematised, 113
Dementia, 159, 253. See also Organic reactions, chronic
  epileptic, 276
  presenile, 266
  senile. See Senile dementia
Denial, 93-94, 170, 245, 388-389, 430, 475
Departure, unauthorised, 455-456
Dependence, 144-145
  as a defence, 100, 433
  in psychiatric hospital, 383, 388, 390, 400-401, 431
  normal, 34, 36, 62, 66

Dependence—contd.
  problems concerning, 144-145, 147, 177, 186, 187, 213, 218, 246, 321, 353-354, 400, 501
  resulting from illness, 100, 137, 321, 378, 390, 473-474
Depersonalisation, 183, 222, 244, 336
Depression, 2, 70, 121-122, 193-194, 222, 225, 243, 266, 276, 314, 368, 389, 420, 449, 454
  as a result of illness, 314, 326, 386, 393
  bodily effects of, 315
  diagnosis of, 246-248
  dynamics of, 102, 131, 194, 209, 334-335
  'endogenous', 121-122, 244-245
  infantile, 40, 385
  management of, 248-251, 356, 363, 364, 371-373, 376, 447-451, 497-498
Depressive reactions, 2, 72, 192, 243-251, 354, 393, 447
  causation of, 244-245
  diagnosis of, 246-248
  neurotic, 193-194, 211, 247-248, 356, 370
  psychotic, 117, 122, 160, 193, 241-251, 356, 371
  'reactive', 193
  symptoms of, 106, 108, 114, 115, 117, 118, 129, 181, 183, 193, 199, 243-244, 247, 449
  treatment of, 215, 248-251, 356, 363, 364, 371-373, 376, 447-451
Destructiveness, 210, 236, 329, 388, 393, 403, 451, 453, 454
  in children, 178, 263, 310, 386
  management of, 270, 331, 367
Devil, 4
'Dexedrine', 280, 295, 371
  dependence on, 201-202
  psychosis due to, 202
Diabetes mellitus, 31, 129, 257, 318, 321
Diagnosis, 153-157, 335
  difficulty of, 18, 166-167, 178, 210, 506
  social, 496
'Diamox', 280
Diarrhoea, 314, 318
Digby, Thomas, 15
Digitalis, 137, 257
Dignity, maintenance of, 21, 442, 446
'Dilantin', 279, 280
Dirt, fear of, 188, 190
Discipline, 310
  ward, 345

INDEX

Disillusionment, 63
Dislocations, 363
Disorientation, 128, 129, 254, 261, 262, 268, 273, 362, 421
Displacement, *97*, 100, 119-120, 187, 189
Dissociation, *98*, 118, 129, 181-183, 184, 211, 274
Dissociative reactions, 181-183, 211
Distractibility, 127, 290
Diversion, 358, 458
Domiciliary service, 8, 484-487
Dominant genes, 302
Double bind, 152
Double-blind trial, 354
Double personality, 182-183
Down's Syndrome, 106, *303*, 307
Dreams, *79*, 96, 119, 155, 180, 332, 351
Drowning, 267
Drug dependence, 72, 173, *196-203*, 215, 218, 225, 370
   dynamics of, 38, 197-198
   treatment of, 201, 337, 364
Drug registers, 375
Drug trials, 353-355
Dryness of mouth, 369
Dull-normal intelligence, 301, 306
Duodenal ulcer, 318, 321

E

Eccentrics, 222, 228
Echolalia, 109, 223
Echopraxia, 109, 223
Ecstasy, 119, 122, 242
Eczema, 289, 319
Educational activities, 463
   special, 295, 299, 301, 311
Ego, *82-84*, 89, 91, 164-165, 167
   development of, 82-83, 149, 204, 483
   disturbances of function of, 113, 117, 149-150, 204, *221*, 228, 291
Ego defences, *90-103*, 132, 143, 152, 154, 207, 262, 378, 388-396, 508
Elation, 122, 225, 242, 389, 420
Electro-convulsive therapy. *See* Electrotherapy
Electroencephalography, 79, 227, 258, *278-279*, 289
Electrotherapy, 12, *355-363*, 510
   complications of, 362-363
   contraindications, 357-358
   indications for, 215, 230-231, 240, 248, 251, 276, *356-357*, 371

Electrotherapy—*contd.*
   technique of, 358-362
   unilateral, 361-362
Emotionally unstable personality, 210
Emotions, 119, 121, 329, 333, 336, 342-344, 379, 380, 387, 420, 451, 508
   bodily effects of, 313-320, 322
   development of, 35-36
Encephalitis, 129, 256, 263, 287, 304
Encopresis, 286
Endocrine glands, 56, 226-227, 267, 314, 318
'Endogenous', 121-122, 244-245
Enuresis, 178, *286*, 295, 341, 386
Environment
   adaptation to, 163, 167
   as therapeutic factor, 234, 250, 259-260, 268, 294-298, *398-399*, 407-411, 438, 440-442, 452, 459, 472
   influence of, 53, 60, 304-305, 402-403, 452, 471
   isolation from, 223, 304
   stress in, 30
Envy, 47, 148-149
Epilepsy, *270-282*, 310, 451
   causes of, 201, 263, 264, 266, 271, 274-275
   diagnosis of, 184, 277-278
   focal, 271, 273-274
   generalised, 271, 272-273
   idiopathic, 275
   psychiatric complications of, 108, 126, *275-277*, 451
   symptomatic, 274-275
   temporal lobe, 118, 127, 271, *273-274*, 275-276, 280
   treatment of, 30, *279-281*, 295, 310, 310, 356-357
   types of, 271-274
'Epileptic personality', 276
Epiloia, 302
'Epontol', 360
Euphoria, 94, *122*, 242, 389
Evil spirits, 1
Excitement, catatonic, 223, 231
Exercise, 444, 452, 464-466
Exhibitionism, 148, 208
Exteriorisation, 50

F

Facial expression, 106, 419
Facial hair, 116-117
Faeces, 42-44
Faith-healing, 4, 353

Family, 67-72, 74-75, 175, 428-437, 471-472, 476
  attitudes of, 43-48, 55, 61-62, 429-437, 476, 495-498
  child's relationship with, 42-49
  of disturbed child, 283, 285, 288, 291, *292-294*
  of mentally retarded, 306, 307-308
  of schizophrenic, 151-152, 227-228, 291, 430-431
  pride, 431
  separation from, 380-381, 385-387, 432
  treatment for, 283, 294-295, 298, 306, 472, 497-498
Fantasy, 50-52, 220-221, 388, 391-392
Father, *46-49*, 55, 58, 68-69, 430
  substitute, 329, 342, 347
Fatigue, 108, 193, 247, 445
Feeding. *See also* Anorexia; Meals
  disturbances of, 38, 285-286, 444
  significance of, 35-39, 321
Fetishism, 208-209
Fever, 256, 275, 280, 369
  artificial, 11
  psychogenic, 290
Fire, 445, 455
First-aid, 455
Fitness, physical, 464-466
Fixation, 147
Flight of ideas, 110, 242
Floors, 441
Folie du doute, 191
Follow up, 478-479
Food, 382-383, 394, 402, 403, 404
Footdrop, 269
Foster-home, 294, 296
Fractures, 357, 363, 446
Frankness, pathological, 221
Freedom, 404-407, 408-445
Freud, Sigmund, *10*, 19, 34, 47, 78-80, 147-148, 327-328, 329
Frigidity, 48
Frontal lobe, 266, 376
Frustration, 42, 145
Fugue, 182
  epileptic, 274
Functional psychotic reactions, 158, 160-161, *219-252*
Furnishings, 402-403, 440
Furor, epileptic, 274

G

Gait, 109, 201, 223, 266, 280, 419
Gastritis, 199, 259
General hospital, 322-326, 388, 410
  acute organic reactions, 253, 260-261, 268

General hospital—*contd.*
  psychiatric units in, 9, 406
  psychosomatic patients in, 320-322
  regime of, 268, 326, 382-383, 408-409
General paralysis of the insane, 11, 159, 263
General practitioners, 483, 484
Genes, 302
Geriatric centres, 439
German measles, 304
Gladesville Hospital, 15
Globus hystericus, 184
Grand mal, *272-273*, 274, 275, 279, 355, 361
Grief, 141
Group psychotherapy, *336-340*, 409-410, 472, 503
Groups
  activities in, 231, 234, 241, 409-410, 426-427, 442, *466-468*, 503
  closed, 337
  for mental retardates, 308-309
  in adolescence, 63, 503
  mixed sex, 234, 405-406, 442, 466-468
  observation of, 426-427, 466-468
  open, 338
Guilt, 59, 89, 331, 333, 335, 343, 390, 420, 508
  delusions of, 113-114
  development of, 52, 83-84
  lack of, 204
  of relatives, 306, 431
  resulting from illness, 380, 393
  significance in illness, 192, 293

H

Habit disturbances, 285
  primary, 285
  secondary, 286-287
Habits, 382
  deterioration in, 223, 236, 262-263, 376, 443-444
  gratification, 286-287, 291
  neurotic symptoms as, 340
  tension, 287
Habit training, 443-444
Hair-pulling, 287
Halfway house, 478
Hallucinations, 3, *117-119*, 129, 222, 223-224, 238, 239, 244, 254-255, 257, 260, 272, 274, 336, 420, 423
  auditory, 101, *117*, 202, 224, 238, 244, 255, 274, 447
  behaviour influenced by, 223, 260, 447-448, 451
  dynamics of, 100

INDEX

Hallucinations—*contd.*
  gustatory, 118
  management of, 260
  olfactory, 118, 274
  tactile, 118
  visual, *118*, 202, 254-255, 274, 447-448
Handwashing, compulsive, 168, 188, 190
Hashish. *See* Marihuana
Hatred. *See* Aggression
Headache, 180, 264, 265, 289, 314, 362, 372
Head-banging, 287
Head injury, 183, 275
  organic reactions due to, 126, 129, 136, 257, *264*, 304
  psychological significance of, 136, 264
Hebephrenia. *See* Schizophrenic reactions, hebephrenic
Hellebore, 3
Hemp. *See* Marihuana
Heredity, 3, 35, 78, 134, *142-143*, 176, 204, 226, 244, 265, 266, 275, 291, 302-303, 316
Heroin, 200
Hippocrates, 2, 3
Hobbies, 66-67, 443, 463
Home. *See also* Family
  consultation in, 8
  mentally retarded child in, 307-308, 311
  psychiatric hospital as, 440
Home-making duties, 440-442
Homer, 2
Homesickness, 380
Home visits, 485-486, 502
Homosexuality, 48, *207-208*, 341, 406
  in adolescence, 58
  repressed, 88, 100-101, 141, 207, 240
Hospital staff, activities with, 28, 398, 464, 467
Hospitalisation, 331, 378-396
  avoidance of, 8, 484
  in adult life, 380-385
  in old age, 76, 268, 326
  of children, 51, 137, 294, 296-298, 323, *385-387*, 484
  problems of, 137, 322-326, 382-385, 474
  psychiatric. *See* Psychiatric hospital
  reactions to, 100, 213, 214, *378-396*, 430-432
  transition from, 386, 473-478
Hostels, 8, 296, 478, 488
  for mentally retarded, 299

Hostility. *See* Aggression
Humility, 20-21
Huntington's chorea, 266, 302
Hygiene, 107, 199, 419, 444
Hyperglycaemia, 257
Hypermnesia, 126
Hypertension, 318, 372
Hyperventilation syndrome, 318
Hypnoanalysis, 335
Hypnosis, 10, 334-335, 391
Hypnotic drugs, 252, 364, *365-366*, 465
Hypochondriacal
  delusions, *114-115*, 120-121, 221
  reaction, 120, *194-195*
Hypochondriasis, 120-121, 289, 420
Hypoglycaemia, 257, 275, 280, 363-364
Hypomania, 243, 251
Hypothalamus, 318
Hysterectomy, 3, 138
Hysteria, 3, 10. *See also* Conversion reactions; Dissociative reactions
Hysterical personality, *187*, 210, 212, 217, 325

I

Id, *82*, 84, 88, 164, 221
Ideas of reference, *113*, 223, 420, 448
Identification, 49, 101, 475
  of patient with nurse, 237
Illegitimacy, 307
Illusions, 119, 254-255
Imagination, 117
Impotence, 247, 319
Impulsiveness, 205, 221, 290, 397, 405
Incoherence, 111, 220
Incontinence, 223, 262-263, 272, 278, 310
  dynamics of, 44, 390, 443-444
Independence, 43, 62, 66, 400, 408, 441, 458, 473-474
Indifférence, la belle, 124, 184
Indigestion, 314
Individuality, 403-404, 408, 441
  development of, 34-36, 40-41, 62
Industrial officers, 24
Industrial programmes, 464
Infancy, 34-41
  acute organic reactions in, 253, 256
Infantile depression. *See* Depression
Infantile sexuality, 147-148, 206-207
Infection, 3, 129, 137, *256*, 258, *263*
Inferiority, 210, 228, 293, 395
Information, recording of, 417-422
Injuries to patients, 278, 362, 441, 445, 446, 455
In-laws, 68

523

Insanity, fear of, 179, 189
Insight, *130-131*, 328, 332, 336, 421
Insomnia, 179, 180, 193, 202, 242-243, 244, 247, 256, 365-366
  in children, 38, 286
  management of, 249, 252, 270, 364, *365-366*, 465
Instincts, 87, 123, 163, 165, 167, 204
Insulin coma therapy, 12, 231
Intellectual deterioration, 130, 262, 389, 421, 442, 507
Intellectually handicapped person, 300
Intelligence, 130, 163, 421
  decline of, 73-74
  development of, 53-56, 60, 304-305
  disorder of, 128, 130, 262, 299-312, 421
  of nurse, 21
  tests, 299, 306, 507
Intelligence quotient, 306, 507
Interpersonal relationships, 22
  defective, 151, 197, 203-204, 220, 222, 227, 234-235, 291, 471
  importance of 17, *150-152*
  reconstruction of, 151, 234-237, 497, 504
Interpretation, 19, 332, 343, 351
Interview skills, 499
Intoxication, 256-257, 263-264
Intravenous therapy, 259, 359, 361
Introjection, 101-102, 194
Involutional melancholia, 246, 356
Irritability, 242, 252, 276, 290, 314
Isolation, 99

J

Jacksonian epilepsy, 271, 273
Jaundice, 369
Jealousy, 45, 47, 210
Jones, Maxwell, 409

K

'Kemadrin', 270
Kinsey, Alfred, 58, 162
Kleptomania, 205-206
Korsakow's psychosis, 127, *264*, 269
Kraepelin, Emil, 10

L

Lability, *125*, 263, 420
Lady Macbeth, 192
Laing, R. D., 11, 151-152
'Largactil', 12, 200, 232, 251, 267, *367-370*
Latent content, 79
Lead, 257
Learning theory, 340

Lesbianism, 208
Leucotomy, 259. *See also* Surgery, cerebral
'Librium', 215, 370
Light sensitivity, 369
Listening, 350, 499
Lithium, 248, 354, 365, 370
Liver
  damage due to drugs, 369, 372
  failure, 137, 199, 257
Love, 67, 86, 141-142, 146, 148, 328-329, 331, 386
  capacity for, 37, 163
  loss of, 86, 141-142, 194
  of mother for child, 36
Love-making, 38, 206
'Lunacy', 5
Lupus erythematosus, disseminated, 267
Lying, 263, 287
Lysergic acid diethylamide, 156, *203*, 336

M

Malingering, 186
Manhandling, 453
Mania, acute, 243
Manic-depressive reactions, 3, 10, 149-150, 160, *241-252*. *See also* Depressive reaction, psychotic
Manic reactions, 108, 115, 122, 126, *242-243*, 389
  treatment of, *251-252*, 356, 367, 370
Manifest content, 79
Manipulation, 343-344, 350-351, 390-391
Mannerisms, 106, 222, 223, 419
Marihuana, 202-203
'Marplan', 372
Marriage, *67-68*, 72, 139-140, 208
'Marsilid', 372
Masculine protest, 47, 148-149
Masochism, 209, 325
Masturbation, 5, 58-59, 168, *286-287*, 406
Maternal rejection, 292-294
Meals, 280, 444
Measles, 256
Medicine men, 1
'Melleril', 232, 367, 369
Memory, 41, 73, *125-127*
  disturbance of, 126-127, 128, 201, 262, 263-264, 362-363, 389, 420, 442
Meningitis, 129, 256, 304
Menopause, 70, 138, 139

INDEX

Menstruation, 56, 58, 275, 314
  disorders of, 315, 317, 319
Mental age, 306, 507
Mental deficiency. *See* Mental retardation
Mental health, 163-165, 284, 400
Mental retardation, 158, 160, 275, 290, 291, *299-312*, 507
  behavioural patterns in, 112, 287, 300-311, 451
  causation of, 301-305
  definition of, 300-301
  diagnosis of, 305-307, 507
  frequency of, 301
  management of, 303, 307-312, 458, 464, 478, 509
  relatives' problems, 30-31, 306, 307-308
  secondary, 304-305
'Mesantoin', 279
Mescaline, 156
'Methedrine', 201, 336, 371
Middle age, 70-72, 138
Migraine, 289-290, 318, 322
Migrants, 479
'Milontin', 280
Mind, 313
Mind-body relationships, 134, 313-315, 320, 326
Miscarriage, threatened, 304
Modesty, 401
Modified insulin therapy, 215, 248, *363-364*
Money, 381-442
Mongolism. *See* Down's syndrome
Monoamine-oxidase inhibitors, 372
Mood, 106, *121-125*, 199, 221-222, 241-242, 243, 420
  appropriate, 121, 238, 239
  inappropriate, *124*, 221, 222, 224, 229, 376
'Moral treatment', 7
Mother, *36-41*, 44, 45, 48, 49, 58, 139, 151-152, 163, 430
  age of, 303
  anger towards, 39, 146, 347
  emotional problems of, 39-40, 68-69, 144, 204, *292-294*
  of schizophrenic, 151-152, 227-228
  substitute, 298, 329, 342
Mother-child relationship
  importance of, 36-41, 82-83, 85, 149, 483-484
  problems in, 39-40, 68-69, 139, 144, 151-152, 172, 197, 204, 227-228, 285, *291-294*, 305, 347, 385, 491-492
Mothering, 36, 38, 69, 85, 149, 231
  deprivation of, 288, 292-293, 305

Mourning, 141
Mouth gag, 279, 359-360, 361
Multiple personality, 182-183
Multiple sclerosis, 136
Mumps, 304
Muscular pain, 319
Mutism, 110, 223, 244, 247
Myocardial infarction. *See* Coronary occlusion
Myoclonic jerks, 271, 273
'Mysoline', 279
Mystification, 151
Myxoedema, 267

N

Nail-biting, 178, 287, 386
Narcissism, 107
Narcoanalysis, 335
'Nardil', 372
Needs
  of mentally retarded children, 307
  of patients, 18-19, 235-237, 444-446, 459
Negativism, 108, 223, 290, 395
Neologisms, 111, 220, 420
'Nervous breakdown', 131
'Nervous disorders', 285
Neuritis, peripheral, 199, 264, 269
Neurodermatitis, 319
Neurotic reactions, 2, 10, 131, 158, 161-162, *168-218*, 264, 324, 447
  causes of, 176-178
  clinical pictures, 120, 126, 178-210
  course of, 211-213, 354
  general characteristics of, 167-170
  in childhood, 289
  meaning of, 168
  nursing problems in, 187, 195, 216-218
  treatment of, *213-216*, 331, 334-335, 356, 364, 370, 376
Nicole, Sister, 13
Nightingale, Florence, 14, 427, 481
Nightmares, 51, 96, 181, 286, 386
Night-nursing, 262, 366, 444, 448
Night terrors, 286
Nocturnal emissions, 56
'Normal person', 65-66, 155, *162-165*
Notes, nurses', 422-423, 427
Nurse, baby health centre, 483, 489
Nurse, general, 21-24
  in psychiatric unit, 22, 410
  role in psychosomatic reactions, 320-322
  training of, 14
Nurse-patient relationship
  closeness in, 16, 17, 236-237, 336, 386-387, 400, 415

525

PSYCHIATRIC NURSING

Nurse-patient relationship—*contd.*
 significance of, 12-16, 233, 324, *342-351,* 377, 398-399, 412, 414-417, 421-422, 449
 understanding of, 216, 347-349, 414
 varieties of, 16, 235-238, 240-241, 249-251, 297-298, 320-322, 342-344, 346-351, 372-373, 390-391, 404, 457
Nurse, psychiatric
 as health teacher, 16-17, 435, 437, 486
 as research worker, 422
 attitudes of, *20-21,* 216-218, 235-237, 250, 251-252, 297-298, 344-351, 353, 366, 400, 401, 410, 414, 433, 454
 consultative role of, 487-490
 domiciliary role of, 485-487
 education of, 14-15, 21-22, 411-412
 general aspects of role of, 12-13, *16-24,* 79-80, 398-399, 400, 404, 410, 412
 health of, 21, 435
 participation by, 426-427, 448, 467-468
 preventive role of, 490-492
 relationship to occupational therapist, 27-28, 470
 relationship to psychiatric social worker, 27, 494, 495-496, 501-502
 relationship to psychiatrist, *25-26,* 216, 217, 344-346, 349, 413, 425, 436
 relationship to psychologist, 26, 510-511
 reports of, 277-278, 279, 358, 366, 374, 418, *422-423,* 446, 447, 454, 456
 role in acute organic reactions, 259-260
 role in child psychiatry, 297-298
 role in chronic organic reactions, 268-269, 270, 439-447
 role in community, 481-493
 role in occupational and recreational therapies, 457, 460, 462, 464-470
 role in physical treatments, 353, 354, 355, 358-362, 364, 366, 369, 372-373, 374-375, 377
 role in psychotherapy, 336, 338, *342-346,* 346-351
 role in rehabilitation, 475-480
 role in depressed patients, 249-251, 447-451
 role with epileptic patients, 276, 277-278, 280-281

Nurse, psychiatric—*contd.*
 role with long-stay patients, 439-447, 467
 role with manic patients, 251-252
 role with mental retardates, 308-312
 role with neurotic patients, 216-218
 role with paranoid patients, 240-241
 role with relatives, 428-437, 446, 452-453
 role with schizophrenic patients, 235-238
 role in therapeutic community, 407-411
 status of, 14-15, 410
 uniform of, 410-411
Nurse, public health, 483
'Nurse-therapists', 346
Nursing, general
 compared with psychiatric nursing, 21-24
 history of, 14
 in psychosomatic reactions, 320-322
 psychiatric experience during, 21
Nursing plans, 424-425, 427
Nursing, psychiatric. *See also* Nurse, psychiatric
 compared with general nursing, 21-24
 history of, 13-15
Nutrition, 199, 256, 260

O

Obesity, 318
Obscenity, 236, 242, 406, 451
Observation, 3, 155, 366, *413-417,* 426-427, 448-449, 467-468, 485
 objective, 414-415
 of relatives, 429-430, 434
 subjective, 415
Obsessions, 109, *115-116,* 172, 189-193, 212, 225, 420
 in childhood, 191-192, 289, 290
Obsessive-compulsive reaction, 51, 181, 188, *189-193,* 211, 212
Occupation, 130, 234, 308, 358, 365, 419, 449, 452, 470, 474, 485
 defensive use of, 389, 460
 used for hospital's benefit, 234, 308, 462, 470
Occupational therapist, 24, 27-28
Occupational therapy, 27-28, 248, 252, 281, 373, 405, 443, *457-470,* 478
Oedipus complex, *47-49,* 57-58, 68, 143, 148

INDEX

Old age, 2, *72-76*, 123, 126, *139*, *261*, 265-266, 268, 363, 365, 466
 physical illness in, 73, 325-326, 445
Open door policy, 407
Opiates, 200-201
Oral hygiene, 260, 280, 444
Oral phase, *37*, 42, 147
 later significance of, 37-38, 101, 353-354
 regression to, 100
Organic reactions, 10, 133, 157-158, 159-160, 211, *253-282*, 389
 acute, 118, 119, 159, *253-261*
 causes of, 256-258, 263-267, 326
 characteristic symptoms of, 112, 115, 117, 118, 119, 122, 126, 127, 129, 181, 211, 220, 247, *253-256*, *261-263*, 271, 389, 443, 447, 507
 chronic, 159-160, 253, *261-270*
 in childhood, 287, 290
 management of, 258-260, 267-270, 331, 357, 368, 458
 nursing care in, 259-260, 268-269, 270, 439-447
Orgasm, 317
Orientation, 129, 262, 440
Outpatient treatment, 8, 215, 439, *479*, 482, 485, 500-501
Overactivity, 108, 242-243, 255, 367, 419, 461
Over-conforming, 394
Overdependency, 391
Overeating, 285, 289
Overprotection, 39-40, 227, 293
Overvalued ideas, 115, 116
Overwork, 140, 390
Oxycephaly, 302
Oxygen, 279, 359, 361

P

Paedophilia, 209, 261
Pain, 138, 209, 258, 335, 363
 pelvic, 317, 319
 psychogenic, 184
Panic, 123, 180, 254, 335
'Paradione', 279
Paraldehyde, 270
Paralysis, 98, 184, 263, 264, 361
 agitans. *See* Parkinson's disease
Paranoia, 238
Paranoid personality 210, 212, *239*
Paranoid reactions, 149, 161, *238-241*, 266, 276
Paraphrenia, 238
Paraplegia, 138
Parkinson's disease, *266-267*, 270, 369-370

'Parnate', 372
Passive-aggressive personality, 210
Passivity feelings, 113, 224
Patient government, 337, 409
'Peeping Tom', 208
Pellagra, 267
Penicillin, 11, 257, 269
Penis, 47, 208
Pensions, 187
Pentothal sodium, 336, 360
Perception, 117
Perfectionism, 289, 293
Permissiveness, 13, 459
Perseveration, 112, 420
Personality
 complexity of, 17, 33, 154-155, 156
 definition of, 34
 deterioration following psychosurgery, 376
 development of, 34, 65, 77-78
 of nurse, *18*, 154-155, 216-218, 298, 344-351, 364, 415, 468
 relationship to psychiatric illness, 17, 136, 154-155, 261, 404
 tests, 508-509
Persuasion, 333-334
'Pertofran', 371
'Pethidine', 372
Petit mal, 271, *273*, 275, 279-280
Phallic stage, 46-49, 147
Phenobarbitone, 279, 365
Phenylketonuria, 303, 305
Phobias, 81, 114-115, *119-120*, 175, 188-189, 207-208, 212, 213, 225, 420
 dynamics of, 81, *97*, 119-120
 in childhood, 120, 188, 285, 290
 school, 284
Phobic reactions, 120, 172, 179, 181, *187-189*, 211, 498
Physical illness, 442
 as precipitant of psychiatric illness, 134-135, 142, 254-255, 264, 301, 383, 386, 391
 denial of, 386-387
 detection of, 443
 in old age, 323, 443
 reactions to, 314, 322-326, *378-396*
 secondary gains from, 185-186, 209, 324-325
Piaget, Jean, 34, 40-41
Pick's disease, 160
Pinel, Philippe, 7, 8
Placebo effect, 327, 353, 354
Plans, nursing, 424-425, 427
Play, 51-52, 191-192, 289
Play therapy, 52, 296
Pleasure principle, *35*, 39, 43, 44, 82, 146

527

Pneumonia, 137, 256, 445
Policemen, 483
Porphyria, 267
Positive conditioning, 340-341
Possessions, 237, 442
Posture, 106, 223, 266, 419
 for electrotherapy, 360
'Pot'. *See* Marihuana
Preconscious, 81
Pregnancy, 68, 139, 211, 304, 357
Pressure of talk, 110, 242
Prevention, 260-261, 284, 465, 484, *490-492*
 primary, 491
 secondary, 491
 tertiary, 490
Privacy, 401, 408
'Privilege patients', 405
Probation officers, 483
Professionalism, 21, 468
Projection, 50, *100-101*, 113, 117, 144, 170, 239-240, 390, 395-396, 431-432
Projective tests, 508
'Prominal', 279
Prostitution, 172, 222
Protection
 of community, 31, 300, 397
 of patient, 30-31, 260, 397
 long-term, 31-32, 300, 439-447
Protriptyline. *See* 'Concordin'
Proverb test, 220
Pruritus, 319
Psychiatric hospital
 admission to, 8, 354, 378-379, 433-434, 438-439, 449
 as therapeutic community, 397-412, 457
 atmosphere of, 7, 8, 234-235, 398
 children's unit in, 296-298
 community services of, 481-493
 development of, 6-9
 emergencies in, 454-456
 for mental retardates, 299, 308-311
 long-stay patients in, 31-32, 234-235, 439-447, 458, 467, 478
 objectives of care in, 29-32, 397-398
 relationship to other units, 8-9, 478-479
 social structure of, 234-235, 407-411, 412
 undesirable effects of, 31, 229, 234-235, 382-383, 399-407
Psychiatric illness
 amount of, 481
 causes of. *See* Causes
 classification of, 153-162
 community attitudes towards, 5, 6, 378, 387, 388, 477-478

Psychiatric illness—*contd.*
 denial of, 388-389
 early detection of, 482-483, 491
 effects on relatives of, 430-432
 forms of, 157-162
 patient's attitude towards, *130-131*, 247, 265, 384, 387, 389, 473
Psychiatric social worker, 24, 27, 283, 295, 351, 424, 435, 436, 472, 479, *494-504*
Psychiatrist, 24, 330, 332-333, 399, 410, 422, 458
 nurse's relationship to, *25-26*, 217, 343-346, 349, 413, 423, 436
Psychoanalysis, 10, 215, 322, *327-330*, 505
Psychoanalyst, 328-505
Psychogenic reactions, 158-159, 160-162
Psychological tests, 323, 506-509
 intelligence, 306, 507
 personality, 508-509
 preparation for, 26, 511
Psychologist, 351, 505
 clinical, 24, 26, *505-511*
Psychomotor epilepsy, 274
Psychopathic personality, 204-205
Psychosomatic reactions, 159, 162, 194, *313-326*
 causes of, 315-320
 in childhood, 289-290
 management of, 320-322, 331, 337
Psychosurgery. *See* Surgery, cerebral
Psychotherapy, 281, 295, *327-351*, 354, 373, 479, 509
 group, 281, *336-340*
 hospitalisation for, 30, 331
 in childhood, 295-296
 in neurotic reactions, 215, 217, 331
 in psychosomatic reactions, 321-322, 331
 in schizophrenic reactions, 233, 331
 nurse's problems with, 217, 342-346
 on the ward, 342-351
 psychoanalytic, 330
 role of nurse in, 336, 338, 342-351
 special varieties of, 334-342
 suitability for, 215-216, 331, 507
 supportive, 214, 333
Psychotic, 158, 366-367, 390
Puberty, 55-56
Puerperium. *See* Child-birth
Punishment
 failure to respond to, 205, 206
 illness seen as, 381, 385
 of children, 46, 52, 83, 294, 297
 of patients, 6-7, 8, 357
Pussin, Jean-Baptiste, 7

INDEX

Pyknic build, 230
Pyromania, 205

Q

Queen Elizabeth I, 5
Questionnaires, 508

R

Radiotherapy, 269
Rationalisation, 99, 199, 390
Reaction formation, *95-97,* 120, 144, 189, 193, 394
Reality
  attitude towards, 158, 164, 169-170
  nurse as representative of, 235-237, 441
  withdrawal from, 220-221, 222, 229, 235-237, 460
Reality principle, 44, 83
Recessive genes, 302-303
Reciprocal inhibition, 340
Recreation, 234, 248 252 281, 338, 365, 373, 404, 443, 452, *457-470,* 478, 485
Recreational therapist, 24, 28, 465
Regression, 46, *99-100,* 294, 298, 321, 443
  in hospital, 386, 390-391
Rehabilitation, 308, 376, 392, 424, 430, 432, 436, *471-480,* 491, 499
  centres, 8
Rejection, 380, 386, 431, 476
  maternal, 40, 292-293
Relatives
  attitude to patient's illness, 227, 228, 430-432, 468
  nurse's relationship to, 428-437, 446
  relief for, 30-31, 397
Relaxant drugs, 355-356, 357, 360, 363
Reliability, 20
REM Sleep, 79
Renal disease, 137, 258
Repression, 49, *94-95,* 98, 125, 207, 328, 333, 335, 336, 475
Research, 133, 134, 481, 502-503, 510-511
Responsibility, 20, 448, 451
  taken by patients, 409, 469
Restlessness, 108, 179, 200, 201, 202, 223, 244, 255, 257
  in childhood, 285, 290, 292
  management of, 251-252, 259, 270, 364, 368
Restraint, 7, 9, 13, 362, 453-454

Retardation, *108,* 110, 122, 243, 247, 419
Retirement, 74
Rh negative, 304
Rheumatoid arthritis, 319
Rituals, 190-193, 291
Rorschach test, 508
Rumination, 190
Rush, Benjamin, 7

S

Sadism, 209
St John of God, 13-14
St Mary of Bethlehem, 6
St Thomas's Hospital, 14
Scapegoating, 396
Schizoid personality, 121, 203, 210, 212, 226, *228-229*
Schizophrenic reactions, 10, 161, 202, 212, *219-238,* 243, 276, 335, 447
  acute undifferentiated, 225
  catatonic type, *223,* 228, 229, 230, 231, 356
  causation of, 151-152, 203, *226-228,* 258, 264, 291
  chronic undifferentiated, 225
  clinical picture of, 106, 108-109, 110-111, 114, 115, 117, 118, 122, 124, 125, 127, 128, 181, 183, 194-195, *219-226,* 242, 246, 447, 507
  deteriorated, 223, 229, 234, 235
  dynamics of, 100, 149, 155, 221, 227-228, 471-472
  hebephrenic type, *222-223,* 224, 229, 231
  in childhood, 225-226, 228, *290-291*
  nature of, 156-157, 219
  onset and course, 228-230
  paranoid type, *223-224,* 228, 230, 238-239, 356
  residual type, 225
  schizo-affective type, *224-225,* 228, 229, 230, 231
  simple, 222, 231
  treatment of, *230-238,* 331, 356, 358, 367-368, 376, 377, 472
  types of, 161, 222-226
School, 53-55, 283-284, 295
  consultation within, 9
  difficulties at, 178, 291, 301
  phobia, 284
  special, 296, 301, 307, 311
School teachers, 54-55
'Scoline', 360
Seclusion, 7, 259, 453
Seclusiveness, 392, 401

Secondary gain, *185-186*, 187, 218, 294
Sedatives, 214, 258, 259, 295, 322, 358, *365*
Seizures
 charting of, 281
 diagnosis of, 277-278
 during electrotherapy, 355, 360-361
 epileptic. *See* Epilepsy
 management of, 279
 precipitants of, 275
 psychogenic, 184, 278
Self-esteem, 134, 235, 464
Self-mutilation, 244, 250, 287
Senile dementia, 30, 107, 125, 126, 137, *265-266*, 357, 368
Sensation, disturbance of, 184
Sensitivity, 57, 239
Separation, 71, 139
 due to hospitalisation, 268, 380-382, 386-387, 393
 of child from mother, 40, 144, 145, 204, 283, *288*, 381, 386-387
Septicaemia, 137
'Serenace', 368, 370
Sex, 143, *147-149*, 162, 177-178, 206, 317, 329
 confusion re, 148, 227-228
 curiosity about, 46-47, 87
 education, 59
 in adolescence, 56-60, 88, 92, 285
 lessening of inhibitions re, 221, 242, 261-262, 263, 290, 376, 406, 443
 play in childhood, 287
 problems concerning, 3, 70, 81, 138, 139, *147-149*, 177-178, 189, 206-209, 227-228, 287, 317, 319, 340, 508-509
 reduction of interest in, 70, 179, 224
 relationship, 67, 206
 secondary characteristics, 56
Sexual deviation, 31, 150, 169, *206-209*, 225
Sexual revolution, 58-59
Sharing, 45
Shock treatment. *See* Electrotherapy
Shyness, 178, 210, 228, 284, 285, 466
Sibling rivalry, *44-46*, 54, 68-69, 100, 146, 381
 seen in psychiatric patients, 46, 54
Signs, 104-105
 of psychiatric illness, 104-132
Skin, disorders of, 280, 319, 369, 446
Sleep disturbance. *See* Insomnia
Slips and errors, 80
Smoking, 38, 320

Social activities, 338, 452, 457-470, 474
Social development, 53, 57, 62-63, 65
Social history, 495
Social groupwork, 503-504
Social therapy, 234-235, 373, 443, 457-470
Social withdrawal, 220, 244, 392, 419, 457, 466-467
Social work, 494-495
 psychiatric, 27, *494-504*
Society, demands of, 59, 77-78, 92, 102-103, 144, 163, 164, 177-178, 378, 400
Sodium chloride, 259
Speech, abnormalities of, *110-121*, 219-220, 242, 244, 247, 254, 263, 280, 291, 305, 420
'Spoilt child', 39-40, 293
Sport, 54, 66-67, 465
Stanford-Binet intelligence scale, 507
Status epilepticus, 274, 279
Stealing, 172, 199, 205-206, 209, 287
'Stelazine', 232, 267, 367, 370
Stereotypy, 108, 223, 419
Stomach, 314, 315
Strokes. *See* Cerebral vascular accidents
Stupor, 108, *129*, 243, 255
 catatonic, 223, 231
Subarachnoid haemorrhage, 372
Sublimation, 60, *91-93*, 144, 146, 167, 206, 234
Subnormality, 300
Suggestion, 296, 333, 334
Suicide, 121, 193-194, 243, 245, 335, 420, *447-451*
 attempted, 150, 193, 210, 449, 500
 dynamics of, 102, 150, 447
 prevention of, 31, 249, 411, 448-449
 threats of, 391, 449-450
Sullivan, Harry Stack, 11, 150-151
Superego, *83-84*, 89, 164, 204, 288
Superiority, 394-395
Supernatural, 1, 5
Superstition, 51, 193, 271, 282
Support, 142, 214, 333, 374, 459, 461, 479, 500-501, 504
 from nurse, 336, 343, 350, 441, 466, 467, 468, 475, 486
Suppression, 90, 333, 389
Surgery
 cerebral, 136, 248, 269, 280, *375-377*
 effects of, 122-123, 258, 323, *325-326*, 389, 393
'Surmontil', 371

INDEX

Symptom neurosis, 158, 161, 173, *179-195*, 207, 209, 336
  course of, 211-212
Symptoms, 104-105, 334-335, 339-340
  meaning of, 131-132, 150
  of psychiatric illness, 104-132
Syphilis, 137, 263, 271, 275
  congenital, 304
  fear of, 189
  treatment of, 11, 269

T

Tattooing, 107, 115
Team approach, *23-29*, 32, 216, 418, 425, 473, 504, 511
Teething, 39
Temper tantrums, 147, 178, 285, 290, 292, 310, 386
Temporal lobe, 118, 127, 271, *273-274*, 275-276, 280
Thematic apperception test, 508
Therapeutic community, 235, 337-338, *397-412*, 473
Thinking
  abstract, 217
  autistic, 217
  concrete, 217
  egocentric, 49
  magical, 50-52, 93, 193, 385
'Thorazine'. *See* Largactil'
Thought disorder, *111*, 219-220, 222, 224, 335, 420
'Three Faces of Eve', 183
Thrombosis, 445
  cerebral, 265
Thumb-sucking, 37-38, 286
Thyrotoxicosis, 137, 318, 321
'Tofranil', 371
Toilets, 402, 441
Toilet-training, 42-44, 87, 286
Tolerance, 297, 386, 442, 459
  drug, 196
'Tom', 315
Tonic phase, 272, 277
Toxic factors, 128, 137, 256-257, 263-264, 304
Toxic psychosis. *See* Organic reactions, acute
Training programmes
  for mental retardates, 299, 306, 308-310
Tranquillising drugs, 12-13, 231-232, 240, 251, 259, 269-270, 295, 322, 353, *364-370*, 372, 453
  complications of, 267, 369-370
  major, 366-370
  minor, 214, 365, 370
  misuse of, 12-13, 232, 358

Transference, *329*, 331, 341, 347-349, 383
Transsexualism, 209
Transvestism, 209
Traumatic neurosis, 181, 186
Treatment, 6-7, 22-23, 151, *327-377*, 397, 472
  causal, 215-216
  in child psychiatry, 294-298
  of acute organic reactions, 258-260
  of chronic organic reactions, 267-270
  of depressive reactions, 248-251
  of manic reactions, 251-252
  of mental retardation, 305-312
  of neurotic reactions, 213-216
  of paranoid reactions, 240-241
  of schizophrenic reactions, 230-238
  supportive, 214
  symptomatic, 29, 214-215
Treatment, physical, 11-13, 327, *352-377*
  dangers of, 12-13, 215, 232, 233, 362-363, 365, 369-370, 376
  in depressive reactions, 248, 356
  in manic reactions, 251
  in neurotic reactions, 214-215, 356, 364
  in paranoid reactions, 240
  in schizophrenic reactions, 230-233, 356
  limitations of, 233, 354
Treatment, psychological. *See* Psychotherapy
Tremor, 256, 263, 266, 369
'Tridione', 279
'Trilafon', 368
'Truancy', 287
'Truth drugs', 335, 391
'Tryptanol', 371
Tube-feeding, 258-259
Tuberculosis, 31, 319
Tuberous sclerosis, 302
Tuke, William, 7
Twilight state, epileptic, 273
Twin studies, 226

U

Ulcerative colitis, 318, 320
Unconscious, 11, 19, *78-82*, 94, 97, 103, 119, 125, 207, 296, 330, 332, 334, 354, 381, 387
Uncovering, 328, 330
Underactivity, 108, 243
Understanding, *20*, 297, 348, 417, 427, 433, 438, 442, 497
  of self, 66, 328, 333, 337, 344
  of self by nurse, 18, 345, 348-349, 415, 468

Undoing, 192-193
Uniforms, 410-411
'Unpardonable sin', 113
Uraemia, 258
Urine testing, 258, 303
Urticaria, 319

V

Vagrants, 204, 222
'Valium', 215, 370
Ventilation, 322, 323, 333, 350
Verbigeration, 111
Violence, 108, 146, 205, 210, 221, 223, 236, 240, 241, 242, 255, 273, 274, 276, 348
   management of, 252, 451-454
Visiting, 259-260, 429-430, 434-435, 452-453, 476
   of children, 386
Vitamins
   deficiency of, 137, 199
   treatment with, 259, 260, 269
Vocational guidance, 61, 477
Volunteers, 24, 469
Vomiting, 373, 374
Voyeurism, 208

W

Ward, psychiatric
   activities within, 463
   atmosphere of, 250, 392, 398-399, 438, 452
   for children, 297-298
   furnishing of, 402-403
   management of, 395- 403-404, 407, 450
   tension, on, 391, 452

Waxy flexibility, 106, 223
Weaning, 39, 474
Wechsler Adult Intelligence Scale (WAIS), 507
Wechsler Intelligence Scale for Children (WISC), 507
Weight, loss of, 107, 215, 243, 247, 249, 266, 364
Will-power, 135, 168
Witchcraft, 4
Withdrawal symptoms, 200, 201
'Woolliness', 220
'Word salad', 111
Work, 163, 381, 464, 476-478
   attitude towards, 60-61, 66, 67, 72
   for psychiatric patients, 311, 459, 462, 464
   interference with, 137, 186, 204, 271, 381
   stresses at, 140, 464
Work settlements, 439
Workshops
   sheltered, 24, 299, 311, 439, 464, 477
   terminal, 311
   training, 311

X

X-rays, 258, 304

Y

York Retreat, 7

Z

Zarontin', 280